UNDERSTANDING AND MANAGING CHOLESTEROL

A Guide for Wellness Professionals

Kevin P. Byrne, MD, MPH
Rose Medical Center, Denver

Human Kinetics Books
Champaign, Illinois

Library of Congress Cataloging-in-Publication Data

Byrne, Kevin P., 1952-
   Understanding and managing cholesterol : a guide for wellness
professionals / by Kevin P. Byrne.
      p.   cm.
   Includes index.
   ISBN 0-87322-309-8
   1. Hypercholesteremia--Diet therapy.   2. Hypercholesteremia-
-Prevention.   3. Atherosclerosis--Etiology.   4. Atherosclerosis-
-Prevention.   5. Blood cholesterol.   I. Title.
   [DNLM: 1. Arteriosclerosis.   2. Cholesterol.   3. Diet.   4. Health
Promotion.   5. Nutrition.   QU 95 B995u]
   RC632.H83B97   1991
   616.1'360654--dc20
   DNLM/DLC
   for Library of Congress   90-5195
                                                                           CIP

ISBN: 0-87322-309-8

Copyright © 1991 by Kevin P. Byrne, MD, MPH

Cover Photo: The digital subtraction angiogram on the cover shows a human heart with an obstructive lesion of the mid left anterior descending coronary artery (LAD) (top center of heart), and another high-grade obstruction of the diagonal branch of the LAD (top right). Photograph courtesy of the BAYER Company, Glenbrook Laboratories, Division of Sterling Drug Inc.

For consultation on health promotion or cost containment, Dr. Byrne may be reached at Rose Medical Center at Peoria, 4955 Peoria St., Suite C, Denver CO 80239, or by phone: (303) 375-0363.

Printed in the United States of America

10 9 8 7 6 5 4 3 2 1

Human Kinetics Books   UK Office:
A Division of Human Kinetics Publishers, Inc. Human Kinetics Publishers (UK) Ltd.
Box 5076, Champaign, IL 61825-5076   PO Box 18
1-800-747-4HKP   Rawdon, Leeds LS19 6TG
                                               England
                                               (0532) 504211

Contents

Preface

Every year in the United States, cholesterol-clogged arteries cause a staggering 700,000 deaths. Families are disrupted, corporations are crippled, and millions are left disabled. More than 7 million Americans are presently afflicted, and the total annual cost to our society is approaching a staggering $100 billion—yet nearly all of this is preventable!

Two avenues of approach exist in attacking the cholesterol epidemic: targeting only those persons at highest risk, and targeting our population as a whole. The traditional medical system takes the high-risk patient-based approach to identify persons who need intensive therapy. These individuals are clearly on a collision course with cholesterol and, from a cost-effectiveness standpoint, stand to gain the most from cholesterol control. However, the majority of individuals who suffer heart attacks and strokes have cholesterol levels in the middle range and are thus omitted from a focus on only the high-risk group. For this reason, *Understanding and Managing Cholesterol* emphasizes the population or public health approach. The ultimate objective is to help shift our society's average cholesterol level toward that of countries with low rates of heart attacks and strokes. Virtually unknown a century ago, atherosclerosis, or hardening of the arteries, now kills nearly half of us. Heart attacks could be rare once again if we learn to control our blood cholesterol levels.

I have taken the high-risk patient-based recommendations of the National Cholesterol Education Program and the medical community one step further. This book provides information not only for those with dangerously high serum cholesterol values, but also for those 60 million Americans who have "borderline high" or "undesirable" levels. If there are differences between the recommendations here and those published by the government, it is because my goal is promoting *optimal* health, not simply postponing death and premature disability.

This book is divided into four parts. The first part presents the necessary background information about blood cholesterol—how it contributes to arterial plaque and how it is controlled. Part II introduces the other contributors to atherosclerosis. Part III gives the theoretical background and rationale behind dietary changes, the mainstay of cholesterol control. Part IV is designed to help health professionals design and implement a cholesterol-lowering program, particularly doing screenings and teaching classes about cholesterol reduction.

Integral to this book is my belief that the control of cholesterol, and indeed of one's life, should be the responsibility of the individual rather than the medical system. Only by taking charge of our own health can we eliminate devastating arterial diseases. Self-responsibility, supplemented by health education, engenders a healthy, productive, and enjoyable life. I hope that the information and techniques presented in this book will enhance your health and that of your clients and loved ones.

Kevin P. Byrne, MD, MPH
Denver, CO

Acknowledgments

This project could not have attained its scope and depth without the assistance of many friends and colleagues in the Denver area. I'm particularly indebted to Dr. Robert Eckel and Dr. Cecil (Buz) Birchfiel who gave generously of their knowledge and support during the developmental stages. A number of registered dieticians offered much-needed guidance, especially Dan Rifkin, Mary Montgomery, Louise Downey, and Betty Cochran. I also appreciate Mike Byrne for providing the graphics and Joyce Bickel for help with the seemingly endless clerical details.

Staff Acknowledgments

Developmental Editor: Peggy Rupert
Managing Editor: Robert King
Assistant Editors: Dawn Levy, Julia Anderson
Copyeditor: Barbara Walsh
Proofreader: Laurie McGee
Indexer: Barb Cohen
Production Director: Ernie Noa
Typesetter: Brad Colson
Text Design: Keith Blomberg
Text Layout: Denise Lowry
Cover Design: Jack Davis
Illustrations: Ed Zilberts
Computer Graphics: David Gregory
Printer: Braun-Brumfield

PART

I

THE CHOLESTEROL STORY

☐

For Herb Shearer, the crushing chest pain came as a complete surprise. As he leaned on his golf clubs, he couldn't seem to get enough air. He was losing consciousness. Fortunately, the spell passed after a minute or so. Later he remembered that his doctor had warned him about his high cholesterol level. He had altered his diet for a while, only to slip back into a typical American diet of fried foods, large portions of red meat, and rich sauces and creams.

Over the next few weeks, Herb had several more episodes of chest pain, each brought on by less and less exertion. Finally, Herb conceded that the pain needed investigation. His doctor determined that his chest pain did have a serious cause: Tests revealed that his cholesterol problem had caused severe narrowing of an artery supplying his heart muscle. Luckily the blockage was not yet severe enough to have caused an actual heart attack. His pain was due to angina pectoris, a condition signaling that his heart muscle was deprived of oxygen.

Herb immediately began to investigate cholesterol and its critical role in health and disease. Cholesterol had literally become a matter of life and death for him. The prospect of a heart attack was as frightening to Herb's wife as to Herb, so together they pored over all the information they could find. At 60 years of age they came to recognize the importance of preventing heart disease through nutrition and exercise.

The Shearers gradually changed their diet to include more fish and poultry, fruit, vegetables, beans, and grains. Their meals were anything but bland or austere; rather, Herb and his wife enjoyed their new food choices. They had distinctly more energy after eating, and, without trying, both lost enough weight to receive compliments from their friends. Also, Herb's wife noticed that their grocery bills were actually lower than before because of the infrequent purchases of rich, gourmet foods.

Another enjoyable lifestyle change was engaging in daily exercise instead of an occasional round of golf. Although the two were skeptical at first, their brisk morning walk became a delight rather than drudgery. They were spending more time together and had more hope for the future.

After several months of controlling his cholesterol, Herb began to lead a pain-free life that was more active and spirited. Friends commented that he looked years younger. More importantly, he felt younger. Herb was fortunate to have been forewarned of his cholesterol problem; over eighty thousand Americans a year succumb to sudden cardiac death without any prior symptoms. The first sign of atherosclerosis in 70% of afflicted middle-aged men is either a heart attack or sudden cardiac death.

As Herb's story illustrates, the cholesterol problem has solutions. Plaque growth is not an inexorable consequence of aging. With risk factor control it can be arrested or even reduced, though to a limited extent. Developing the heart-saving lifestyle habits to do so, both as individuals and as a society, remains our greatest health challenge.

In Part I of this book, the cholesterol story is sketched from its molecular roots to its effect on our population. The first chapter presents cholesterol physiology and describes the tremendous scope of its associated diseases. Chapter 2 details the cellular destruction that cholesterol wreaks on arteries, a condition that becomes quite severe before external symptoms appear. The third chapter describes the basics of controlling cholesterol, including a preview of the nutritional approach, exercise, weight control, and finally the cholesterol-lowering-drug and surgical approaches.

Chapter

1

Cholesterol's Role in Atherosclerosis

Cholesterol plays the key role in the development of atherosclerosis, which literally means "hardening of the arteries." This is by far the major health problem in the United States and other Western industrialized countries (1). Since the 1940s, atherosclerosis has been responsible for nearly half of all deaths in the United States. One in three men and one in six women develop serious heart disease by the age of 65 (2). Heart attacks, just one result of atherosclerosis, kill 550,000 Americans each year—more than any other disease, including all forms of cancer and accidents combined (3). Figure 1.1 shows the leading causes of death in the United States in 1988, with cardiovascular diseases leading the list (4).

The Research

Although until recently there has been much controversy in this area, indisputable evidence now implicates elevated blood cholesterol (hypercholesterolemia) as a major cause of atherosclerosis (5). Strong and consistent proof of this connection has come from a variety of sources, including animal and metabolic ward experiments, population studies, autopsy reports, dietary research, genetic and biochemical studies, and clinical trials (6).

Since the turn of the century, scientists have been inducing atherosclerosis in over a dozen different animal species by feeding them diets high in cholesterol and fat. Some of the experimental diets were virtually identical to those typically eaten in America. The higher the level of blood cholesterol achieved, the more the plaque formation in the animals' arteries was accelerated. The fatty tumors even formed with little or no rise in their blood cholesterol levels (7).

3

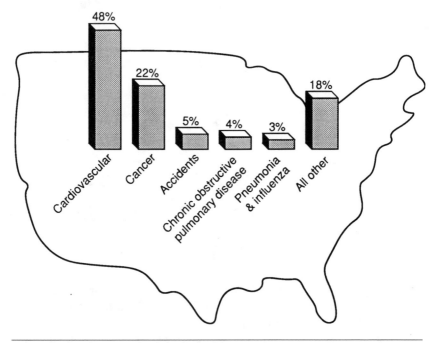

Figure 1.1 Major causes of death in the United States in 1988.
Note. Adapted from the National Center for Health Statistics, U.S. Public Health Service, Department of Health and Human Services.

The cholesterol-heart link in man has been more difficult to demonstrate because of difficulties in obtaining adequate dietary histories (a 7-day eating log seems to be a minimum), the complexity of interacting dietary elements, individual variation, and the long time frame required to notice "hard endpoints" such as heart attack or stroke. Since 1980, five studies in humans have demonstrated that dietary cholesterol, in and of itself, promotes heart attack (7, 8). The studies indicate that the hazard of excessive dietary cholesterol is so great that its impact can be noticed independently of its effect on blood cholesterol. If blood cholesterol also rises, the consequence is compounded.

The relationship of blood cholesterol to atherosclerosis is more direct and has been easier to demonstrate. Testimony supporting this comes chiefly from studies that follow groups of individuals over time, keeping track of their blood cholesterol to determine if people with lower levels lived longer or suffered fewer heart attacks and strokes. These prospective studies not only show an intimate association between blood cholesterol and heart disease, but also demonstrate that hypercholesterolemia is a direct cause of atherosclerosis.

One of the most distinguished prospective studies of cardiovascular disease is the Framingham Heart Study, which continues today (9).

Thousands of residents of Framingham, Massachusetts, have been followed since 1948. Every 2 years they are questioned about their current lifestyles and examined for evidence of cardiovascular disease. Blood samples are taken for a wide array of tests. The Framingham study has spawned hundreds of scientific articles that have greatly enhanced our understanding of the various cardiovascular risk factors and enabled us to sort out their independent and combined effects on atherosclerosis.

Clinical trials, another type of prospective study, have provided the most convincing evidence of cholesterol's intimate connection to atherosclerosis (10-14). These have used cholesterol-lowering diets, drugs, or both to counter arterial plaque. They have shown that not only does high blood cholesterol cause atherosclerosis, but also that intervening with diet, drugs, or both will lower cholesterol levels and subsequently reduce the risk of disease.

Validation that changing cholesterol levels will in turn promote health or prevent disease has not come easily. Physicians have been reluctant to encourage dietary changes or prescribe cholesterol-lowering drugs because of uncertainty that these interventions were both safe and effective in reducing the risk of heart attack. In the Coronary Drug Project, for example, men who were given estrogen or thyroid hormone actually had higher rates of heart attacks (15).

The most distinguished clinical trial to date has been the Lipid Research Clinics Study sponsored by the National Institutes of Health (13). This pivotal study finally proved that lowering cholesterol prevents subsequent heart attacks and strokes. Its results are still sending shock waves through the medical community and have mandated a new and aggressive approach toward cholesterol control.

A wealth of data has now firmly established that elevated blood cholesterol is the *sine qua non* of arterial plaque formation (16). In its absence, little atherosclerosis would be present. The Japanese, who have blood cholesterol levels averaging only 160 mg/dl (4.1 mmol/L), seldom have heart attacks in spite of their rates of hypertension and smoking that are among the highest in the world.

Risks Associated With Atherosclerosis

Cholesterol is a major component of atherosclerotic plaque, which has been simplistically compared to a film coating on the inside of affected arteries, like lime deposits in a pipe. But a much more accurate description is that plaque is a thickening or tumor within the artery wall itself. It has a three-dimensional structure, making treatment difficult once clinical disease is apparent.

Although death can occur instantly from a single blocked artery, atherosclerosis progresses at a slow and fairly predictable pace, gradually developing over decades. Its rate depends on the individual's level of blood cholesterol and blood pressure, and the presence of smoking and other risk factors (17). By middle age, nearly all Americans have worrisome amounts of atherosclerosis throughout their bodies, even though they may have no symptoms. Regardless of age, at least 60% of the victim's entire vascular surface must be impregnated with atherosclerotic plaque before a heart attack can occur (17). A lengthwise section of such an artery and a normal artery are illustrated in Figure 1.2.

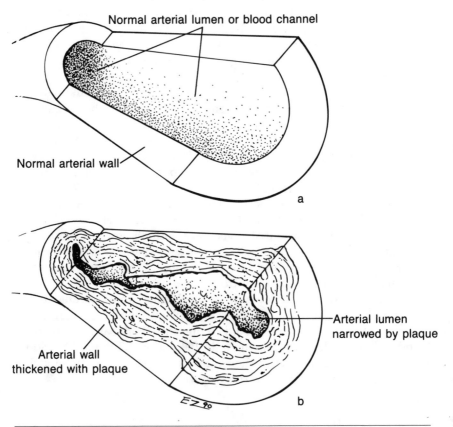

Figure 1.2   Lengthwise section of a normal artery (a) and a blocked artery (b).

Atherosclerotic plaque results in an increased risk for three potentially fatal diseases—coronary heart disease, stroke, and peripheral vascular disease.

Heart attack, angina pectoris, and sudden cardiac death are collectively referred to as **coronary heart disease** (CHD) because they are caused by plaque accumulation within the heart's coronary arteries. CHD has been our nation's number-one cause of death for 40 years and is predicted to remain such well into the next century (18). Its total annual cost to our society, including direct medical care and lost productivity, is estimated to be more than $60 million (3, 19).

A heart attack, or *myocardial infarction* (MI), occurs when one of the coronary arteries supplying the heart muscle (myocardium) becomes totally blocked with atherosclerotic plaque. This section of the heart dies and can never again assist in pumping blood. If the loss of heart tissue is extensive or if multiple attacks occur, the viable heart muscle that remains cannot keep pace with the body's needs. Blood then backs up into the lungs and/or the extremities in a condition termed *congestive heart failure*.

The squeezing chest pain of *angina pectoris* results when the coronary arteries are so severely narrowed that insufficient blood reaches the heart muscle in times of mental or physical stress. A person experiencing angina is on the very brink of having a full-blown heart attack.

Sudden cardiac death, the third manifestation of CHD, is as lethal as its name implies. A victim succumbs to the condition within one hour and is usually found lifeless by a family member. Because the victim dies before reaching a hospital, traditional diagnostic techniques cannot confirm the exact mechanism, but a fatal heart arrhythmia (due to atherosclerosis) is presumed to be responsible. A total of 330,000 Americans die each year from sudden cardiac death, making this the single most common cause of death in the United States.

Hypercholesterolemia is probably the most important factor in the development of CHD, accounting for nearly half of the cases (16, 20-22). High blood pressure is also important, followed by smoking, heredity, diabetes, obesity, stress, and lack of exercise. An estimated 90% of CHD is preventable by healthy lifestyle habits (16).

A **stroke** results when part of the brain dies as a result of blood vessel disease, usually atherosclerosis, in one of the cerebral arteries of the brain or the carotid arteries of the neck. This may be from thrombosis (a stationary clot), embolism (migrating pieces of clot), or hemorrhage. Although not as common as heart attacks, strokes are still our third-leading cause of death and a major source of disability. Approximately 500,000 Americans have strokes each year; 150,000 of these victims die. The remainder are often left with severe disabilities. The cost of their medical care and loss of productivity now total about $10 billion a year (23).

In **peripheral vascular disease** (PVD), the third major atherosclerotic disease, arteries in the legs are severely affected by cholesterol deposits. The early warning signs and symptoms of PVD are subtle, such as diminished pulses in the feet and behind the knee. If PVD progresses, a characteristic cramp-like claudication pain occurs in one or both calf muscles with walking. Eventually gangrene develops, often requiring amputation of all or part of the extremity. An estimated 200,000 Americans are afflicted with PVD.

Dietary Sources of Cholesterol

Animal tissue is the only source of cholesterol, and all animal products contain some cholesterol. Organ meats, such as sweetbreads and liver, are heavily concentrated with it. For example, a 3-ounce piece of liver contains 400 mg of cholesterol, compared to 60 to 90 mg in a similar amount of lean meat, fish, or poultry. In general, blood cholesterol levels rise 8 to 10 mg/dl (.25 mmol/L) for every 100 mg of cholesterol in the diet.

Most Americans need to cut their dietary cholesterol in half. The average intake is 450 to 500 mg for men and about 300 mg for women (24). Fortunately for most Americans, not all of the cholesterol in food is absorbed. When the cholesterol intake exceeds 500 mg per day—not an uncommon amount in affluent societies—only about 30% to 35% is absorbed. Most people ingesting 450 mg of cholesterol per day absorb roughly half that amount. When the dietary intake is relatively small, absorption is quite efficient, perhaps reaching 70%. In other words, adding another egg or two to a diet rich in meats will not increase an individual's blood cholesterol as

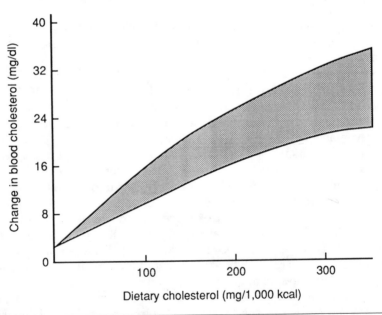

Figure 1.3 Blood cholesterol rises as greater amounts of cholesterol are consumed, but at a progressively slower rate. The relationship is represented by the shaded area because it varies considerably from one individual to another and is influenced by other dietary factors such as fiber.

Note. From ''The Plasma Lipids, Lipoproteins, and Diet of the Tarahumara Indians of Mexico'' by W.E. Connor, 1978, *American Journal of Clinical Nutrition*, **31**, p. 1136. Copyright 1978 by American Society for Clinical Nutrition. Reprinted by permission.

much as if those eggs were added to a vegetarian diet. Figure 1.3 illustrates this relationship (25-27).

A rich diet affects blood cholesterol directly by increasing the amount absorbed and indirectly by boosting cholesterol production and inhibiting its removal by the liver. Only 20% to 40% of blood cholesterol is derived from dietary sources. Thus, the liver is the body's major cholesterol source, producing about 1,000 mg a day.

The distinction between dietary cholesterol and blood cholesterol must be kept clear. Many food components influence blood levels, especially the amount and types of fats and fiber. Although plant products contain no cholesterol, some highly saturated vegetable fats, such as coconut and palm oils, tend to raise cholesterol levels in the circulation. This distinction is crucial because it is the level of cholesterol in the blood that is especially dangerous, much more so than the amount consumed. Specifically, laboratories measure the cholesterol concentration in the plasma (blood minus its cells) and in serum (plasma minus clotting elements).

In addition to blood cholesterol, factors such as blood pressure and smoking promote cholesterol infiltration into arterial walls as plaque. Stress, obesity, and diabetes are important risk factors for CHD because they not only may raise blood cholesterol levels, but each can also contribute directly to the formation of plaque and heart disease. Figure 1.4 places the risk factors of this process in perspective.

Cholesterol's Natural Function in the Body

Cholesterol is the greatest health problem in our society—yet it's also essential to life. Cholesterol is not a deadly fat floating around in our arteries, waiting to do us in. Actually, it's not a fat at all, but rather an alcohol-wax that at times behaves like a fat. Cholesterol is a natural compound found in all animal tissues and is important for many structures and functions, including the following.

Cell Membranes.   Cholesterol is one of the most important components of cell membranes, imparting stability and other properties. Most of the body's 10-gram store of cholesterol is contained in cell membranes, 25% of which is held in the central nervous system alone. Abundant cholesterol in the specialized membranes of nerve fibers allows electrical impulses to travel quickly—in some nerves at speeds of 100 yards per second. Only 7% of the body's cholesterol is found in the plasma and is therefore potentially dangerous.

Hormone Production.   Cholesterol is also the precursor molecule for the synthesis of steroids, the largest group of hormones. These include estrogen and progesterone in women, testosterone in men, and many

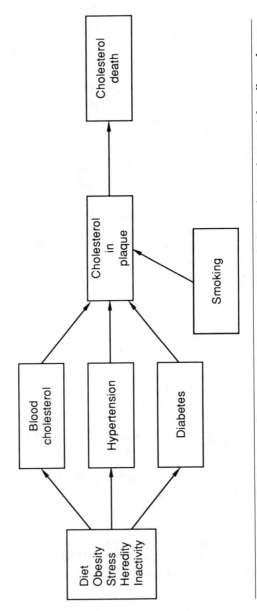

Figure 1.4 Cardiovascular risk factors act in concert to drive cholesterol into the arterial wall as plaque.

others. They regulate a myriad of metabolic processes and sexual characteristics. Cholesterol is also the initial compound used for the production of vitamin D.

Bile.   The liver modifies cholesterol to produce bile, then stores it in the gall bladder. The greenish liquid is then released into the small intestine to aid in the digestion of fat. Figure 1.5 shows the chemical structure of cholesterol and its molecular relatives.

Although cholesterol is necessary for life, we need absolutely none from food. Because it is such as essential molecule, every cell in the body has the ability to synthesize all the cholesterol it needs (though most is produced by the liver). There is no Recommended Dietary Allowance (RDA) for cholesterol, and doctors recognize no diseases of cholesterol

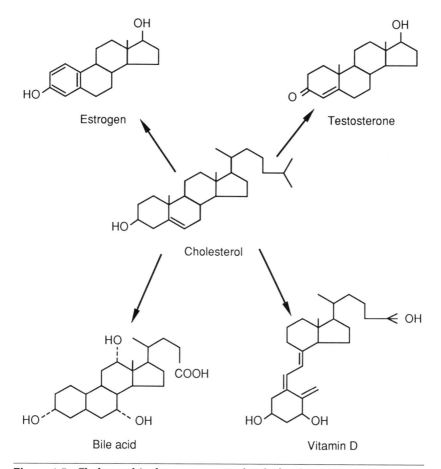

Figure 1.5   Cholesterol is the precursor molecule for the synthesis of steroid hormones, vitamin D, and bile.

deficiency. But the reverse is overwhelmingly true. Many of us have too much of it—in our diets, in our bloodstreams, and in our arteries.

This is the crux of our major health problem: The human body is physiologically unprepared for the heavy load of fat and cholesterol that the traditional American diet provides. Cholesterol is not a toxin, and so it is not chemically degraded and excreted like most other substances. On the contrary, it's actually conserved. For example, 98% of bile is reabsorbed in the large intestine and sent back to the liver for reprocessing. It is a sad paradox indeed that such a vital substance should contribute to such tremendous amounts of death and disability.

What Is a Normal Cholesterol Level?

Considerable confusion and debate surround the level of blood cholesterol that should be considered normal. Until recently, many people were told that their cholesterol of 300 mg/dl (7.8 mmol/L) was normal or slightly high. Yet today they learn that this value is dangerously high. Many laboratories still report cholesterol results of 330 to 350 mg/dl (8.5-9.05 mmol/L) within normal limits (28), even though a healthy or physiologically normal cholesterol level is below 180 mg/dl (4.7 mmol/L) (19, 29).

This apparent inconsistency can be reconciled by reviewing the laboratory criteria for setting normal values for blood tests. A range of numbers is generally interpreted as being within normal limits if it falls within two standard deviations from the mean, or average. Ninety-five percent of the population being tested will be within this range. This convention does not function well for cholesterol because average cholesterol levels are not synonymous with normal or healthy levels. In the United States, where heart attacks are common, the average cholesterol level is 215 mg/dl (24).

As a result of these antiquated cholesterol standards, many physicians (including some cardiologists) do not get concerned until the cholesterol level is close to 300 mg/dl (7.8 mmol/L). Meanwhile, over half of all heart attack victims have cholesterol levels under 225 mg/dl (5.8 mmol/L) (30). These are well within the traditional range of "normal." Individuals with an ideal cholesterol level of under 160 mg/dl (4.1 mmol/L) are among the lowest 5% to 10% of our population. At this level, an individual might paradoxically be labeled as having "abnormally" low cholesterol.

Another difference between cholesterol and many other blood constituents is that with cholesterol, any elevation above the optimal level can cause harm. This is especially true for low-density lipoprotein (LDL) cholesterol, discussed in the next section. Cholesterol screening of the 356,000 men in the Multiple Risk Factor Intervention Trial (MRFIT) study clearly demonstrated that cholesterol levels well below the U.S. average still carried an increased risk of heart attack. Early analysis of the MRFIT data suggested that lower levels of cholesterol might be associated with an increased risk of death. But when participants with preexisting cancer were excluded from the analysis, this relationship disappeared. In other words, cancer and other wasting diseases cause a lowering of serum cholesterol, but the reverse is not true.

Thus, the MRFIT study, which was several times larger than any other of its type, convincingly showed that the lower the serum cholesterol, the better: "These data of high precision show that the relationship between serum cholesterol and coronary heart disease is not a threshold one [plateaulike] . . . but rather a continuously graded one that powerfully

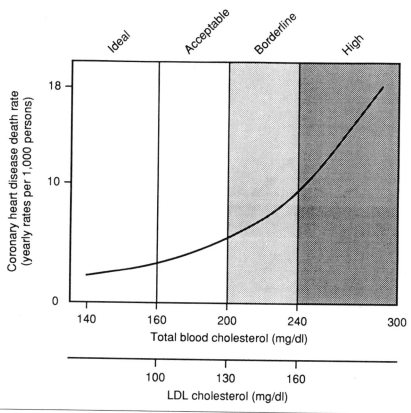

Figure 1.6 The relationship of total blood cholesterol and low density lipoproteins (LDL) to coronary heart disease. Persons within a given zone according to their cholesterol level should be reclassified into the next higher category if they have already existent atherosclerosis, i.e., a personal history of heart attack, angina pectoris, or stroke, or if they have two or more of the following additional risk factors: male gender, smoking, high blood pressure, diabetes, severe obesity, HDL-cholesterol less than 35, or a history of heart attack before age 55 in an immediate family member.

Note. From "Serum Cholesterol, Blood Pressure, and Mortality: Implications From a Cohort of 361,662 Men" by M.J. Martin, W.S. Browner, S.B. Hulley, L.H. Kuller, and D. Wentworth, 1986, Lancet, 2, p. 934. Copyright 1986 by The Lancet Ltd. Adapted by permission.

affects risk for the great majority of American men" (20, p. 2823). Figure 1.6 illustrates this graded relationship between cholesterol levels and death from coronary heart disease (31).

Experts in preventive cardiology have stated that physiologically normal cholesterol levels are in the range of 140 to 180 mg/dl (3.6 to 4.7 mmol/L) (29, 32, 33). In the 40-year experience of the Framingham Heart Study, no person with a cholesterol level of 150 mg/dl (3.9 mmol/L) or below has had a heart attack (30). To lend further support, a compilation of large autopsy studies has indicated that if blood cholesterol remained under 150 mg/dl, heart attacks would be virtually eliminated (16).

Average cholesterol levels this low do exist in developing countries, and CHD in those countries is indeed rare. Heart attacks are essentially unknown among vegetarian groups such as the Tarahumara Indians of Mexico and the Yanomano Indians of Brazil. Only about 15% to 20% of their total calories come from fat, and blood cholesterol levels average 130 mg/dl (3.36 mmol/L), even in adult men (25, 34).

In reviewing the evidence now amassed, expert panels in Europe and the U.S. have concluded that ideal cholesterol levels are in the range of 160 to 180 mg/dl (4.1 to 4.7 mmol/L) and below (5, 19, 74). By this definition, at least 80% of our adult population have elevated cholesterol levels. Fully 60 million Americans are at high risk for CHD and definitely need dietary or drug intervention to reduce their levels into a safer range. Another 40 million Americans are at borderline high risk with levels in the 200 to 240 mg/dl (5.2 to 6.2 mmol/L) range. These levels will cause problems in advanced age or even earlier if accompanied by smoking, diabetes, or high blood pressure.

Truly normal cholesterol levels, though far below average values, are nonetheless attainable for most people in our society if they select generally available foods and prepare them in a heart-healthy manner. (See Part III and chapter 11 for more information.)

Lipoproteins: Structure and Function

Cholesterol and other blood lipids (fats and fat-like substances) are fat-soluble and thus cannot float around freely in the water-like medium of the blood. For this reason they are packaged into lipoproteins—spherical molecular complexes that transport and regulate blood lipids. Nearly all of the cholesterol in the blood is carried by low-density and high-density lipoproteins, or LDL and HDL, respectively. Chylomicrons and very low–density lipoproteins (VLDL) are the largest lipoproteins and carry primarily triglycerides.

Lipoproteins are marvelously constructed with a thin outer shell surrounding a central area of fat molecules. The shell contains proteins, phospholipids, and free cholesterol lined up in a parallel array, one molecule thick (see Figure 1.7 a and b) (35). The free cholesterol and phospholipids have detergent-like properties that make the particle soluble in the blood. They are oriented with their water-soluble ends facing outward and the fat-soluble ends facing the lipoprotein core. The apoproteins, a type of protein, are imbedded in the shell with a similar polar arrangement. They are instrumental in the regulation and ultimate metabolic fate of these floating cholesterol carriers.

The center of the lipoprotein sphere contains the two predominant forms of fat in the bloodstream: triglycerides and cholesterol ester. They must be contained within the lipoprotein core for transport because they are completely insoluble in the blood.

Cholesterol ester is constructed from free (non-esterified) cholesterol linked to a fatty acid molecule via a chemical (ester) bond. Most of the

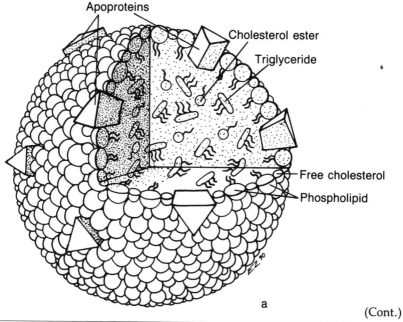

a

(Cont.)

Figure 1.7 A composite lipoprotein (a). Free cholesterol and phospholipids provide support to the lipoprotein shell. The water-soluble ends face outward and help make the lipoprotein soluble in the blood. The other ends are immersed in the triglycerides and cholesterol esters of the lipoprotein's fatty core. The relative proportion of cholesterol, protein, triglyceride, and phospholipid in lipoproteins (b). VLDL = very low density lipoprotein; LDL = low density lipoprotein, and HDL = high density lipoprotein.

Note. Adapted from information appearing in *New England Journal of Medicine.* "Pathogenesis and Management of Lipoprotein Disorders" by E.J. Schaefer and R.I. Levy, 1985, *New England Journal of Medicine,* **312,** pp. 1300-1310.

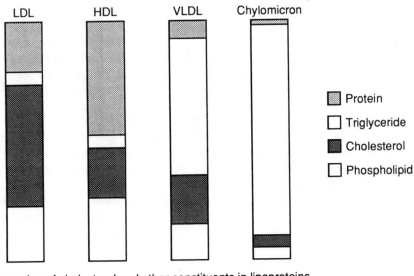

Proportion of cholesterol and other constituents in lipoproteins

b

Figure 1.7   (Continued)

cholesterol contained in food is nonesterified. Because this form is water-soluble, it is easier for the body to transport it. Once non-esterified cholesterol enters arterial plaque, most of it becomes esterified. It is then extremely difficult to remove because it cannot be moved easily across cell membranes. Thus, primary prevention—arresting atherosclerosis in its early stages—is much preferred to relying on the reverse cholesterol transport system to extract it later.

The apoproteins on the lipoprotein surface are essential in regulating the transport of lipids and the complex interactions between the different lipoprotein classes. At least 16 apoproteins have been discovered to date, and most act as cofactors, activating enzymes that in turn speed up chemical reactions. Others assist structurally in the stability of the lipoprotein sphere. Elevated levels of *apoprotein B-100, E* and *lipoprotein a* (Lp[a]) are associated with an increased risk of CHD. Measuring these blood components is becoming clinically useful in select cases.

Low-Density Lipoprotein

Low-density lipoprotein (LDL) is the major cholesterol-carrying lipoprotein and the villain in the cholesterol drama. Elevated LDL levels herald a strong predisposition to CHD, stroke, and peripheral vascular disease. The LDL particle is half cholesterol; this is more than is found in any other lipoprotein type. LDL particles transport approximately three fourths of the total blood cholesterol, delivering cholesterol to tissues throughout the body for a variety of functions. If the LDL concentration in the bloodstream rises above 100 to 130 mg/dl (2.6-3.36 mmol/L), some of its cholesterol is deposited into arterial walls as plaque (see Figure 1.6).

The concentration of LDL in the blood is determined by its rates of production and removal, both of which are dramatically affected by diet. Dietary saturated fat and cholesterol increase the liver's production of very low-density lipoproteins (VLDL), some of which are transformed into LDL particles within the bloodstream (17). Saturated fat and cholesterol also suppress the withdrawal of LDL by the liver, which boosts LDL levels even further.

Recent research has indicated that certain "modified" forms of LDL are especially menacing. The most important instance occurs when LDL combines with oxygen to form a chemically reactive oxidized LDL (36). A diet rich in citrus fruits, whole grains, and beans provides the body with vitamins C, E, and selenium, all of which have antioxidant properties. Supplementation with antioxidants, though, cannot be generally recommended. Selenium in particular can be toxic to arteries when taken in doses higher than the RDA—70 µg/day for adult males and 55 µg/day for adult females (37).

LDL Receptors. The outer membranes of liver cells contain numerous LDL receptors, the molecular "gates" central to cholesterol control. The LDL apoprotein (B-100) fits into the three-dimensional structure of the LDL receptor much like a key into a lock (see Figure 1.8). The cell

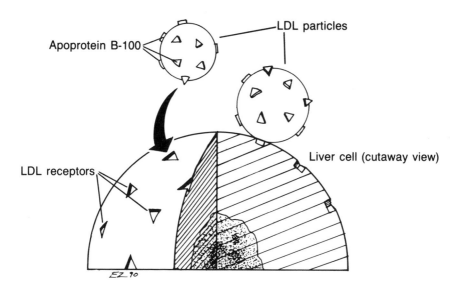

Figure 1.8 The LDL receptors, which are most numerous in the liver, attract and snare the LDL particles by binding to the apoprotein known as B-100.

recognizes LDL and binds it, then absorbs the particle with its cholesterol payload and "digests" it (35).

Apoprotein B-100 is also found on another atherogenic particle termed the intermediate-density lipoprotein, or IDL. Smaller than LDL, it is formed from the partial breakdown of triglyceride-carrying VLDL particles. IDLs are cleared from the blood by the same receptor mechanism as are LDL particles. If not cleared by the liver, they may go on to form LDL particles within the bloodstream.

The number of LDL receptors a cell displays varies with the cell's need for cholesterol. Liver cell membranes are dense with LDL receptors because they remove most of the LDL and IDL from the bloodstream, using the cholesterol to produce bile. The adrenal glands, ovaries, and testes also have many LDL receptors because these organs use cholesterol to produce steroid hormones.

Within most cells the LDL-delivered cholesterol exerts two important effects: It inhibits cholesterol synthesis within the cell and also decreases the manufacturing of LDL receptors. By these two negative feedback mechanisms, the individual cell protects itself from excessive accumulation of cholesterol, yet simultaneously promotes a backlog of LDL particles in the bloodstream.

Unfortunately, the LDL receptors of the "scavenger cells" in the arterial wall, the monocytes and smooth muscle cells, cannot reduce their LDL receptors. Thus they continue to act as cholesterol sponges, swelling with fat droplets and eventually dying. This process results in the progressive formation of plaque, described in detail in chapter 2.

LDL receptors, primarily in the liver, remove two thirds to three fourths of the circulating LDL particles; the remainder is cleared by another, unknown pathway. Accordingly, the major cause of elevated blood LDL is diminished LDL-receptor activity. The LDL receptor is so fundamental to our knowledge of the present-day atherosclerotic epidemic that its discoverers, Drs. Joseph Goldstein and Michael Brown of the University of Texas, were awarded the Nobel prize in medicine in 1985 (38).

Medical Conditions Affecting LDL. Medical conditions that may raise LDL levels include hypothyroidism, obstructive liver disease (such as biliary stones), nephrosis, and, rarely, the blood diseases porphyria and dysproteinemia. Medications that tend to elevate LDL are thiazide diuretics, commonly used for high blood pressure, phenytoin, anabolic steroids, and progestins. Psychological stress, obesity, and an inherited tendency may also elevate LDL in some individuals.

Thyroid hormone is important for the proper synthesis of LDL receptors. Estrogen increases the number of functioning LDL receptors on the cell surface, perhaps accounting for some of the protection women have against high cholesterol levels and CHD (39).

A medical evaluation is indicated for persons with high blood cholesterol (total cholesterol over 240 mg/dl or over 6.2 mmol/L) or those with borderline cholesterol (200 to 240 mg/dl or 5.2 to 6.2 mmol/L) who have other risk factors or who do not respond to a healthy diet. The workup should include a urinalysis, a complete blood count, thyroid studies, and a blood panel including at least glucose, albumin, creatinine, and alkaline phosphatase.

High-Density Lipoprotein

High-density lipoprotein (HDL) has been aptly called the "good" cholesterol because high levels of it reduce an individual's tendency to develop atherosclerosis. HDL protects the blood vessels by removing some of the cholesterol from the arterial walls (17) and possibly by slowing cholesterol's entry into tissues (40). HDL also promotes the production of *prostacyclin*, a substance that inhibits clotting along the inner walls of arteries.

Studies of human populations since the early 1950s have shown that higher levels of HDL are associated with a lower incidence of CHD (41). Numerous studies have confirmed that these lipoproteins can protect arteries, at least in advanced, Western societies (11, 42-45). In general, a 10 mg/dl increase in HDL nearly halves the risk for developing one of the manifestations of CHD. A similar inverse relationship between HDL and stroke or peripheral vascular disease is also present but is weaker than for CHD (46).

HDL is the smallest and densest class of lipoproteins; an HDL particle is only half the size of an LDL particle. The HDL particle is half protein; this is more than is found in any other lipoprotein. These proteins control a variety of interactions with other classes of lipoproteins in which lipids and other components are exchanged.

Most HDL particles are synthesized by the liver and small intestine, but they can also be generated within the bloodstream from VLDL and chylomicrons (35). Newly formed HDLs have a disc-like shape. As they acquire more and more cholesterol from the tissues and arterial walls, they assume a spherical shape like the other lipoproteins.

HDL has two major subtypes, HDL-2 and HDL-3, and several minor subtypes. HDL-2 is thought to be more protective against atherosclerosis and is increased by exercise and weight loss. Women have more than three times the concentration of HDL-2 as men, making this the most striking lipoprotein difference between the sexes (47).

Diet has surprisingly little effect on HDL levels for most individuals (48). A boost in HDL level will take many months to occur (49) and may follow an initial drop (50). Perhaps the most effective means for boosting HDL levels is regular exercise and weight reduction (51).

Moderate use of alcohol tends to raise HDL by about 5 mg/dl (52). "Moderate" refers to three beers or two glasses of wine, or 2 ounces (60 ml) of 100-proof whiskey per day. The alcohol-induced HDL boost may resist atherosclerosis, but this is somewhat conjectural, because alcohol primarily increases HDL-3, which is less important in CHD protection. Because of its unproven benefit and the tremendous health cost when it is abused, consumption of alcohol cannot be recommended to the general public as a preventive measure. In addition, raising HDL levels by any means will not necessarily guarantee protection against CHD. After all, pesticides are known to raise HDL, yet no sane person would suggest taking supplements of these as a health aid. Table 1.1 lists factors that affect HDL levels.

Table 1.1   Factors Influencing Blood HDL Levels

Factors associated with higher HDL	Factors associated with lower HDL
Low triglyceride levels	High triglyceride levels
Female gender	Male gender or postmenopausal female
Leanness	
Regular vigorous exercise	Overweight
Certain medications such as estrogen, prazosin, niacin, and gemfibrozil	Sedentary lifestyle
Pharmacologic levels of vitamin B₆ (pyridoxine)	Certain medications such as androgens, beta blockers, progestins
Low intake of refined sugars	Diabetes, kidney failure
Alcohol consumption	Zinc supplementation (in doses higher than the RDA)
	High intake of refined sugars
	Smoking

How HDL Causes Plaque to Shrink.   HDL is central to the *reverse cholesterol transport system*, the body's mechanism to heal atherosclerosis. Excess cholesterol from tissues, including the artery walls, is returned to the liver for excretion into the bile. HDL accepts free (non-esterified) cholesterol from peripheral tissues, including the arterial walls (53). The free cholesterol that is taken up by HDL is quickly altered to cholesterol ester, which prevents it from reentering the arterial wall.[1]

HDL then carries the cholesterol ester to the liver, or transfers it to LDL or to the partially metabolized remnant particles of VLDL or chylomicrons, which do likewise. Remarkably, the liver is able to selectively remove only

---

[1]Apoprotein A-I on the HDL surface triggers an enzyme called lecithin-cholesterol acyl transferase (LCAT) to convert free cholesterol taken up from plaque into cholesterol ester so that it cannot reenter the arterial wall. Apoprotein D then helps transfer the ester to chylomicron remnants and VLDL remnants (IDL), which ferry cholesterol to the liver.

the cholesterol from HDL, leaving the remaining particle intact to absorb more cholesterol from arteries and tissues. The other lipoproteins are completely absorbed by the liver. Figure 1.9 is a schematic illustration of the basic cholesterol transport system.

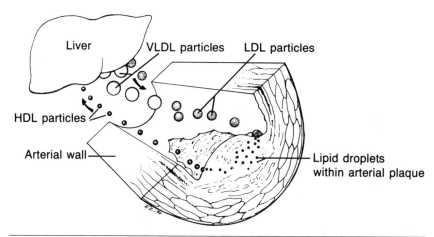

Figure 1.9   Cholesterol transport. The liver synthesizes and releases VLDL particles (large spheres) into the circulation, some of which are transformed into the atherogenic LDL particles (intermediate spheres) which can deposit cholesterol in plaque. Some of the cholesterol in plaque can be absorbed by HDL particles (small spheres) and returned to the liver in the process of reverse cholesterol transport.

Evidence for plaque regression was first demonstrated by animal experiments with pigeons, rabbits, and monkeys (54). The animals' food was packed full of cholesterol, saturated fat, or both to raise the animals' blood cholesterol levels and induce atherosclerosis. When the animals were later switched to normal feed (55, 56) or allowed to exercise, the plaque subsided (57).

Solid clinical evidence for the protective role of HDL has been obtained using angiography, special X-ray pictures of the coronary arteries. Subjects with the most severe narrowing of their arteries have the lowest HDL concentrations. Although women in general have higher HDL levels, the HDL levels of men and women with the same degree of atherosclerosis is surprisingly similar (58). In autopsy studies as well, higher HDL levels are highly correlated with the extent of atherosclerosis.

Stronger evidence has recently come from prospective studies in the United States and Europe. People with higher HDL levels were found to have less progression and more regression of plaque in their arteries. Some studies followed the subjects' clinical courses, noting fewer heart attacks (12, 59), whereas others looked at the actual condition of the arteries with angiography (60, 61).

In an elegant human regression study released in 1987, the Cholesterol Lowering Atherosclerosis Study (CLAS), patients who had undergone coronary bypass surgery were randomly assigned to either a diet-alone group or a diet-plus-drug (colestipol and niacin) group. The latter group achieved a 26% decrease in total cholesterol, a 43% decrease in LDL, and a 37% increase in HDL. These patients, who already had severe CHD, achieved a 16% reversal of atherosclerosis through diet and medication (10).

Counterpoint: Too Much Emphasis on HDL?   Although high HDL levels seem to be beneficial for most people in advanced Western societies, they should not be viewed as a prerequisite for good health. Vegetarians in the United States have HDL values 9 mg/dl (.23 mmol/L) lower than the national average yet have CHD rates one third to one eighth of the national average (62, 63).

Many primitive groups, such as the Tarahumara Indians of Mexico and the African Masai, have low HDL levels yet virtually no CHD. Their HDL levels are at or below 40 mg/dl (1.03 mmol/L) even though the typical adult is thin, exercises daily, and eats a low-fat diet (25). Perhaps these people do not need higher HDL levels because their diets are so low in fat and cholesterol and high in fiber. If cholesterol is not accumulating in their arterial walls, they may require less reverse cholesterol transport. Thus, although an HDL level of 60 mg/dl (1.55 mmol/L) or above tends to be protective, it should not lure one into complacency about LDL. Cholesterol deposition is caused by the LDL particle and may well be occurring concurrently. The primary goal in cholesterol management is to maintain LDL concentration as low as possible.

Very Low–Density Lipoproteins

Triglycerides are carried primarily by two lipoproteins, chylomicrons and VLDL. Chylomicrons transport absorbed dietary fat from the intestine to the liver whereas VLDL carry triglycerides constructed in the liver to the rest of the body.

Chylomicrons, or chylos for short, are the largest of the lipoproteins and do not bear any relationship to atherosclerosis. Intestinal cells package the fat absorbed from a meal into chylos and send them on their way to the liver. En route they give up some of their triglycerides, thus shrinking into chylomicron remnants, which are rapidly cleared by the liver.

Normally, chylomicrons are present for only a few hours after a meal. In the fasting state nearly all the triglyceride present in the blood is contained in VLDL (negligible amounts are also present in LDL and HDL). Thus, *triglycerides* in this book will refer only to VLDL triglycerides, because an individual's blood test (lipid profile) should be drawn after an overnight fast.

VLDL particles are the second-largest of the lipoproteins. The VLDL core contains little cholesterol but large amounts of triglyceride, the body's major energy-storage molecule. Being overweight and consuming too much alcohol or refined sugar can cause a person's VLDL levels to escalate. Medical conditions that increase triglycerides are kidney failure and poor control of diabetes. Many common blood pressure medications (the beta blockers and diuretics) and some steroids have adverse effects on triglycerides. Women with a predisposition to high triglycerides frequently encounter a more serious elevation when they use oral contraceptives.

Unlike the cellular control for cholesterol, triglycerides have a complex regulatory system mediated by hormones throughout the body. VLDL give up most of their triglycerides to cells, thus shrinking into LDL particles one fourth their previous size. This process occurs in the presence of an enzyme called lipoprotein lipase, which is present along the arterial walls. The activity of lipoprotein lipase is modulated by a number of hormones such as insulin, thyroxin (thyroid hormone), cortisol, and oral contraceptives. Unlike cholesterol, triglycerides do not tend to accumulate in the bloodstream because they can be broken down into carbon dioxide and water, releasing stored energy.

VLDL pass through an intermediate stage called VLDL remnants, or intermediate-density lipoproteins (IDL), which are removed by the same LDL receptor mechanism as LDL. In general, 30% of the IDL that is not cleared by the liver is transformed in the blood to LDL (64). About half of the circulating LDL particles are formed in this way; the remainder are synthesized and released by the liver. By reducing LDL receptors, dietary saturated fats and cholesterol suppress the clearance of both LDL and VLDL remnants, causing more of the latter to end up as LDL particles.

In spite of this physiological link to LDL cholesterol, the health risk of having elevated VLDL triglycerides remains controversial. In general, triglyceride levels of 250 mg/dl (2.8 mmol/L) and higher are associated with a twofold increase in CHD. These high concentrations are particularly ominous for diabetics and women, as well as those with low levels of HDL, high levels of apoprotein B, or a family history of CHD before age 55 (65, 66). In some people, high triglyceride levels may be the only clue to a diagnosis of familial combined hyperlipidemia, an inherited disorder that promotes CHD. The risk of CHD with elevated triglyceride levels is minimally increased for individuals without these conditions.

Epidemiological studies using univariate analysis suggest that people with hypertriglyceridemia (high blood triglyceride levels) seem to have a greater risk of heart attack. However, this statistical method does not take into account that triglyceride levels are higher in people who are diabetic and/or overweight—conditions that in themselves present higher risks.

Using multivariate analysis, which adjusts for other confounding risk factors such as low HDL, obesity, diabetes, and smoking, the risk of high triglycerides is difficult to demonstrate (67). Triglycerides may only indirectly damage the arteries by being degraded to LDL particles or by suppressing HDL. (Triglycerides tend to have an inverse relationship with HDL; as VLDL increases, HDL decreases.) If HDL and LDL levels are normal, people with mildly elevated VLDL levels in the range of 150 to 250 mg/dl (1.7 to 2.8 mmol/L) may not be at increased risk for CHD.

To clarify the independent role of triglycerides, Carlson and Bottiger in Sweden followed 6,224 men and women for 19 years (68). The results of their study implicated triglycerides in heart attacks, though not in other forms of coronary heart disease such as angina or sudden cardiac death. The European Consensus Recommendations on hyperlipidemia states that a fasting triglyceride of higher than 200 (2.3 mmol/L) is considered to represent increased risk of CHD (69).

Risk Ratios for Coronary Heart Disease

In most advanced societies, the relative proportion of LDL to HDL cholesterol is a more sensitive and specific indicator of an individual's risk of developing coronary heart disease than is the total cholesterol level alone (9, 70). In an individual with an acceptable total cholesterol (TC) but very little HDL, the TC/HDL ratio can indicate an increased risk of CHD. Alternatively, an active person may have slightly higher total cholesterol due to high HDL levels but will still maintain a healthy TC/HDL ratio.

Obtaining a cholesterol ratio requires a *lipid panel* or *coronary risk profile*. This test, which requires a 12-hour fast, measures total cholesterol as well as triglycerides, HDL, and LDL. A lipid panel is especially valuable for individuals over age 55, when HDL measurement greatly improves the accuracy of the test to predict the risk for CHD. Others who definitely require a lipid panel are those whose total cholesterol is higher than 240 mg/dl (6.2 mmol/L) or whose LDL is higher than 160 mg/dl (4.1 mmol/L) (5). These cutoff points should be much lower for children, adolescents, and those with additional CHD risk factors (71). A low HDL value (less than 35 mg/dl or 0.9 mmol/L) should be repeated because laboratory measurements of HDL tend to be less accurate than for total cholesterol or LDL.

Many labs calculate the ratio of total cholesterol to HDL and translate this into a risk category—low, average, or high risk. An average TC/HDL ratio in the United States is about 5, which is not very healthy. People with a ratio of 3.5 have about half the average risk of CHD. Those with ratios of 9.6 have twice the average risk of heart attack, angina pectoris, or sudden cardiac death. A ratio of 23.4 imparts a threefold higher risk (72).[2]

Figure 1.10 is an example of a standard printout from a hospital laboratory. Patient identification information is at the top, followed by the

Rose Medical Center

Patient Name: Byrne, Kevin

Age: 36   Sex: Male   Date: 5/29/89   Time: 23:34

———————————————— CHEMISTRY ————————————————

| Lipid Profile | | Normals | | |
		Low	High	Units
Cholesterol	135.	110.	232.	mg/dl
LDL-calc	88.	70.	152.	mg/dl
HDL chol	39.	35.	70.	mg/dl
Triglyceride	40.	45.	190.	mg/dl
Chol/HDL	3.46		See Table 1	

Table 1.   Cholesterol/HDL Ratio and Risk of Coronary Heart Disease

	Male	Female
1/2 risk	3.43	3.27
Normal risk	4.97	4.44
2X risk	9.55	7.05
3X risk	23.39	11.04

Table 2.   Cholesterol Normal Ranges and Treatment Goals Recommended by the National Cholesterol Education Program (NIH)

Total Cholesterol Normal Range		LDL Cholesterol Normal Range	
Desirable:	<200 mg/dl	Desirable:	<130 mg/dl
Borderline high:	200-239 mg/dl	Borderline high:	130-159 mg/dl
High:	>239 mg/dl	High:	>159 mg/dl

Figure 1.10   Sample lipid profile. A lipid panel report should list the total blood cholesterol, LDL (which is calculated), HDL, triglycerides, and the ratio of total cholesterol to HDL. A table is frequently used to assist the clinician in interpreting the ratio value.

———————

[2]Some labs calculate the ratio of LDL to HDL with the following results: A value of 1.0 corresponds to half the average CHD risk; 3.6 is average; 6.3 is twice average; and 8.0 is three times the average risk of CHD in the United States. These ratios apply to lipoproteins whether measured in mg/dl or mmol/L.

lipoprotein values and the ranges the lab considers normal. Values to help interpret the TC/HDL ratio (Table 1 in figure) are now usually given on the report.

TC includes the cholesterol contained in LDL, HDL, and VLDL. HDL and VLDL are measured directly, whereas LDL is usually calculated. If triglycerides are lower than 400 mg/dl, the following formula is used (73) to calculate LDL:

$$LDL = total\ cholesterol - [(HDL + triglycerides/5)]$$

To convert to the international lipid units, millimoles per liter (mmol/L), use these conversion formulas:

cholesterol in mg/dl × .02586 = cholesterol in mmol/L
triglycerides in mg/dl × .01129 = triglycerides in mmol/L

Conversely, to derive cholesterol values in mg/dl, multiply the cholesterol level in mmol/L by 38.67 or the triglyceride level in mmol/L by 88.57.

To convert from serum to plasma cholesterol values, multiply serum levels by 0.954. To convert plasma cholesterol to the larger serum values, multiply by 1.048. The basic unit, mg/dl (or mmol/L), remains the same.

References

1. Stamler, J. (1979). Population studies. In R.I. Levy, B.M. Rifkind, B.H. Dennis, & N. Ernst (Eds.), *Nutrition, lipids, and coronary disease: A global view* (pp. 25-88). New York: Raven Press.
2. Kannel, W.B., McGee, D., & Gordon, T. (1976). A general cardio-vascular risk profile: The Framingham Study. *American Journal of Cardiology*, **38**, 46-52.
3. American Heart Association. (1987). *1987 heart facts*. Dallas: Author.
4. Vital Statistics of the United States, 1987. (1989). National Center for Health Statistics, U.S. Department of Health & Human Services, Public Health Service, Centers for Disease Control. Publication No. (PHS) 89-1102, Hyattsville, MD.
5. Expert Panel of the National Cholesterol Education Program. (1988). Report of the National Cholesterol Education Program Expert Panel on detection, evaluation, and treatment of high blood cholesterol in adults. *Archives of Internal Medicine*, **148**, 36-39. (Also available as NIH Publication No. 88-2925, January 1988.)
6. Stamler, J. (1978). Lifestyles, major risk factors, proof and public policy. *Circulation*, **58**, 3.
7. Stamler, J., & Shekelle, R.B. (1988). Dietary cholesterol and human

coronary heart disease. *Archives of Pathology and Laboratory Medicine,* **112,** 1032-1040.

8. Shekelle, R.B., & Stamler, J. (1989). Dietary cholesterol and ischaemic heart disease. *Lancet,* **I,** 1177-1179.

9. Anderson, K.M., Castelli, W.P., & Levy, D. (1987). Cholesterol and mortality: 30 years of follow-up from the Framingham study. *Journal of the American Medical Association,* **257,** 2176-2180.

10. Blankenhorn, D.H., Nessim, S.A., Johnson, R.L., San Marco, M.E., Azen, S.P., & Cashin-Hemphill, L. (1987). Beneficial effects of combined colestipol-niacin therapy on coronary atherosclerosis and coronary venous bypass grafts. *Journal of the American Medical Association,* **257,** 3233-3240.

11. Frick, M.H., Elo, O., Haapa, K., Heinonen, O., Heinsalmi, P., Helo, P., Huttunen, J.K., Kaitaniemi, P., Koskinen, P., Manninen, V., Mäenpää, H., Mälkönen, M., Mänttäri, M., Norola, S., Pasternack, A., Pikkarainen, J., Romo, M., Sjöblom, T., & Nikkilä, E. (1987). Helsinki Heart Study. Primary-prevention trial with gemfibrozil in middle-aged men with dyslipidemia: Safety of treatment, changes in risk factors, and incidence of coronary heart disease. *New England Journal of Medicine,* **317,** 1237-1245.

12. Arntzenius, A.C., Kromhout, D., Barth, J.D., Reiber, J.H., Bruschke, A.V., Buis, B., vanGent, C.M., Kempen-Voogd, N., Strikwerda, S., & Van der Velde, E.A. (1985). Diet, lipoproteins, and the progression of coronary atherosclerosis: The Leiden Intervention Trial. *New England Journal of Medicine,* **312,** 805-811.

13. Lipid Research Clinics Program. (1984). The Lipid Research Clinics Coronary Primary Prevention Trial results. I. Reduction in incidence of coronary heart disease. *Journal of the American Medical Association,* **251,** 351-364.

14. Hjermann, I., Byre, K.V., Holme, I., & Leren, P. (1981, December 12). Effect of diet and smoking intervention on the incidence of coronary heart disease. *Lancet,* **2,** 1303-1310.

15. Coronary Drug Project Research Group. (1975). Clofibrate and niacin in coronary heart disease. *Journal of the American Medical Association,* **231,** 360-381.

16. Hopkins, P.N., & Williams, R.R. (1986). Identification and relative weight of cardiovascular risk factors. *Cardiology Clinics,* **4,** 3-32.

17. Grundy, S.M. (1986). Cholesterol and coronary heart disease. *Journal of the American Medical Association,* **256,** 2849-2858.

18. Weinstein, M.C., Coxson, P.G., Williams, L.W., Pass, T.M., Stason, W.B., & Goldman, L. (1986). Coronary heart disease morbidity, mortality, and cost for the next quarter century. Abstract from *Clinical Research,* **34,** 386A.

19. Consensus Development Conference. (1985). Lowering blood

cholesterol to prevent heart disease. *Journal of the American Medical Association*, **253**, 2080-2086.

20. Stamler, J., Wentworth, D., & Neaton, J.D. (1986). Is relationship between serum cholesterol and risk of premature death from coronary heart disease continuous and graded? Findings from 356,222 primary screenees in the Multiple Risk Factor Intervention Trial (MRFIT). *Journal of the American Medical Association*, **256**, 2823-2828.

21. Solberg, L.A., & Strong, J.P. (1983). Risk factors and atherosclerotic lesions. A review of autopsy studies. *Arteriosclerosis*, **3**, 187-198.

22. Holme, I., Enger, S.C., Helgeland, A., Hjermann, I., Leren, P., Lund-Larsen, P.G., Solberg, L.A., & Strong, J.P. (1981). Risk factors and raised atherosclerotic lesions in coronary and cerebral arteries. *Arteriosclerosis*, **1**, 250-256.

23. American Heart Association. (1986). 1986 stroke facts. Dallas: Author.

24. Grundy, S.M., Bilheimer, D., Blackburn, H., Brown, W.V., Kwiterovich, P.O., Matterson, F., Schonfeld, G., & Weidman, W.H. (1982). Rationale of the Diet-Heart Statement of the American Heart Association. *Circulation*, **65**, 839A-854A.

25. Connor, W.E., Cerqueira, M.T., Connor, R.W., Wallace, R.B., Malinow, M.R., & Casdorph, H.R. (1988). The plasma lipids, lipoproteins, and diet of the Tarahumara Indians of Mexico. *American Journal of Clinical Nutrition*, **31**, 1131.

26. Mattson, F.H., Erickson, B.A., & Kligman, A.M. (1972). Effect of dietary cholesterol on serum cholesterol in man. *American Journal of Clinical Nutrition*, **25**, 589-594.

27. Keys, A., Anderson, J.T., & Grande, F. (1965). Serum cholesterol responses to changes in the diet. II. The effect of cholesterol in the diet. *Metabolism*, **14**, 759.

28. Laboratory Standardization Panel of the National Cholesterol Education Program. (1988). Current status of blood cholesterol measurement in clinical laboratories in the United States (NIH Publication No. 88-2928). Washington, DC: U.S. Department of Health and Human Services.

29. Kannel, W.B. (Chairman), Doyle, J.T., Ostfeld, A.M., Jenkins, C.D., Kuller, L., Podell, R.N., & Stamler, J. (1984). Atherosclerosis Study Group. Optimal resources for primary prevention of atherosclerotic diseases. *Circulation*, **70**, 155A-205A.

30. Castelli, W.P., & Anderson, K. (1986). A population at risk. Prevalence of high cholesterol levels in hypertensive patients in the Framingham Study. *American Journal of Medicine*, **80**(Suppl. 2A), 23-32.

31. Martin, M.J., Hulley, S.B., Browner, W.S., Kuller, L.H., & Wentworth, D. (1986). Serum cholesterol, blood pressure, and mortality: Implications from a cohort of 361,662 men. *Lancet*, **2**, 933-936.

32. Rifkind, B.M., & Lenfant, C. (1986). Cholesterol lowering and the

reduction of coronary heart disease risk [Editorial]. *Journal of the American Medical Association, 256*, 2872-2873.

33. Keys, A. (1969). Serum cholesterol and the question of "normal." In E.S. Benson & P.E. Strandjord (Eds.), *Multiple laboratory screening* (pp. 147-170). New York: Academic Press.

34. Mancilha-Carvalho, J.J., & Crews, D.E. (1988, November). *Lipid profiles of Yanomono Indians in Brazil.* Presented at Poster Session 2, First National Cholesterol Conference, Washington, DC.

35. Schaefer, E.J., & Levy, R.I. (1985). Pathogenesis and management of lipoprotein disorders. *New England Journal of Medicine, 312*, 1300-1310.

36. Steinberg, D., Parthasarathy, S., Carew, T.E., Khoo, J.C., & Witztum, J.L. (1989). Beyond cholesterol. Modifications of low-density lipoprotein that increase its atherogenicity. *New England Journal of Medicine, 320*, 915-924.

37. Subcommittee on Recommended Dietary Allowances, Food and Nutrition Board (1989). *Recommended Dietary Allowances* (10th ed.). Washington, DC: National Academy Press.

38. Brown, M.S., & Goldstein, J.L. (1983). Lipoprotein receptors in the liver: Control signals for plasma cholesterol traffic. *Journal of Clinical Investigation, 72*, 743-747.

39. Weinberg, R.B. (1987). Lipoprotein metabolism: Hormonal regulation. *Hospital Practice, 22*, 223-243.

40. Mahley, R.W., Weisgraber, K.H., Bergot, T.P., & Innerarity, T.L. (1978). Effects of cholesterol feeding on human and animal high density lipoproteins. In A.M. Gotto, N.E. Miller, & M.F. Oliver (Eds.), *High density lipoproteins and atherosclerosis* (pp. 149-176). Amsterdam: Elsevier-North Holland.

41. Barr, D.P., Russ, E.M., & Eder, H.A. (1951). Protein-lipid relationships in human plasma. *American Journal of Medicine, 11*, 480-493.

42. Castelli, W.P., Garrison, R.J., Wilson, P.F., Abbott, R.D., Kalovsdian, S., & Kannel, W.B. (1986). Incidence of coronary heart disease and lipoprotein cholesterol levels. The Framingham Study. *Journal of the American Medical Association, 256*, 2835-2838.

43. Goldbourt, U., & Medazlie, J.H. (1979). High density lipoprotein cholesterol and incidence of coronary heart disease—the Israeli ischaemic heart disease study. *American Journal of Epidemiology, 109*, 296.

44. Hulley, S.B., Ashman, P., Kuller, L., Lasser, N., & Sherwin, R. (1979). HDL-cholesterol levels in the Multiple Risk Factor Intervention Trial (MRFIT) by the MRFIT Research Group. *Lipids, 14*, 119.

45. Gordon, T., Castelli, W.P., Hjortland, M.C., Kannel, W.B., & Dawber, T.R. (1977). High density lipoprotein as a protective factor against coronary heart disease. *American Journal of Medicine, 62*, 707-713.

46. Kannel, W.B. (1983). High-density lipoproteins: Epidemiologic profile and risks of coronary artery disease. *American Journal of Cardiology*, 52, 9B-12B.

47. Gotto, A.M. (1983). High-density lipoproteins: Biochemical and metabolic factors. *American Journal of Cardiology*, 52, 2B-4B.

48. Schwandt, P., Janetschek, P., & Weisweiler, P. (1982). High density lipoproteins unaffected by dietary fat modification. *Atherosclerosis*, 44, 9-17.

49. Hjermann, I., Enger, S.C., Helgeland, A., Holme, I., Leren, P., & Trygg, K. (1979). The effect of dietary changes on high density lipoprotein cholesterol. The Oslo study. *American Journal of Medicine*, 66, 105-109.

50. Ehnholm, C., Huttunen, J.K., Pietinen, P., Leino, U., Mutanen, M., Kostiainen, E., Pikkarainen, J., Dougherty, R., Iacono, J., & Puska, P. (1982). Effect of diet on serum lipoproteins in a population with a high risk of coronary heart disease. *New England Journal of Medicine*, 307, 850-855.

51. Cowan, G.O. (1983). Influence of exercise on high-density lipoproteins. *American Journal of Cardiology*, 52, 13B.

52. Castelli, W.P., Gordon, T., Hjortland, M.C., Kagan, A., Doyle, J.T., Hames, C.G., Hulley, S.B., & Zukel, W.J. (1977). Alcohol and blood lipids. *Lancet*, 2, 153-155, 8030.

53. Stein, O., Vanderhoek, J., Friedman, G., & Stein, Y. (1976). Deposition and mobilization of cholesterol ester in cultured human skin fibroblasts. *Biochimica Biophysica Acta*, 450, 367.

54. Wissler, R.W., & Vesselinovitch, D. (1977). Regression of atherosclerosis in experimental animals and man. *Modern Concepts Cardiovascular Disease*, 26, 27.

55. St. Clair, R.W. (1983). Atherosclerosis regression in animal models: Current concepts of cellular and biochemical mechanisms. *Progress in Cardiovascular Diseases*, 26, 109-132.

56. Armstrong, M.L. (1976). Regression of atherosclerosis. In R. Paoletti & A.M. Gotto (Eds.), *Atherosclerosis* (p. 137). New York: Raven Press.

57. Kramsch, D.M., Aspen, A.J., Abramowitz, B.M., Kreimendahl, T., & Hood, W.B. (1981). Reduction of coronary atherosclerosis by moderate conditioning exercise in monkeys on an atherogenic diet. *New England Journal of Medicine*, 305, 1483-1489.

58. Pearson, T.A., Bulkley, B.H., Achuff, S.C., Kwiterovich, P.O., & Gordis, L. (1979). The association of low levels of HDL cholesterol and arteriographically defined coronary artery disease. *American Journal of Epidemiology*, 109, 285-295.

59. Manninen, V., Elo, O., Frick, M.H., Haapa, J., Heinonen, O.P., Heinsalmi, P., Helo, P., Huttunen, J.K., Kaitaniemi, P., Koskinen, P., Mäenpää, H., Mälkönen, M., Mänttäri, M., Norola, S., Pasternack, A., Pikkarainen, J., Romo, M., Sjöblom, T., & Nikkilä, E.A. (1988).

Lipid alterations and decline in the incidence of coronary heart disease in the Helsinki Heart Study. *Journal of the American Medical Association*, **260**, 641-651.

60. Levy, R.I., Brensike, J.F., Epstein, S.E., Kelsey, S.F., Passaman, E.R., Richardson, J.M., Loh, I.K., Stone, N.J., Aldrich, R.F., Battaglini, J.W., Moriarty, D.J., Fisher, M.L., Friedman, L., Friedewald, W., & Detre, K.M. (1984). The influence of changes in lipid values induced by cholestyramine and diet on progression of coronary artery disease: Results of NHLBI Type II Coronary Intervention Study. *Circulation*, **69**, 325-327.

61. Nikkila, E.A., Viikinkoski, P., Valle, M., & Frick, M.H. (1984). Prevention of progression of coronary atherosclerosis by treatment of hyperlipidaemia: A seven year prospective angiographic study. *British Medical Journal*, **289**, 220-223.

62. Philips, R.L., Lemmon, F.R., Beeson, W.L., & Kuzman, J.W. (1978). Coronary heart disease among Seventh-Day Adventists with differing habits: A preliminary report. *American Journal of Clinical Nutrition*, **31**, S191-S198.

63. Sacks, F.M., Castelli, W.P., Donner, A., & Kass, E.H. (1975). Plasma lipids and lipoproteins in vegetarians and controls. *New England Journal of Medicine*, **292**, 1148.

64. Krauss, R.M., Lindgren, F.T., Williams, P.T., Brensike, J., Detre, K.M., Lindgren, F.T., Kelsey, S.F., Vranizan, K., & Levy, R.I. (1987). Intermediate-density lipoproteins and progression of coronary artery disease in hypercholesterolemic men. *Lancet*, **2**, 62-66.

65. Grundy, S.M. (1988). Lessons from the Helsinki Heart Study. *Postgraduate Medicine*, **84**, 217-231.

66. Miller, V., & LaRosa, J.C. (1988). Hypercholesterolemia in women: What are the special considerations? *Female Patient*, **13**, 22-32.

67. Hulley, S.B., Rosenman, R.H., Bawol, R.D., & Brand, R.J. (1980). Epidemiology as a guide to clinical decisions: The association between triglyceride and coronary heart disease. *New England Journal of Medicine*, **302**, 1383-1389.

68. Carlson, L.A., Böttiger, L.E., & Åhfeld, P.E. (1979). Risk factors for myocardial infarction in the Stockholm prospective study: A 14-year follow-up focussing on the role of plasma triglycerides and cholesterol. *Acta Medica Scandinavica*, **206**, 351-360.

69. Study Group, European Atherosclerosis Society. (1987). Strategies for the prevention of coronary heart disease: A policy statement of the European Atherosclerosis Society. *European Heart Journal*, **8**, 77-88.

70. Castelli, W.P., Abbott, R.D., & McNamara, P.M. (1983). Summary estimates of cholesterol used to predict coronary heart disease. *Circulation*, **67**, 730-734.

71. Berenson, G.S., & Epstein, R.H. (Chairmen) (1983). Conference on blood lipids in children: Optimal levels for early prevention of

coronary artery disease. Workshop report: epidemiologic section, American Health Foundation. *Preventive Medicine, 12,* 741-797.
72. Atherosclerosis Study Group. (1984). Optimal resources for primary prevention of atherosclerotic diseases. *Circulation, 70,* 157A-205A.
73. Friedewald, W.T., Levy, R.I., & Frederickson, D.S. (1972). Estimation of the concentration of low-density lipoprotein cholesterol in plasma, without use of the preparative ultracentrifuge. *Clinical Chemistry, 18,* 499.
74. Expert Committee on Prevention of Coronary Heart Disease. (1982). Prevention of coronary heart disease. *Technical Report Series 678.* Geneva: World Health Organization.

Suggested Readings

Committee on Diet and Health, Food and Nutrition Board, Commission on Life Sciences, National Research Council. (1989). *Diet and health. Implications for reducing chronic disease risk.* Washington, DC: National Academy Press.

Fraser, G.E. (1986). *Preventive cardiology.* New York: Oxford.

Kaplan, N.M., & Stamler, J. (1983). *Prevention of coronary heart disease.* Philadelphia: W.B. Saunders.

U.S. Department of Health and Human Services, Public Health Service. (1990). Healthy people 2000: National health promotion and disease prevention objectives. [DHHS, PHS Publication No. 017-001-00474-0 (full report) or 017-001-00473-1 (summary report)]. Washington, DC: U.S. Government Printing Office.

Chapter

2

Plaque and Arterial Destruction

The first steps in any health promotion and disease prevention program are education, awareness, and motivation. Developing and maintaining the healthy lifestyle habits to control cholesterol are easier if we realize the subtle dangers of atherosclerosis. Advanced atherosclerosis has no medical or surgical cure, and none is likely to be developed in the near future. The only way this process can be reversed is by our own internal healing mechanism.

Primary, or early, prevention is crucial to cardiovascular health because plaque is not simply a veneer along the artery's inner lining. It's more like a tumor mass that thickens and destroys the arterial wall. As it expands in all directions, it becomes more dangerous and more difficult to treat. A brief look at the structure of arteries will facilitate our discussion of *atherogenesis*, or plaque formation.

Artery Structure

Arteries have three distinct layers: the endothelium (or intima), the media, and the adventitia. The most critical layer for atherogenesis is the endothelium, which faces the bloodstream (see Figure 2.1). It consists mainly of a single layer of flat endothelial cells arranged in a patchwork pattern. Encircling these cells is a thin tube of noncellular supporting material called the basement membrane. Plaque growth originates in the subintimal space, just under the endothelial cells.

The endothelium is critical for normal arterial function. It allows nutrients to pass through into deeper layers. These cells also act as "gatekeepers" to exclude toxins from the deeper regions of the wall. If this delicate mosaic is injured in any way, plaque formation can begin.

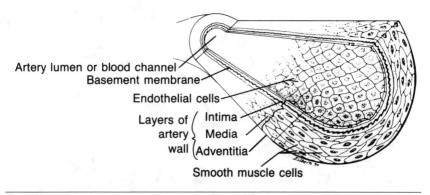

Artery lumen or blood channel
Basement membrane
Endothelial cells
Layers of / Intima
artery \ Media
wall (Adventitia
Smooth muscle cells

Figure 2.1 The normal structure of arteries includes three distinct layers: the endothelium, or intima, which faces the bloodstream, the media, and the adventitia.

Surrounding the endothelium is the media, which contains spindle-shaped smooth muscle cells (SMCs) arranged in concentric layers. This is the thickest section of the artery and one that serves an important function in health. The resiliency of the media allows for expansion and contraction of the artery's diameter as a pulse of blood flows through it. The rebound constriction following the pulse aids in the forward propulsion of the blood. Normally, these cells are shielded from cholesterol by the endothelium. If this protection is lost because of endothelial damage, SMCs become active participants in atherogenesis by multiplying and absorbing cholesterol.

The third layer, the adventitia, is an outer sheath of tough, fibrous connective tissue. It does not regularly play a role in atherosclerosis, except in complications that develop when the disease is in advanced stages. Weaving through this layer are tiny blood vessels that supply the SMCs with nutrients. The arterial wall also contains minute nerves that regulate SMC level of contraction, or tone. Unfortunately, these nerves do not send pain messages to the brain, allowing us to unwittingly destroy our arteries.

Atherogenesis

Atherogenesis begins with damage to the endothelium layer. As early as 1852, the German scientist Von Rokitansky suggested that atherosclerosis (then a rare disease) was caused by "recurrent deposition of elements derived from the blood mass" (1). Support for the critical role of the endothelium has mounted steadily, particularly in recent years. According to the generally accepted "response-to-injury" hypothesis, endothelial damage may result from a variety of insults, primarily border-line or high blood cholesterol, high blood pressure, and smoking (2, 3). An individual without one or more of these major risk factors to initiate endothelial injury will experience little if any atherosclerosis.

Once the endothelial barrier is disrupted, cholesterol from the harmful LDL (low-density lipoprotein) particles can infiltrate the arterial wall. If the endothelial damage is severe, as in people with several risk factors, even mild elevations of LDL can be problematic. When high concentrations of LDL cholesterol are present, the plaque grows even more quickly. As cholesterol collects beneath the endothelium, the developing plaque thickens the arterial wall and narrows its channel.

Types of Injury to Endothelial Cells

Cholesterol plays a dual role in atherogenesis. First, it may be sufficient in itself to harm the artery's intimal layer (4). Second, cholesterol carried by the LDL fraction passes through and collects in the subintimal space. Cholesterol molecules and crystals comprise a fourth of the plaque's bulk. As more cholesterol accumulates, the plaque swells.

Chemically modified low-density lipoproteins, especially oxidized LDL, and small, dense LDL are particularly toxic to the endothelium (5). They interfere with this layer's gatekeeper role, allowing substances, including more cholesterol, to pass through the disrupted cell barrier. Modified LDL particles also promote the growth of plaque from within, by attracting more scavenger cells (discussed below).

Smoking damages the endothelium layer either by direct chemical irritation or by inducing a mild allergic reaction (6). Nicotine, carbon monoxide, and cadmium are most frequently incriminated as the endothelial poisons that initiate cholesterol influx. Tobacco seems to alter the endothelium's production of prostacyclin, a substance that keeps the arterial lining smooth. (Higher levels of HDL, on the other hand, are thought to improve the endothelium's production of prostacyclin.) Tobacco also increases the synthesis of thromboxane by platelets, making them more sticky (7). Platelets have a shortened survival time in smokers, an effect that is reversed when smoking ceases.

Hypertension is thought to damage the endothelium either by sheer forces or increased turbulence. The forces weaken the endothelial cells, increasing their permeability to blood cholesterol. Sustained hypertension may eventually tear them off their supporting basement membrane, exposing the underlying collagen fibers (8). The cellular injury resulting from diabetes is poorly understood but probably involves a modified (glycosylated) form of LDL. Diabetes is a much less important factor for endothelial injury than high cholesterol, hypertension, or smoking.

Stages in Plaque Formation

Plaque is formed in three overlapping steps: the fatty streak of childhood, the fibrous plaque of adolescence, and the complicated plaque of middle age and older. Though these distinctions are useful for describing and understanding atherogenesis, no abrupt changes occur between the categories. Instead, one type of lesion gradually phases into the next. Virtually all adults in advanced societies have more than one stage present at any one time (9).

Stage 1: Fatty Streak Formation

The initial phase of plaque development is the appearance of the fatty streak. Cholesterol and fat accumulation beneath the endothelium result in flat, slightly raised areas that can just be seen with the naked eye. They arise in rows, arranged lengthwise along the artery, and take on a yellow hue. As they increase in size and number, they coalesce to form yellow streaks, hence the name (see Figure 2.2).

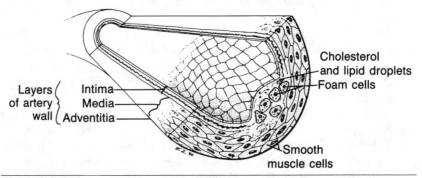

Figure 2.2   The earliest sign of atherosclerosis is the fatty streak, which results from cholesterol deposits accumulating in the subintimal space, imparting a yellowish hue to the endothelial surface.

This early stage in atherogenesis actually begins in infancy. Autopsies of children one month to one year of age have verified that nearly half of them had begun to form fatty streaks in the aorta, the largest artery in the body (10, 11). Streaks begin to appear around puberty in the coronary arteries that supply the heart muscle (12).

Because of their low profile and smooth surface, fatty streaks in themselves are not dangerous. They occur in all cultures worldwide and are slightly more prevalent in females. In people who consume a heart-healthy diet, such as those in less developed countries, fatty streaks stabilize or even disappear completely.

In Western societies, however, fatty streaks seem to herald future problems. Fatty streaks are found in the same locations in children as the more advanced plaque is in adults (13, 14). And like older, established plaque, fatty streaks contain the same scavenger cells that engulf cholesterol droplets. When these cells cannot keep up with the cholesterol influx, the fatty streak converts from a mere blemish to more serious plaque.

The two most important cell types in the growth of plaque are the SMCs of the artery's media layer, and monocytes, which originate in the blood. Both have a basic function to remove foreign substances and bacteria throughout the body. They are referred to as scavenger cells because they kill and digest microbes (bacteria and viruses) and absorb toxic and foreign substances. In the endangered artery, they act as cholesterol sponges, surrounding and engulfing the cholesterol droplets (2).

As previously noted, hypercholesterolemia alone can be sufficient to injure the endothelium, permitting cholesterol entry into the arterial wall. Following in pursuit of the cholesterol are the monocytes, squeezing through the junctions between the endothelial cells. High cholesterol levels increase the invasiveness of the monocytes and also lessen the ability of the endothelial cells to resist their entry.[1]

Smooth muscle cells enter the intima from the surrounding media in response to the cholesterol invasion and chemical "messages" from monocytes and epithelial cells (15). Once they arrive beneath the endothelium, SMCs and monocytes multiply and begin the process of cholesterol cleanup and containment. Eventually, both cell types become so filled with fat globules that they are indistinguishable from one another. Because of their appearance, the SMCs and monocytes are then called foam cells.

Although functionally impaired, the endothelium is still intact in the fatty streak stage, completely covering the incipient plaque beneath it. If the injury and cholesterol ingress stop soon enough, the artery can heal itself. HDL cholesterol particles play the major role in this process of reverse cholesterol transport.

If arterial injury continues beyond this stage, as it typically does in people from developed societies, fatty streaks begin to show signs of decay. The foam cells start to disintegrate and release chemically modified cholesterol and enzymes into the surrounding subintimal space. These substances further damage the overlying endothelium, accelerating the seepage of cholesterol, the migration of SMCs and monocytes, and the overall growth of the plaque. In brief, the death of foam cells starts a chain of events leading to fibrous plaque.

---

[1]Technically, once the monocyte is within the arterial wall (or any tissue) it is called a macrophage. For simplicity here, the former term is retained.

Stage 2: Fibrous Plaque

Beginning at about the time of puberty, fatty streaks in larger arteries commonly progress to become fibrous plaques, so named because of their abundance of collagen fibers, molecular strands produced by SMCs that provide the strength for ligaments, tendons, and scar tissue (12). Just under the endothelium, the SMCs form the fibrous cap, a dense canopy of collagen fibers. The cap is a distinguishing feature of fibrous plaque, though its thickness is variable.

The SMCs also lay collagen fibers along the sides and base of the plaque to encapsulate it, like the walls of a cyst. Saturated fats entering the intima promote more of the undesired fibrous reaction than polyunsaturated fats do, resulting in a thicker shell around the plaque.

Elsewhere in the body, this tactic of "surround and contain" works well, whether the offending agent is bacteria or a piece of foreign material. In the arterial wall, however, this shell eventually becomes scar-like and calcified, making subsequent regression, or shrinkage of the plaque, more difficult. The lesson we learn from this is that the longer we let atherogenesis continue, the more irreversible it becomes.

SMCs also form proteoglycans, long molecules composed of protein and carbohydrate. These substances have a high affinity for LDL cholesterol, a relationship that accelerates LDL cholesterol deposition within the intima. The beneficial HDL cholesterol is thought to block the attachment of LDL to the proteoglycans, thus reducing cholesterol accumulation (16, 17).

Unlike the fatty streak stage, when little cholesterol is found outside monocytes and SMCs, in the fibrous stage cholesterol now accumulates faster than the struggling cells can control it. The foam cells have become so overloaded with fat that they die, releasing toxic compounds into the arterial wall. This results in the formation of even more collagen fibers and further damages the overlying endothelium, inducing more LDL particles to enter.

Another distinction from fatty streaks is that fibrous plaques are raised considerably above the surface of the surrounding intima. Like tiny abscess cavities, the lesions expand in three dimensions, pushing upward against the intima. The plaque bulges into the artery's lumen (channel), causing turbulence in the blood flow that further damages the endothelium.

This expansion also stretches the endothelium thin, creating gaps called stomata between the cells. Endothelial cells that are unable to withstand the stress retract at their edges and are swept away by the blood. Adjacent endothelial cells can divide to replace some of those lost, but eventually bare areas persist over the fibrous cap. Now the arterial wall is even more susceptible to the influx of fats, cholesterol, and monocytes (see Figure 2.3).

Dead and disintegrating foam cells, cholesterol globules, and crystals form a sludge that sinks to the base of the plaque, furthest from the blood-

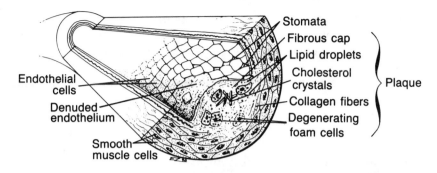

Figure 2.3   The fibrous plaque protrudes into and narrows the artery's inner diameter, or lumen. The lesion expands from the multiplication of foam cells and causes separation (stomata) and loss of the overlying epithelial cells.

stream. This accumulated debris has attracted the attention of scientists for more than a century. Early researchers in the field likened the appearance of the plaque's central area to that of porridge. In fact, the term "atherosclerosis" was derived from the Greek word "athero" for porridge or gruel combined with "sclerosis," which means scar. The porridge-like core content is called an atheroma.

The exposed fibrous cap is now a prime area for the formation of microscopic clots. The disrupted epithelial surface attracts platelets, which are the blood cells involved in clotting. These small cells affix to the edges of stomata and to exposed collagen fibers. They then release chemicals that cause other platelets to attach to the injured wall and to each other. This aggregation or clumping of platelets is the first step in clot formation.

Platelets do not normally bind to undamaged endothelium. Healthy endothelial cells have a very smooth surface and produce chemical substances such as prostacyclin and heparin that retard platelet adhesion. In the presence of elevated blood cholesterol, however, endothelial cells have less ability to form these chemicals (4). In addition, hypercholesterolemia increases the "stickiness" of the platelets, allowing them to aggregate more easily and the clot to grow more quickly (18). The disrupted endothelial surface, then, together with reduced antiplatelet coating and increased platelet stickiness, fosters clotting.

At the fibrous plaque stage, the platelets form only minute clots called microthrombi. These remain attached for a period of minutes to hours before they are carried off in the blood or condensed into a thin layer that becomes indistinguishable from the fibrous cap. Some investigators believe that the formation and consolidation of microthrombi is decisive for the progression to complicated plaque (19).

From the microthrombi, platelets release growth factors such as platelet-derived growth factor (PDGF) that stimulate more SMCs to migrate into the region, multiply, and produce collagen. Also, microthrombi cause more endothelial cells to die, uncovering more of the rough fibrous cap. The loss of endothelial cells is another crucial turning point in atherogenesis because it hastens the development of the menacing conditions of complicated plaque.

Fibrous plaque, then, can be likened to the body's response to inflammation in general. SMCs and monocytes migrate to the troubled area to remove the offending substance, which in this case is cholesterol. SMCs produce collagen fibers that surround a central core of fat globules, cholesterol crystals, and cellular debris. By middle age, the majority of Americans have formed countless micro-abscesses along their medium- and large-sized arteries. The fate of these cholesterol pus pockets determines the course of the final stage in atherogenesis, complicated plaque.

Stage 3: Complicated Plaque

Just as the death of foam cells begins the transition from fatty streak to fibrous plaque, the next major step in atherogenesis occurs when the endothelial cells die. Assaulted from both sides and stretched thin by an expanding plaque, these vital cells finally succumb to the blasting force of blood pressure. Once the endothelium is denuded, the fibrous cap is directly exposed to the circulation. Some very serious complications can then develop: calcification, hemorrhage, rupture, ulceration, and clot formation.

Calcification. With time, calcium accumulates among the collagen fibers, presenting an impediment to repair mechanisms that could heal the artery. The human body has difficulty reducing plaque that is surrounded by a hard, dense mineral shell. Even in an individual with high HDL levels and excellent control of cardiovascular risk factors, it is nearly impossible to break down thick layers of calcified collagen fibers. The rigid fibrous cap may then split, making possible two other serious sequelae—hemorrhage and rupture.

Hemorrhage. When calcified and brittle, the fibrous cap is much less resilient to the pulsation of blood, and it commonly fractures. Blood can then rush through the fissure to enter the central area of the plaque. With this sudden and fierce expansion, the plaque may completely occlude the artery's lumen above it.

Another possibility is that a break may occur at the base of the plaque. In this case, blood enters the core from one of the tiny arteries in the surrounding adventitia layer. The blood dissects through to accumulate between the media and the adventitia, creating an aneurysm. This occurs most commonly along the aorta, the major artery within the chest and abdomen. When an aneurysm expands rapidly, it is excruciatingly painful and presents a surgical emergency. Surprisingly, aneurysms usually advance gradually and without symptoms. A calcified aneurysm is often first detected by a chest or abdominal X ray performed for another problem.

Rupture, Ulceration, and Clot Formation. The steady growth of the plaque's core progressively distends and splits the overlying fibrous cap, creating fissures (see Figure 2.4). Already made brittle by calcium, the cap further deteriorates from the enzymes and toxic chemicals released by the monocytes beneath it. Eventually the cap may rupture, spilling the contents of the atheroma into the bloodstream, like a boil that has burst. Immediate and complete blockage of the artery can occur at the site if sufficient atheromatous material is exuded. Or smaller amounts of debris can be carried downstream by the blood to lodge in smaller arteries. A recent Scottish autopsy study found that 64% of sudden cardiac death victims had evidence of acute plaque rupture (20).

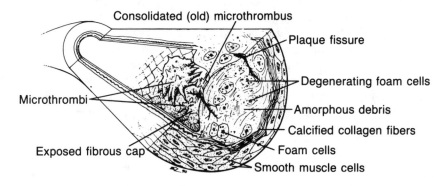

Consolidated (old) microthrombus
Plaque fissure
Degenerating foam cells
Microthrombi
Amorphous debris
Calcified collagen fibers
Exposed fibrous cap
Foam cells
Smooth muscle cells

Figure 2.4 Complicated plaque, the most severe stage of atherogenesis, can take a variety of courses, including calcification and hemorrhage. The tiny cholesterol tumor may rupture, presenting the constant threat of clot formation over the resultant ulcer or fissure.

If death does not occur immediately, the ruptured plaque now presents an open fissure or crater to the circulation, inviting clot formation. Attachment of platelets to the exposed collagen fibers occurs virtually instantaneously. Within seconds the aggregated platelets attract clotting factors in the blood and form a thrombus, a stationary clot. A majority of heart attacks result from a thrombus forming in one of the coronary arteries and fracture of the fibrous cap is estimated to initiate about 40% of the blood clots (21).

If the individual survives the immediate crisis of plaque rupture and thrombosis, the ulcer will continue to be a ready target for subsequent clots. Unless it totally blocks the artery and causes a heart attack, each thrombus is gradually converted into a dense layer of fibrous material. With repeated thrombus formation and resolution, layer upon layer is deposited over the ulcerated fibrous cap. This of course progressively reduces the diameter of the lumen. If the individual's risk factors are not reduced, the artery may eventually become totally occluded.

Another possibility is for pieces of clot and debris from the ulcer to dislodge and be carried downstream as an embolus, a moving clot. As the artery narrows, the clot eventually becomes wedged, obstructing blood flow. This complication commonly causes strokes, with the embolus typically originating along plaque-riddled arteries in the neck. (Often the source of blockage, whether thrombus or embolus, cannot be determined, and thus the disease process is referred to as thromboembolism.)

The expanding plaque progressively reduces blood flow, which causes gradual wasting of the organs supplied. In the heart, this often results in congestive heart failure, a condition in which insufficient heart muscle remains to adequately pump the blood. Blood may then collect in the legs, causing them to swell (peripheral edema), or may accumulate in the lungs, causing breathing difficulty (pulmonary edema).

Slow death of brain tissue can also occur and is easier to demonstrate. Advanced brain scanners have revealed that many persons have had multiple small strokes that leave empty spaces called *lacunae* within the brain. As a result of the thrombosis or embolism, areas of devitalized (infarcted) brain are gradually resorbed, leaving cavities. Eventually the gradually diminishing mental function and personality changes of atherosclerotic dementia are apparent.

Predicting Plaque Formation

Depending on the presence of the cardiovascular risk factors, atherogenesis is fairly predictable and allows a rough estimation of plaque progression. Beginning in adolescence, plaque growth extends to cover about 1% of the arterial surface area each year.

Scott Grundy of the University of Texas developed an age-dependent approach to calculate when atherosclerosis has reached a dangerous level (22). Using data from large autopsy studies (23), he pointed out that a heart attack or stroke seldom occurs unless at least 60% of the arterial surface is covered with plaque. Once this degree of atherosclerosis has developed, the individual can develop a fatal complication. A heart attack or stroke may not happen for years, or even at all, but at this point it may occur at any second.

If a person has a cholesterol level of 200 mg/dl (5.2 mmol/L) and no other risk factors, the critical 60% surface area coverage will occur at about age 70. If the cholesterol level is 220 mg/dl (5.7 mmol/L) the danger zone is reached at about age 60; if 240 mg/dl (6.2 mmol/L), age 50. This relationship is illustrated in Figure 2.5. The horizontal line indicates when

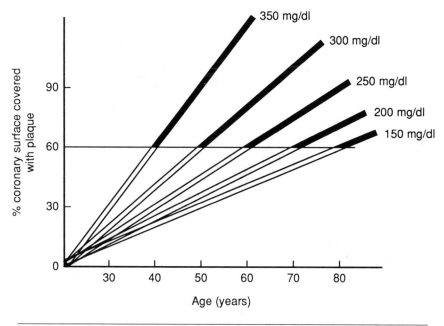

Figure 2.5 The diagonal bars represent the progressive amount of plaque coverage along the arterial walls at different cholesterol levels (mg/dl). The horizontal line indicates a critical point in atherosclerosis when 60% of the arterial surface area is covered with plaque and a heart attack can occur. Higher levels of blood cholesterol confer steeper slopes because the plaque buildup is faster. Blood cholesterol of 150 mg/dl = 3.9 mmol/L; 200 mg/dl = 5.2 mmol/L; 250 mg/dl = 6.5 mmol/L; 300 mg/dl = 7.8 mmol/L; 350 mg/dl = 9.0 mmol/L.

Note. From "Cholesterol and CHD: A New Era" by S.M. Grundy, 1986, *Journal of the American Medical Association,* **256**, pp. 2855-2856. Copyright 1986 by American Medical Association. Adapted by permission.

atherosclerotic plaque involves 60% of the arterial surface area. Again, this graph assumes that no other risk factors, such as smoking or high blood pressure, are present (22).

The presence of high blood pressure, smoking, or symptomatic diabetes hastens the onset of critical atherosclerosis by about 10 years at any given cholesterol level. For example, a person with a cholesterol level of 200 mg/dl (5.2 mmol/L) will cross into the danger zone at about age 70. If he or she is also a smoker, this is reduced to age 60. Subtract another 10 years for hypertension or diabetes. Again, this does not mean that a heart attack will definitely occur at this age, just that it becomes an ever-present possibility (see Figure 2.6) (22).

To summarize, the process of atherogenesis begins with the formation of fatty streaks in childhood and adolescence. These consist primarily of foam cells, the cholesterol-laden SMCs and monocytes that have migrated

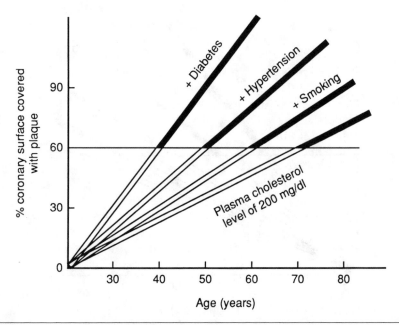

Figure 2.6   A person with a plasma cholesterol of 200 mg/dl (5.2 mmol/L) would enter the danger zone at about age 70. However, the presence of each additional risk factor (hypertension, smoking, or diabetes) hastens this situation by approximately 10 years.

Note. From "Cholesterol and CHD: A New Era" by S.M. Grundy, 1986, *Journal of the American Medical Association*, **256**, pp. 2855-2856. Copyright 1986 by American Medical Association. Adapted by permission.

beneath the artery's endothelium layer. The fate of fatty streaks is to stabilize, disappear, or progress further to fibrous and complicated plaque.

In the fibrous plaque stage, the protective layer of endothelium is overcome by various chemical (smoke), physical (high blood pressure), and metabolic (cholesterol) insults. With the endothelium's gatekeeper function impaired, cholesterol accumulates within the arterial wall more rapidly than the foam cells can digest it.

Once the foam cells begin to disintegrate, a vicious cycle of events hastens the formation of more serious plaque. Remaining foam cells struggle to absorb the LDL cholesterol that now intrudes more easily through the damaged endothelium. Growth factors are released by the endothelium, monocytes, platelets, and SMCs. These chemicals cause additional SMCs and monocytes to enter the area, multiply, and begin to absorb the cholesterol. Collagen fibers encapsulate the plaque in scar tissue, which eventually becomes calcified and brittle.

As the plaque swells, gaps appear between the overlying endothelial cells, inviting platelet attachment and the formation of minute clots. Plaque expansion also pushes the intima out into the arterial lumen, encroaching on the channel and reducing the flow of blood. If plaque expands further, the artery eventually closes off, completely starving the tissue that it supplied. In the coronary vessels, this results in a heart attack. Instead, the fibrous cap may split, releasing the plaque's porridge-like contents into the bloodstream. The ensuing ulcer has a rough and irregular surface that invites clotting. Thrombus formation, embolization, or both are life-threatening complications that may cause heart attack, stroke, or gangrene in the future.

It is appalling but true that this sickening process is occurring right now in nearly every American. By middle age, most Americans have plaque covering a major part of their arterial surface area. Autopsy studies have shown that by age 90, fully 90% of the coronary artery surface is involved in plaque (24). Only 5% of nonsmokers and a mere 0.5% of heavy smokers are free of atherosclerosis at the time of their deaths (25).

Fortunately, diet and lifestyle changes may arrest or even reverse this arterial pollution. The earlier these changes occur, the better, because plaque is more resistant once calcification and scarring develop. The key to prevention is to curb this deadly process before it becomes irreparable. Its first manifestation may be when it imperils or ends one's life.

References

1. Rokitansky, K. Von. (1852). *Handbuch der pathologischen anatomie* [*Handbook of Pathological Anatomy*]. Vienna: Braumuller u Siedel.
2. Ross, R. (1986). The pathogenesis of atherosclerosis—an update. *New England Journal of Medicine, 314*, 488-500.
3. Moore, S. (Ed.) (1981). *Vascular injury and atherosclerosis*. New York: Marcel Dekker.
4. Silkworth, J.B., McLean, B., & Stehbens, W.E. (1975). The effect of hypercholesterolemia on aortic endothelium en face. *Atherosclerosis, 22*, 335.
5. Steenberg, D., Parthasarathy, S., Carew, T.E., Khoo, J.C., & Witztum, J.L. (1989). Beyond cholesterol. Modifications of low-density lipoprotein that increase its atherogenicity. *New England Journal of Medicine, 320*, 915-924.
6. Gleich, G.J., Welsh, P.W., Yunginger, J.W., Hyatt, R.E., & Catlett, J.B. (1980). Allergy to tobacco, an occupational hazard. *New England Journal of Medicine, 302*, 617-619.
7. Nowak, J., Murray, J.J., Oakes, J.A., & Fitzgerald, G.A. (1987). Biochemical evidence of a chronic abnormality in platelet and vascular function in healthy individuals who smoke cigarettes. *Circulation, 76*, 6-14.
8. Payling-Wright, H.P. (1972). Mitosis patterns in aortic endothelium. *Atherosclerosis, 15*, 93-95.

9. McGill, H.C., Jr. (1968). *The geographic pathology of atherosclerosis*. Baltimore: Williams and Wilkins.

10. Newman, W.P., Freedman, D.S., Voors, A.W., Gard, P.D., Srinivasan, S.R., Cresanta, J.L., Williamson, G.D., Webber, L.S., & Berenson, G.S. (1986). Relation of serum lipoprotein levels and systolic blood pressure to early atherosclerosis. The Bogalusa Heart Study. *New England Journal of Medicine*, **314**, 138-144.

11. Swartz, C.J., Ardlie, N.G., Carter, R.F., & Paterson, J.C. (1967). Gross aortic sudanophilia and hemosiderin deposition. *Archives of Pathology*, **83**, 325-332.

12. Strong, J.P, & McGill, J.C. (1969). The pediatric aspects of atherosclerosis. *Journal of Atherosclerosis Research*, **9**, 251-265.

13. McGill, H.C., Jr. (1980). Morphologic development of the atherosclerotic plaque. In R.M. Lauer & R.B. Shekelle (Eds.), *Childhood prevention of atherosclerosis and hypertension*, 41-50. New York: Raven Press.

14. Katz, S.S., Shipley, G.G., & Small, D.M. (1976). Demonstration of a lesion intermediate between fatty streaks and advanced plaques. *Journal of Clinical Investigation*, **58**, 200-211.

15. Martin, B.M., Gimbrone, M.A., Unanue, E.R., & Cotran, R.S. (1981). Stimulation of nonlymphoid mesenchymal cell proliferation by a macrophage-derived growth factor. *Journal of Immunology*, **126**, 1510-1515.

16. Hessler, J.R., Robertson, A.L., & Chisolm, G.M. (1979). LDL-induced cytotoxicity and its inhibition by HDL in human vascular smooth muscle and endothelial cells in culture. *Atherosclerosis*, **32**, 213-229.

17. Weber, G., Fabbrini, P., Resi, L., Sforza, V., & Tanganelli, P. (1979). Effect of glycosaminoglycans on experimental cholesterol atherogenesis. A morphological approach. *Pharmacological Research Communications*, **11**, 311, 341.

18. Armstrong, W.L., Peterson, R.E., Hoak, J.C., Megan, M.B., Cheng, F.H., & Clarke, W. R. (1980). Arterial platelet accumulation in experimental hypercholesterolemia. *Atherosclerosis*, **36**, 89-100.

19. Mustard, J.F., Packham, M.A., & Kinlough-Rathbone, R.L. (1981). Platelets, atherosclerosis, and clinical complications. In S. Moore (Ed.), *Vascular injury and atherosclerosis*, 79-110. New York: Marcel Dekker.

20. El Fawal, M.A., Berg, G.A., Wheatly, D.J., & Harland, W.A. (1987). Sudden coronary death in Glasgow: Nature and frequency of acute coronary lesions. *British Heart Journal*, **57**, 329-335.

21. Bouch, D.C., & Montgomery, D.L. (1970). Cardiac lesions in fatal cases of recent myocardial ischaemia from a coronary care unit. *British Heart Journal*, **32**, 795-803.

22. Grundy, S.M. (1986). Cholesterol and coronary heart disease: A new era. *Journal of the American Medical Association*, **256**, 2855, 2856.

23. Strong, J.P., Solberg, L.A., & Restrepo, C. (1968). Atherosclerosis in persons with coronary heart disease. *Laboratory Investigation, 18,* 527-537.
24. Waller, B., & Roberts, W.C. (1983). Cardiovascular disease in the very elderly—analysis of 40 necropsy patients 90 years of age or older. *American Journal of Cardiology, 51,* 403.
25. U.S. Department of Health, Education, and Welfare, Public Health Service, Center for Disease Control. (1976). *The health consequences of smoking* (DHEW Publication No. (CDC) 78-8357).

Chapter

3

Controlling Cholesterol

Recent scientific breakthroughs have left no room for doubt that nutrition not only plays the pivotal role in causing atherosclerosis, but remains the cornerstone for its prevention and treatment as well. Diet has been shown to reduce blood pressure, cholesterol, triglycerides, and clotting tendencies, and also to help control diabetes and excess weight gain.

The relationship between diet and atherosclerosis is complex, and some key pieces of this giant puzzle have only recently fallen into place. Tracing the evolution of this knowledge base will put cholesterol and the diet-heart picture into perspective.

The Diet-Heart Link:
An Overview of Cholesterol Research

For centuries, anatomists have noted plaque in the arteries of some deceased persons (1). Cholesterol was first isolated from arterial plaque in the mid-19th century (2). The source of the cholesterol was first traced to dietary factors by the Russian pathologist Nikolai Anitschkow (3, 4). But the subject raised little curiosity until the industrialized nations witnessed a dramatic surge in atherosclerosis after World War II.

The first concerted effort to trace the diet-heart link came through population studies that began in the 1950s. Ancel Keys, an epidemiologist at the University of Minnesota, and collaborators around the world studied dietary patterns in Finland, Greece, Italy, Japan, the Netherlands, the United States, and Yugoslavia. In what was to be known as the Seven Countries Study, these scientists surveyed the diets and blood cholesterol levels of thousands of people and later compared the subjects' death rates from cardiovascular diseases (5, 6).

This landmark study was the first to convincingly incriminate diet as a major cause of atherosclerosis. CHD rates in locales where the average serum cholesterol level was 240 to 280 mg/dl (6.2 to 7.2 mmol/L) were 10 times higher than in places where the average level was 160 mg/dl (4.1 mmol/L). A strong correlation of 84% was found between the amount of saturated fat in a country's average diet and the country's CHD rate (5) (see Figure 3.1). A similar correlation of 89% was noted between saturated fat intake and serum cholesterol (6) (see Figure 3.2). A striking correlation of 96% was found between a country's average serum cholesterol and its CHD (7) (see Figure 3.3).

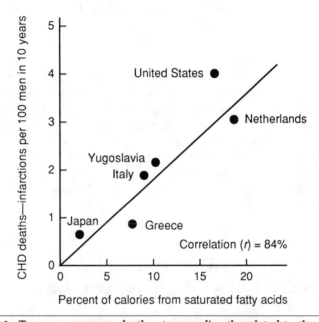

Figure 3.1 Ten-year coronary death rates are directly related to the percent of calories from saturated fat with a correlation factor (r) of 84%.
Note. From "Coronary Heart Disease in Seven Countries" by A. Keys, 1970, *Circulation*, Suppl. 1, p. I-174. Copyright 1970 by American Heart Association. Adapted by permission of the American Heart Association, Inc.

Meanwhile, autopsy studies documented the damage that was occurring within the artery. The International Atherosclerosis Project compiled results of 31,000 autopsies from 15 cities worldwide. The researchers found more atherosclerosis at autopsy in those persons with elevated blood cholesterol, strengthening the causal link between affluent diets and cholesterol death (8). Information from third-world countries is scarce but

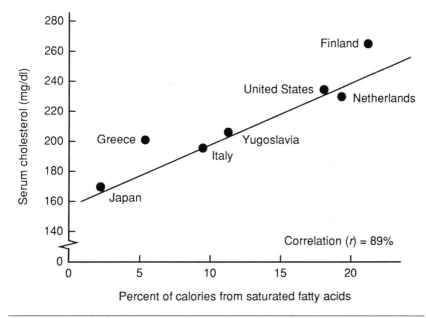

Figure 3.2   Percent of total calories from saturated fatty acids were 89% correlated with serum cholesterol in the Seven Countries Study.
Note. From "Coronary Heart Disease in Seven Countries" by A. Keys, 1970, *Circulation,* Suppl. 1, p. I-170. Copyright 1970 by American Heart Association. Adapted by permission of the American Heart Association, Inc.

indicates that atherosclerosis is negligible except among people from higher socioeconomic groups who consume a rich diet.

Figure 3.4a compares Americans to the Japanese in terms of blood cholesterol levels at various ages. A steady rise with age is seen in Americans that does not occur in Japan (9). Figure 3.4b compares autopsy findings from the two countries in terms of the development of significant narrowing of the coronary arteries (10). The Japanese have traditionally taken in only about 130 mg/day of cholesterol, compared with 400 to 600 mg/day in the United States. Their intake of saturated fat is but a minor percent of total calories, while Americans average 15%.

Physiologists then examined the effect of modifying food sources in the carefully controlled environment of metabolic wards. Scores of such experiments were reported by many researchers (11-13). Dietary cholesterol and saturated fat were shown to consistently raise the subjects' blood cholesterol, whereas unsaturated fat and fiber lowered their levels. Later studies found that dietary cholesterol raises the CHD risk independently of its effect on blood lipids (14-15).

Some investigators thought that heredity explained the differences between the various countries' rates of heart disease. But when diets

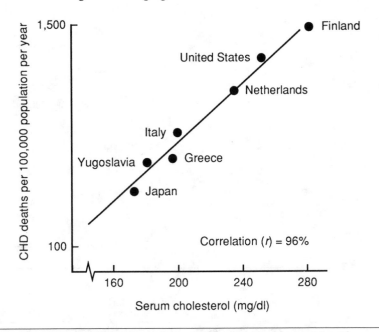

Figure 3.3   CHD deaths had a striking 96% correlation factor (r) with serum cholesterol in a long-term follow-up of the Seven Countries Study.
Note. From "Incubation Period of CHD" by G. Rose, 1982, *British Medical Journal, 284,* p. 1600. Copyright 1982 by *British Medical Journal.* Adapted by permission.

differed within a genetically homogeneous population, atherosclerosis varied as well. Vegetarians in the United States and Europe consume much less cholesterol and saturated fat than those who eat meat. They have significantly lower levels of LDL, triglycerides, and blood pressure (16-20). But inheritance cannot explain why vegetarians' rates of heart attack are 77% lower than those who eat meat.

Migration studies also cast doubt on theories that cholesterol-laden arteries are predestined only for genetically susceptible populations. Japanese who emigrated from Japan to Hawaii and California, Jews from Yemen to Israel, Indians from Asia to South Africa, and Italians from Naples to Boston all quickly attained the same rates of CHD as the locals in their newly adopted homelands (15, 21). The acceleration of atherosclerosis took only one or two generations to surface—much too short a time for genetics to play a part.

The now-classic Ni-Hon-San study followed thousands of men in Nagasaki, Japan, and compared them to Japanese emigrants in Honolulu and San Francisco (22, 23). Their diets, blood cholesterol, and subsequent rates of atherosclerosis were closely monitored over several years. The traditional Japanese diet included much more fish and much less saturated fat and cholesterol than the typical American diet. Blood cholesterol levels in Japan averaged about 180 mg/dl (4.7 mmol/L). Japanese men who had

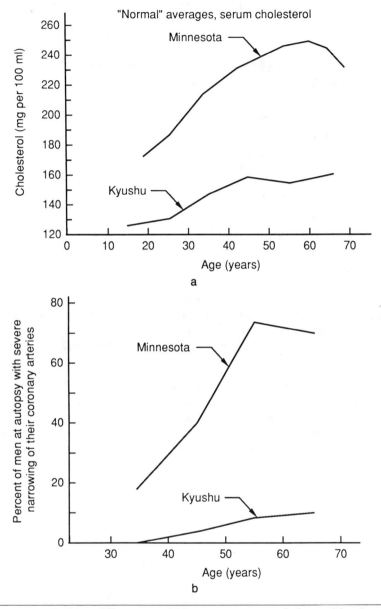

Figure 3.4 Striking differences exist in average serum cholesterol levels between the United States and Japan (a) and in the percentage of persons having significant amounts of atherosclerosis with increased age (b).
Note. Figure 3.4a from "Serum Cholesterol and the Question of 'Normal' " by Ancel Keys. In *Multiple Laboratory Screening*, E.S. Benson, & P.E. Strandjord (Eds.) (p. 169), 1969. Copyright 1969 by Academic Press. Adapted by permission. Figure 3.4b from "Correlations in Coronary Artery Disease" by N.K. White and J.E. Edwards, 1950, *Circulation*, 1, p. 645. Copyright 1950 by the American Heart Association. Adapted by permission of the American Heart Association, Inc.

moved to Hawaii and California had cholesterol levels averaging 218 and 228 mg/dl (5.6 and 5.9 mmol/L), respectively. The California-Japanese men (ages 55 to 59) had rates of heart attack almost 3-1/2 times that of their counterparts who remained in Japan (24). Table 3.1 illustrates the changes in the diets, serum cholesterol, and CHD rates of the Japanese who migrated to Hawaii and to California (25, 26).

Table 3.1 Dietary Fat Differences Among Japanese Men Living in Japan, Hawaii, and California

	Japan	Hawaii	California
Fat (% of total calories)	15%	33%	38%
Saturated fat (% of total calories)	7%	23%	26%
Serum cholesterol (mg/dl)	181	218	228
CHD deaths per 1000 persons	25	35	45

Note. From "Epidemiologic Studies of CHD and Stroke in Japanese Men Living in Japan, Hawaii, and California" by M.G. Marmot, S.L. Syme, A. Kagan, H. Kato, J.B. Cohen, and J. Belsky, 1975, *American Journal of Epidemiology, 102,* p. 514. Copyright 1975 by the *American Journal of Epidemiology.* Adapted by permission.

The publication of these statistics had surprisingly little impact on scientific recommendations or public policy regarding the American diet. Skeptics were reluctant to advise dietary changes until they were convinced that dietary changes were safe and effective in reducing blood cholesterol, and that this cholesterol improvement would in turn reduce the rate of heart attacks, angina, and strokes.

The first concern was satisfied by the Diet Heart Feasibility Study, organized by the NIH in the 1960s (27). In this study, participating Americans demonstrated that they could safely reduce their consumption of saturated fat and cholesterol as a result of nutritional education. Correspondingly, their blood lipid levels were significantly improved.

The latter concern was much more difficult to prove, due to the slow progression of atherosclerosis and the complexity of its contributing risk factors. Proving that widespread dietary changes would be beneficial to the general public required clinical or intervention trials. In these studies, individuals are placed in one of two or more groups that are carefully matched for similar age, sex, lifestyle, and health characteristics. One group receives some form of treatment or intervention that another group does not. Over time, data are collected to determine if the intervention has changed the incidence of disease.

Early reports gave encouraging support for a dietary approach to preventive cardiology. These included the Finnish Mental Hospital Trial

(28) and the Los Angeles Veterans Administration Study (29). Though they implicated diet as a major cause of CHD, these intervention studies still suffered from relatively small numbers of participants—hundreds, not thousands. To irrefutably demonstrate that dietary changes could lower subsequent CHD rates would require enormous funding, massive organization, and many years of follow-up. Until the 1980s, no public or private organization had the resources for such a study.

Because the evidence was so convincing, however, larger and more sophisticated studies were planned and funded. These included the Multiple Risk Factor Intervention Trial (MRFIT) (30), the Oslo Study (31, 32), the Western Electric Study (14, 33), the Leiden Intervention Trial (34), the Ireland-Boston Diet-Heart Study (15), and the Helsinki Heart Study (35, 36). The consistency of their conclusions strengthened the hypothesis that lowering blood cholesterol through diet has a positive effect on cardiovascular health.

The most notable intervention trial to date has been the NIH-sponsored Lipid Research Clinics Study (LRC) (37, 38), also called the Coronary Primary Prevention Trial (CPPT). With the release of the results of this $150-million, 10-year investigation, the evidence supporting dietary intervention to prevent atherosclerosis had finally become indisputable.

The Lipid Research Clinics Study randomly divided hypercholesterolemic men, ages 35 to 59, into two groups. All subjects consumed a moderate cholesterol-lowering diet. In addition, one group received cholestyramine, a cholesterol-lowering drug, while the other group was given an inactive placebo drug. All 3,806 men were closely monitored for changes in lipid values and any sign of atherosclerosis. The study was double-blinded, meaning that neither the subjects nor the investigators knew who actually received the drug until the end of the study.

In the diet-plus-drug group, a 13.4% decrease in total cholesterol (and a 20.3% decrease in LDL) resulted in a 24% reduction in the number of CHD deaths as compared to the diet-plus-placebo group. Additional benefits were a 20% reduction in new-onset angina, 25% fewer positive exercise stress tests, and 21% fewer coronary bypass operations. Because of the chronic nature of atherosclerosis, the cholesterol-lowering benefit needed more than five years to manifest itself (see Figure 3.5).

As might be expected, full compliance with the treatment protocols was only achieved by a small minority of the subjects. (Imagine the reluctance of taking two tablespoons of a sand-like substance with each meal, not knowing if it was an active ingredient.) This in effect diluted the impact of the study and the significance of cholesterol control. When those individuals who complied with the diet and drug recommendations were examined separately, the researchers noted that they had attained a 25% decrease in blood cholesterol and a 50% decline in CHD rates (38). Statistical analysis showed that over a broad range of cholesterol values, the greater the reduction in blood cholesterol by diet, drugs, or both, the greater the reduction in CHD risk (see Figure 3.6).

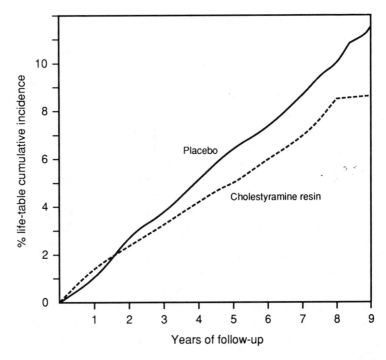

Figure 3.5 The Lipid Research Clinics Program results show the cumulative percent of persons diagnosed with either a first definite heart attack or sudden cardiac death (N = total number of study participants). After two years, the graphs of those taking cholestyramine (dotted line) and those taking a placebo (solid line) began to diverge. After seven years the impact of cholesterol control gained enough strength that the study was terminated. *Note.* From "The Lipid Research Clinics Coronary Primary Prevention Trial Results, I" by Lipid Research Clinics Program, 1984, *Journal of the American Medical Association,* **251,** p. 356.

The Lipid Research Clinics, then, firmly secured the relationship suggested by previous studies that for every 1% reduction in blood cholesterol, there is a corresponding 2% reduction in CHD risk. Even greater protection is afforded if HDL increases significantly, as occurred in the Helsinki Heart Study (36). Other salient findings included the following:

- The health effect of cholesterol is dose-related; that is, the lower the cholesterol, the greater the protection against CHD.
- Whether cholesterol is lowered by diet alone or by diet-plus-drug, the health effects are the same for similar reductions in cholesterol.

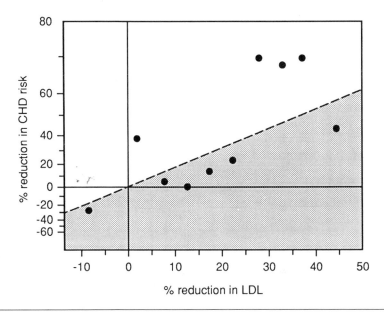

Figure 3.6   Statistical analysis of the Lipid Research Clinics Program demonstrated a 2% lowering of CHD risk for every 1% drop in serum cholesterol, whether the reduction was from taking the bile acid drug, dietary measures, or both. The greater the reduction in cholesterol level, the greater the protection.

Note. From "The Lipid Research Clinics Coronary Primary Prevention Trial Results, II" by Lipid Research Clinics Program, 1984, *Journal of the American Medical Association,* **251**, p. 369.

Taking Action Through Diet

The bottom line to all these studies is an urgent call for prevention. Recent clinical intervention trials have shown conclusively that high-fat, high-cholesterol, low-fiber diets are strongly and consistently linked to atherosclerosis, especially CHD. Moreover, they have finally demonstrated that eating less saturated fat and cholesterol lowers not only a person's blood cholesterol level, but the risk of CHD as well.

Scores of health and nutrition agencies are now calling for heart-healthy diets, not only for those with CHD, but for the general population. Organizations leading the crusade include

- National Cholesterol Education Program (39),
- American Heart Association (40),
- Surgeon General (41),
- Food and Nutrition Board of the National Academy of Sciences (42),

- National Institutes of Health (43),
- Centers for Disease Control,
- American Medical Association,
- National Research Council (44), and
- U.S. Department of Agriculture (45).

The scope of interest of these and other agencies mirrors the immensity of our nation's cholesterol problem. More than three quarters of our population have blood cholesterol levels that place them in need of dietary changes. Only a concerted attack, on a societal level, can reduce the appalling toll of atherosclerosis. To accomplish this, a two-stepped dietary approach to treat high cholesterol was developed by the National Cholesterol Education Program (39), based on earlier recommendations of the American Heart Association (46).

The diet plans, known as the Step One and Step Two diets, do not consist of special fares to be consumed only by the unfortunate high-risk segment of the population. Instead, the plan provides a healthy diet intended to replace average American food choices, which are typically quite unhealthy (47). The Step One diet is simply a healthy diet, not a depriving one. Step Two is a very healthy diet, but is not puritanical. These plans are discussed thoroughly in Part III and summarized in Table 10.1.

Overview of a Heart-Healthy Diet

A heart-healthy diet plan has at least three important features:

1. *It is low in cholesterol and fat, particularly saturated fat.*[1] On the average, Americans need to reduce the cholesterol and saturated fat in their diets to one half the current amount. This change will also reduce calories consumed and thus assist in controlling obesity. The rationale and methods for reducing cholesterol and fat are explained in chapter 7.
2. *It includes more fiber, particularly soluble fiber.* The soluble fiber found in certain fruits, vegetables, and whole grains has been shown to lower blood cholesterol by 20% to 30% (48). It also lowers blood pressure and triglyceride levels and aids in the control of diabetes and excess weight. Most members of Western societies should double their fiber intake. The evidence for the recommendation is reviewed in chapter 8.
3. *It includes more fish because fish is low in fat, especially saturated fat.* The best fish to eat are those caught in cold Northern seas, especially mackerel, salmon, and halibut. The omega-3 fatty acids in these fish lower serum cholesterol and triglyceride levels and inhibit blood clot formation, as discussed in chapter 9.

---

[1]Nothing in the diet increases blood cholesterol more than saturated fat. This relationship is even stronger than the relationship between dietary cholesterol and blood cholesterol.

Few individuals need to radically or instantly alter their diets. Gradually improving food choices over several weeks or months is easier and ensures that the new eating habits become solidly fixed. This is crucial because hypercholesterolemia has no permanent cure; if an individual resumes an unhealthy diet, hazardous cholesterol levels will quickly return.

Finally, diet also has a strong influence on several other risk factors such as hypertension, diabetes, and obesity. Exercise, weight control, drugs, and surgical approaches to the cholesterol epidemic are examined in the following sections.

Taking Action Through Exercise and Weight Control

All parts of the body which have a function, if used in moderation and exercised in labours in which each is accustomed, become thereby healthy, well-developed and age more slowly, but if unused and left idle they become liable to disease, defective in growth, and age quickly.

Hippocrates

The health hazards of obesity and inactivity have been noted since antiquity. Early attempts to study these characteristics more carefully were carried out by Morris and colleagues in England (49, 50). They found that sedentary bus drivers had much higher rates of heart attack than conductors who constantly climbed up and down the stairs of London's double-decked buses. But the drivers were also more likely to be overweight, which had to be accounted for in calculating the health risk.

As Morris and others discovered, the cardiovascular risks attributed to moderate obesity or inactivity are mostly indirect because they promote other cardiovascular risk factors such as hypercholesterolemia, hypertension, and diabetes (51). In the absence of other cardiovascular risk factors, moderate obesity or inactivity impart much less risk for CHD (52).[2] Conversely, exercise and weight loss are beneficial not only in themselves but also in controlling these other risk factors.

To quantify the impact of inactivity on health, Paffenbarger and colleagues conducted an activity survey of 17,000 male Harvard alumni (53, 54). As self-reported activity increased, so did the protection it afforded against CHD, up to about 3,500 calories expended per week. More activity than this only minimally improved the health risks. This relationship is illustrated in Figure 3.7 (54).

---

[2]Severe obesity (greater than 30% above ideal weight) significantly increases CHD risk even if other risk factors are absent (Expert Panel of the NCEP, 1988).

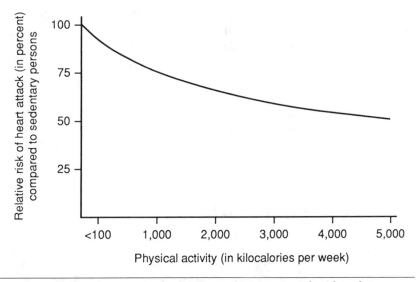

Figure 3.7   The relative risk of a heart attack as compared with sedentary individuals falls with even modest activity. Physical activity is shown as the estimated total kilocalories expended per week in vigorous activity.
Note. From "Physical Activity as an Index of Heart Attack Risk in College Alumni" by R.S. Paffenbarger, 1978, *American Journal of Epidemiology,* **108**, p. 161. Copyright 1978 by *American Journal of Epidemiology.* Adapted by permission.

This report supported the use of vigorous exercise as an effective natural protection against atherosclerosis. The men whose leisure-time exertion burned less than 2,000 calories per week had a 64% higher incidence of coronary heart disease. The authors estimated that if all the Harvard men had expended at least 2,000 calories a week in recreational activity, a quarter of the heart attack deaths could have been prevented. This was true for all age groups from 35 to 74 and was independent of other risk factors such as smoking, hypertension, obesity, or a family history of CHD.

Another important finding of the Harvard Alumni Study is that the level of activity in adulthood, not the activity level in youth, influences atherosclerosis. Former collegiate athletes who had become sedentary were if anything at increased risk of CHD. Those who remained active enjoyed better health, an effect that persisted well into advanced age. We can conclude that a healthy diet and regular exercise should be maintained for life.

Other surveys corroborate Paffenbarger's conclusion that physical activity reduces the risk of CHD by about half (55). The greatest enhancement to well-being accompanies the change from a completely sedentary to a moderately active lifestyle (57-59).

Using a sample of 12,866 men from the MRFIT study, researchers divided the volunteers into three groups according to their activity level (60). After 8 years of follow-up, those who were moderately active had one third fewer heart attacks (and lower overall death rates) than the least active participants. Men in the most active section did only slightly better than the middle third. From a cost effectiveness standpoint of the greatest health gains per energy expended, a target of 2,000 calories per week of leisure-time activity seems best.

What the Overweight and Underactive Have in Common

As with high blood pressure and cholesterol, a medical or genetic cause for obesity is found in only about 5% of cases. The vast majority of overweight people either eat too much, exercise too little, or, more commonly, both. Surprisingly, decreased activity is a more important cause for obesity than overeating for most individuals. The average American today eats fewer calories than did his or her counterpart at the turn of the century in spite of the overwhelming increase in obesity since that time (61). Obese persons *in general* take in fewer calories than thin persons and expend even fewer in daily activities.

Overweight and underactive people also have slightly higher LDL and significantly lower HDL levels than people of normal weight (62, 63). Weight loss and exercise in turn result in a slight average drop in LDL cholesterol (64, 65). The effect on cholesterol is much more pronounced for some individuals than for others (66). The boost to the beneficial HDL fraction is perhaps the most important lipid benefit from exercise and weight loss. Every 5 mg/dl increase in HDL corresponds to a 25% lower risk of CHD (67) (see Table 3.2) (68).

Table 3.2   Lipid Levels of Runners and Nonrunners

Subjects	Total cholesterol	LDL cholesterol	HDL cholesterol	Triglycerides
Runners	200	125	64	70
Nonrunners	210	139	43	146

Note. Values given in mg/dl. LDL = low-density lipoprotein; HDL = high-density lipoprotein. From "The Distribution of Plasma Lipoproteins in Middle-Aged Male Runners" by P. Wood, W. Haskell, H. Klein, S. Lewis, et al., 1976, *Metabolism,* **25**, p. 1253. Copyright 1976 by W.B. Saunders. Adapted by permission.

Improvements in blood lipids, especially the lowering of LDL, requires regular and moderately vigorous aerobic exercise (69, 70).[3] Physiological studies indicate that the minimum amount of exercise needed to impact lipids will consume at least 1,000 calories per week (66, 71, 72). These changes may be evident after only 3 weeks (73) but generally require several months to reach the full benefit (74, 75). Cholesterol levels in men seem to be affected more by exercise than those in women (76).

In general, a sustained exercise program will result in the following lipid changes (66, 77):

- total cholesterol decreases of 4% to 6% (8 to 12 mg/dl)
- LDL decreases of 10% to 15% (13 to 20 mg/dl)
- triglyceride decreases of about 25% (25 to 30 mg/dl)
- HDL cholesterol increases of 20% to 35% (12 to 20 mg/dl)

When combined with a healthy diet, a less strenuous program will still elicit improvements in blood lipids. Jogging as little as 10 miles a week may result in HDL elevation (78). If weight loss occurs simultaneously, it seems to double the exercise-induced drop in LDL and triglycerides as well as the rise in HDL (79).

Exercise and weight loss also improve other CHD risk factors such as blood pressure and diabetes (80-86). (These areas are covered in chapters 4 and 6, respectively.) Finally, exercise and weight loss decrease the stickiness of platelets, lessening the threat of clot formation and the promulgation of plaque (87).

Perhaps as important as all these physiological benefits are those for the psyche (88). Regular exercisers and persons of normal weight report less anxiety, chronic fatigue, and depression and have more of a sense of being "in control." Exercise is enough of a mood-elevator that many psychotherapists suggest it as an alternative to toxic antidepressant drugs. In one study, aerobic workouts were equal to or more effective than traditional psychotherapy and antidepressant drugs (89).

Other quality-of-life returns from regular exercise include more physical and psychological energy; improved self-image, sleep, sexual function, clarity of thinking, and relaxation; and an enjoyable and healthy way to share time and activity with family or friends (90, 91).

Exercise as a Treatment for Obesity

Exercise is an essential component of any program to achieve permanent weight loss (92). The activity need not be vigorous. In fact, activities of lower intensity and longer duration are the most effective in promoting weight loss. More calories are consumed in these activities, and the energy

---

[3]Aerobic movements are rhythmic, dynamic, and continuous and involve major muscle groups. Examples include brisk walking, jogging, swimming, stair climbing, hiking, cycling, rowing, calisthenics, and racket sports such as singles tennis, handball, and squash.

source is largely fat from adipose tissue rather than glycogen stored in muscle.

An invigorating 30-minute walk burns up 150 calories; done daily, it will result in a weight loss of 15 pounds per year. Although important for improving aerobic fitness, increasing the speed or intensity of exercise is of little additional value in weight reduction (see Table 3.3) (93).

Exercise accelerates the basal metabolic rate[4] so that additional calories are expended throughout the day and night, even after exercise has ended (94). This can be invaluable for millions of overweight persons who do not overeat but are inactive and have a slow metabolic rate. Besides burning calories, exercise also helps to reset the body's appestat, or internal hunger meter. When this is set at a lower level, a person desires only as much food as the body needs.

Yet another benefit to exercise is that it helps maintain lean body tissue. When a person diets without exercising, up to 25% of the weight lost is muscle. If the weight is later regained rapidly, nearly all of it becomes fat tissue, thus greatly expanding the person's percent body fat and health risks. Incorporating an exercise program reduces the percent of muscle tissue lost to about 5% and greatly augments the cholesterol-lowering effect (56).

We need no tricks or diets to lose weight. Following the low-fat, high-fiber diet described in Section III will automatically cause weight reduction for a number of reasons. The most obvious is that a gram of fat has more than twice the calories (9) of protein or carbohydrate (4 each). Also, research shows that dietary fat is turned into adipose (fat) tissue more efficiently than other foodstuffs (95-98). Finally, eating more soluble fiber assists weight loss because it increases the feeling of satiety (99) and possibly reduces fat absorption. As with a cholesterol-lowering diet, a weight-reduction diet should be tailored to individual needs and preferences and must include all necessary vitamins and minerals.

Behavioral methods to reduce weight include stimulus control and positive reinforcement (100). Basic methods of stimulus control are purchasing only healthy foods and keeping high-calorie foods out of sight. Eating slowly also helps, because the feeling of satiety emerges about 20 minutes after eating begins. An individual can benefit from positive reinforcement —support and praise from others—or from rewards such as new clothes.

Keeping food records is a helpful technique for initiating diet changes. The type of food eaten, the amount, and the individual's prevailing mood are logged according to the time of day. The highest calorie foods can then be targeted, minimizing the change in weekly menu plans. Sometimes this technique alone is sufficient to achieve weight loss (101).

---

[4]Basal metabolic rate (BMR) is represented by the calories expended at total physical and mental rest at ideal (thermoneutral) room temperature 12 to 18 hours after the last meal. BMR is responsible for the majority of the body's total caloric expenditure.

Table 3.3   Calories Consumed During Various Activities

Kilocalories expended per hour	Occupational activities	Recreational activities
120-150	Desk work, electric typing, auto driving, operating calculating machine	Walking 1 mile/hour, motorcycling, flying, playing cards, sewing, knitting
150-240	Auto repair, radio/TV repair, janitorial work, manual typing, bartending	Level walking 2 miles/hour, level bicycling 5 miles/hour, riding lawn mower, billiards, bowling, shuffleboard, skeet shooting, light woodworking, powerboat driving, golf (power cart), canoeing 2.5 miles/hour, horseback riding (walk), playing piano and many other musical instruments
240-300	Bricklaying, plastering, wheelbarrow (100 lb of load), machine assembly, driving trailer truck in traffic, welding (moderate load), cleaning windows, painting	Walking 3 miles/hour, cycling 6 miles/hour, horseshoe pitching, volleyball (6-person, noncompetitive), golf (pulling bag cart), archery, sailing (handling small boat), swimming (25 yards/min), fly fishing (standing with waders), horseback riding (sitting to trot), badminton (social doubles), pushing light power mower, energetic music playing, softball, snorkeling
300-360	Painting, masonry, paperhanging, light carpentry, raking leaves, hoeing	Walking 3.5 miles/hour, cycling 8 miles/hour, table tennis, golf (carrying clubs), dancing (fox trot), badminton (singles), tennis (doubles), hunting, cross-country hiking, many calisthenics
360-420	Digging garden, shoveling light earth	Walking 4 miles/hour, cycling 10 miles/hour, canoeing 4 miles/hour, horseback riding ("posting" to trot), stream fishing (walking in light current in waders), ice or roller skating 9 miles/hour, backpacking, scuba diving, soccer

Kilocalories expended per hour	Occupational activities	Recreational activities
420-480	Shoveling 10 lb (10 times/min)	Walking 5 miles/hour, cycling 11 miles/hour, badminton (competitive), tennis (singles), splitting wood, snow shoveling, hand lawn-mowing, folk (square) dancing, light downhill skiing, ski touring 2.5 miles/hour, water skiing
480-600	Digging ditches, carrying 80 lb, sawing hardwood	Jogging 5 miles/hour, cycling 12 miles/hour, horseback riding (gallop), vigorous downhill skiing, basketball, mountain climbing, ice hockey, canoeing 5 miles/hour, swimming 50 yards/min, touch football, paddleball
600-660	Shoveling 14 lb (10 times/min)	Running 5.5 miles/hour, cycling 13 miles/hour, ski touring 4 miles/hour, social squash or handball, fencing, basketball (vigorous)
660-plus	Shoveling 16 lb (10 times/min)	Cross-country skiing 6 miles/hour, jumping rope, running: 6 mph = 12.4 kcal/min 7 mph = 14.4 kcal/min 8 mph = 16.9 kcal/min 9 mph = 18.8 kcal/min 10 mph = 21 kcal/min

These calorie counts are based on a 150-pound person and will vary in direct proportion to body weight. For example, if you weight 100 lb, multiply the calories listed by .66 (that is, 100/150) to figure the number of calories expended per hour for your weight. If you weigh 200 lb, multiply by 1.33 (200/150). (1 lb = 0.453 kg.)

Note. From "Physical Activity in Cardiovascular Health: The Exercise Prescription, Frequency, and Type of Activity" by S.M. Fox, 1972, *Modern Concepts of Cardiovascular Disease*, **41**, pp. 27-28. Copyright 1978 by the American Heart Association. Adapted by permission of the American Heart Association, Inc.

In spite of their many health benefits, exercise and weight control cannot invariably prevent the occurrence or progression of CHD. Other risk factors such as high blood pressure or hypercholesterolemia may persist even though an individual exercises regularly. Ninety percent of the people in Finland, for example, are thin and active, yet their blood cholesterol levels and CHD rates are among the highest in the world (5). And the late runner and author Jim Fixx had an LDL cholesterol level of 156 mg/dl (4.1 mmol/L) at the time of his fatal heart attack.

On the other hand, even people who have had heart attacks can safely exercise if they are medically cleared and supervised (102-104). After a year of exercising and maintaining a low-fat diet, a group of coronary patients in Heidelberg, West Germany, were able to increase their work capacity by 21%. Sophisticated techniques (thallium 201 scintigraphy) documented that the areas of heart muscle receiving inadequate blood flow had decreased by more than half (104).

Complications arising from exercise programs continue to decline as more experience is gained in screening participants and in proper initiation and progression of activity (105). Recently a comprehensive review of supervised cardiac rehabilitation programs noted only one fatal heart attack for every 784,000 hours of participation. In such a high-risk group as this, a cardiac death could have been due to chance alone (106). (See Appendix A, Guidelines for Screening Exercise Participants.)

Cholesterol-Lowering Drugs

Drug therapy needs to be considered as an addition to dietary and exercise treatment if LDL cholesterol levels remain high after 6 months of these lifestyle changes. This step is more urgent if atherosclerosis is already symptomatic or if other CHD risk factors are present: high blood pressure, smoking, severe obesity, male gender, diabetes, HDL levels below 35 mg/dl (0.9 mmol/L), or a family history of CHD.

The National Cholesterol Education Program (NCEP) has recently recommended that LDL cholesterol be used as the yardstick for determining when drug therapy should be instituted. If LDL cholesterol levels remain above 190 mg/dl (4.9 mmol/L), even in the absence of other risk factors, medication is indicated. If the individual already has atherosclerosis or more than one other risk factor, an LDL level above 160 mg/dl (4.1 mmol/L) is unacceptable (39).

Drug Therapy Goals

LDL cholesterol should also be used to set goals for therapy. No effort should be spared to get the LDL level below 160 mg/dl. In persons who have already had a heart attack, angina pectoris, bypass surgery, or a stroke, or those who have two or more other risk factors, the goal is to keep LDL below 130 mg/dl (3.4 mmol/L). In these high-risk individuals whose LDL levels persist above 160 mg/dl, medication should at least be given a trial and continued if the benefit to LDL control is worth the side effects (if any) and cost. If the goal is not reached with one drug, another may be added for a greater combined effect (39). Drugs should not be started until secondary causes of hypercholesterolemia have been excluded. These include medical conditions such as hypothyroidism, and liver or kidney disease. Medications that could be responsible include progestins and steroid hormones and the thiazide diuretics that are commonly used for hypertension.

Responses of different individuals to a cholesterol-lowering drug will be quite variable. Some people have dramatic results with a low dose, whereas others experience a minimal effect. Thus, it is essential to recheck cholesterol at one and three months after initiating or changing therapy. Treatment must be continued indefinitely because the response is rapidly lost if the medication is discontinued.

Fortunately we now have safe and effective cholesterol-lowering drugs. First-line medications have traditionally been nicotinic acid (niacin) or the bile acid sequestrants cholestyramine and colestipol. Together with gemfibrozil, they have been shown in clinical trials to lower the incidence of heart attacks. Lovastatin, released in late 1987, is the first of a class of drugs that powerfully curtail the body's own production of cholesterol.

Bile Acid Sequestrants. In many cases, the initial drug of choice will be one of the two bile acid sequestrants, colestipol and cholestyramine. Trade names for these are Colestid and Questran, respectively. They have similar mechanisms, effectiveness, and long-term safety records. Both come in granular powder form rather than pills.

The bile acid sequestrants can be expected to lower LDL by 15% to 30% and total cholesterol by about 20% (37, 107-109). In some studies, cholestyramine also elevated HDL by 5% to 25% (110). These drugs may elevate triglycerides, so triglyceride levels should be followed closely early in treatment.

Colestipol and cholestyramine are fairly safe drugs because they are not absorbed from the intestine. They bind with the bile acids, which contain cholesterol, and carry them out of the body in the feces. By holding onto (sequestering) bile acids within the intestine, they gradually deplete the body of some of its cholesterol and bile that is normally reabsorbed and sent back to the liver. The liver responds with an increase in the number of its LDL receptors, which then pull more cholesterol out of the bloodstream. Because of their mechanism of action that interrupts the enterohepatic circulation, the bile acid drugs must be taken two to four times daily to be effective.

These drugs frequently cause troublesome side effects such as constipation, heartburn, bloating, belching, abdominal pain, gas, nausea, and vomiting. These symptoms often occur when the individual starts taking the drugs but usually decrease with regular usage. Though they are certainly annoyances, these side effects are not dangerous and can be minimized by education and careful usage. Give the patient the following suggestions to minimize side effects and improve compliance:

1. Begin with a small dose and gradually increase as needed. For the first week, take only one scoop or packet 30 minutes after the evening meal. Then, if bloating is not troublesome, the next week increase to two scoops or packets after supper. Increase to three scoops after another week or when the intestine becomes adapted to the medication. Then begin this same gradual dosage at another large meal, either breakfast or lunch. The dose can be increased if necessary to attain a satisfactory cholesterol level to 10 to 15 gm twice daily for colestipol, or 8 to 12 gm twice daily for cholestyramine. Maximum dosage is 30 gm per day for colestipol and 24 gm per day for cholestyramine. If side effects begin later, a reduction in dosage will usually help.

2. Mix the powder with a thin soup, a cold beverage, or a soft, high-water-content food such as applesauce. Do not overdilute or cook the medication.

3. Try using a blender to lessen the medication's grainy consistency and improve its palatability. After mixing, allow the medication to sit in the liquid for several minutes, or preferably overnight.

4. For convenience, try mixing a full day's supply in a blender every morning or every evening. Keep it refrigerated, then briefly stir before each use.

5. Take the medication at least twice daily, 30 minutes before (if side effects are significant), during, or after meals. Drink it slowly to avoid swallowing air. Never skip doses—this undermines your body's adaptation to the drug.

6. Increase dietary fiber and overall fluid intake to prevent constipation.

7. If heartburn becomes a problem, take antacids after and between meals.

8. If difficulties continue, switching to the other drug in this category may be helpful. Or, take the drug 30 minutes or even an hour before meals.

9. If cost is a consideration, the drugs may be purchased by the tin rather than individual packets. Colestipol is slightly less expensive, averaging $46 per month for a full dose, as compared with $56 per month for cholestyramine. The individual packets are convenient when traveling.

Besides combining with bile acids, the sequestrants also bind to some drugs, reducing the amount available to the tissues. This includes digitoxin (digitalis), thyroid hormones, iron preparations, diuretics, anticoagulants (warfarin), tetracycline, phenobarbital, and beta blockers. If these drugs are required, they should be taken at least 1 hour before the bile acid sequestrants or 4 hours afterward. The treating physician may need to adjust the dosage upward. If the sequestrants are discontinued for any reason, the effect of these other drugs will increase temporarily and may cause toxicity. Small amounts of the fat-soluble vitamins A, D, E, and K will also be bound, but these do not generally require supplementation.

Nicotinic Acid (Niacin).   Nicotinic acid, or niacin, is a B vitamin that can lower cholesterol by 20% and triglyceride levels by 40%. When used in high doses of 3 to 6 gm per day, it may also raise HDL as much as 20%, thus conferring additional protection against atherosclerosis (111). It has been used in clinical trials and shown to be effective in reducing heart attacks (112) and in shrinking plaque (113).

Niacin is thought to act by decreasing the body's synthesis of LDL and VLDL rather than by removing them after they are already formed (114). In addition, niacin may decrease the "stickiness" of platelets in the blood, thus reducing the chance for a clot to form within a damaged artery.

Niacin is effective and inexpensive and is the only cholesterol-lowering drug that is available without a prescription. Unfortunately, it has frequent side effects, some of which are dangerous. Most people will experience skin flushing starting about 20 minutes after the niacin dose and persisting for 30 to 60 minutes. Although very uncomfortable and possibly embarrassing, the flushing is not medically serious and tends to diminish or disappear after 2 weeks of regular niacin use. One aspirin tablet each morning tends to minimize the flushing sensation, as does eliminating hot drinks, especially coffee and tea. Other minor side effects that are less common include nausea, vomiting, itching, skin rash, and dizziness.

In the high doses required to significantly lower cholesterol, niacin is considered a drug rather than a vitamin, and consultation with a physician before starting therapy is definitely warranted. Hepatitis occurs in at least one third to one fourth of patients on high-dose niacin. Uric acid levels may also become inflated, causing problems for those with gout. Occasionally, niacin may cause abnormal heart rhythms or may interfere with the control of blood sugar or peptic ulcers. For these reasons, niacin should not be used in people with active liver disease and should be used cautiously in people with ulcers, diabetes, gout, arrhythmias, or bundle branch (heart) block. Blood tests for liver enzymes, uric acid, and glucose are recommended soon after the niacin therapy is initiated.

The initial niacin dose is no more than 100 mg three times daily with meals. For some individuals, dosages of only 1 gm per day give sufficient results. The maximum daily dose of 3 to 6 gm is seldom attained because of side effects. To minimize side effects it is essential the patient take niacin on a regular schedule and increase the dose gradually. Missing even a single dose may cause increased flushing after subsequent doses.

Niacin is available in 100-, 250-, and 500-mg tablets as well as in sustained-release forms, such as Nicobid. The long-acting tablets frequently cause less skin flushing but may also be less effective in controlling cholesterol. Nicotinamide, a closely related compound, is equally effective as a vitamin, but it has no effect on cholesterol or triglycerides. It is sometimes mistakenly recommended as a substitute for niacin because it does not cause flushing. Niacin costs a mere $3 to $10 per month.

Gemfibrozil (Lopid).   Gemfibrozil belongs to a class of drugs called fibric acid derivatives. Initially used to treat elevated triglycerides, gemfibrozil has recently gained favor in hypercholesterolemia as well. In the Helsinki Heart Study, gemfibrozil combined with a heart-healthy diet resulted in an 8% decrease in LDL and total cholesterol, and HDL levels climbed 10%. Triglyceride levels in the subjects dropped 35% (35).

As a group, the 2,000 Finnish men taking Lopid had an impressive 34% decrease in new cases of CHD over 5 years. This study was the first to support drug therapy in treating low HDL levels, because the boost in high-density lipoproteins seemed to account for some of gemfibrozil's cardioprotection (36).

Gemfibrozil's effect on cholesterol is variable, generally lowering LDL in the range of 5% to 15%. The drug lowers VLDL triglycerides up to 40%, and individual gains in HDL levels have been reported as high as 20% (115). Its action is unknown but probably involves stimulation of lipoprotein lipase. This enzyme accelerates the conversion of LDL from VLDL in the circulation. (As a result, some people taking this drug note a temporary and mild increase in LDL.)

Side effects are uncommon and consist of nausea, diarrhea, rash, abnormal heart rhythms, and myositis (inflammation of muscle). Occasionally, abnormalities in liver tests or a decrease in the white blood cell count occur. Gemfibrozil may increase the effect of warfarin (an anticoagulant drug) and cannot be used while a woman is pregnant or breastfeeding.

Clofibrate is an older fibric acid drug that has been used with discouraging results, possibly increasing the incidence of gallstones and cancer in the World Health Organization's Cooperative Trial (116). It is seldom used today.

The usual dose for gemfibrozil is 600 mg twice daily. It costs approximately $45 per month.

Probucol (Lorelco).   Available since 1977, probucol has a modest ability to decrease LDL by 10% to 15%. Unfortunately, it may also lower HDL cholesterol as much as 25%, an effect that may limit its usefulness (110). Its maximal effect on blood lipids may not be present for up to 6 months.

Current research is focusing on probucol's antioxidant properties, which may be its greatest merit (117). (Oxidized LDL is especially damaging to the inner lining of the artery, thereby promoting cholesterol influx and plaque growth.) Probucol is thought to become incorporated within the LDL particles perhaps facilitating their removal by the liver.

Probucol has infrequent side effects other than diarrhea, nausea, and flatulence. It should be avoided by anyone with a recent heart attack or serious heart rhythm disturbances (ventricular arrhythmias or prolonged QT interval).

The dosage for probucol is 500 mg twice daily. It costs about $50 per month.

Lovastatin (Mevacor). Recent developments in pharmacology have brought about a class of drugs that are revolutionizing the treatment of hypercholesterolemia. These are classified as HMG CoA reductase inhibitors. They interfere with a cellular reaction that removes oxygen from hydroxy-methyl-glutaryl Coenzyme A. This is the first and the rate-limiting step of the 26 steps in cholesterol synthesis. Because cells produce less cholesterol on lovastatin, the liver draws more cholesterol out of the circulation for its production of bile and hormones (118).

Research indicates that more than 95% of individuals with hypercholesterolemia who take lovastatin and related drugs will have a marked reduction in LDL accompanied by a modest increase in HDL cholesterol— exactly what is desired. Furthermore, because the mechanism of action is so specific, lovastatin has a very low incidence of side effects or interactions with other drugs. Its effectiveness makes control of even markedly elevated cholesterol a realistic goal (119, 120).

Studies have shown that lovastatin results in an average decrease of 25% to 45% in LDL cholesterol. Total cholesterol decreases about 35% and the triglycerides decline 20% to 30%. An extra bonus is the 8% to 15% average increase in HDL cholesterol (39, 121, 122). Responses are obtained within 2 weeks of therapy, with maximum effects noted after 4 to 6 weeks. Patients with moderate elevations in cholesterol may have adequate control with a convenient regimen of 20 or 40 mg taken once daily at bedtime. Maximum dosage is 40 mg twice daily (123).

Two notes of caution: First, although lovastatin has been shown to dramatically lower blood cholesterol levels, this does not absolutely prove its effectiveness in preventing CHD. Because a full scale clinical trial for lovastatin would cost in the range of $100 million, it has not been and may never be done. (Large-scale studies such as the Coronary Drug Project [124] and the Lipid Research Clinics Study [38] used the drugs available at the time, niacin and cholestyramine, respectively.) Thus, it requires a small but reasonable leap of faith to conclude that the cholesterol-lowering effect of lovastatin will reduce the risk of subsequent heart attacks and strokes.

Second, a diet low in cholesterol and saturated fat is still mandatory. Lovastatin decreases the liver's production of cholesterol but cannot reduce what enters the body via the diet. Taking this or any drug cannot override the harmful effects of a high-fat diet. The combination of good nutrition with lovastatin, however, is a powerful approach to lowering cholesterol levels.

Side effects of drugs in this class are low because of the specific action of the drugs. In comparing six different drug regimens, researchers found lovastatin to be the only treatment without significant adverse effects (107). Mild to moderate stomach and intestinal complaints were the most common symptoms and were usually transient. Fewer than 2% of patients must be withdrawn from lovastatin therapy because of adverse effects. Of these, most have liver problems detected by blood tests. For this reason, a liver profile of the patient is suggested with cholesterol testing every 3 to 4 months for the first 15 months of therapy.

A painful inflammation of muscles (myositis) occurs in approximately 1% of persons on lovastatin. These persons must be followed closely and possibly withdrawn from the drug if muscle pain and elevations in muscle enzymes (CPK) persist. The chances an individual will develop myositis are enhanced if he or she is also taking gemfibrozil, niacin, or cyclosporine (the latter is a drug frequently used in transplant recipients) (125).

Another potential problem is clouding of the eye lens. In early trials, subtle lens changes that were not detected before treatment were noted after therapy. However, in an even greater number of persons, lens clouding noted at the onset of therapy was not found on the posttreatment exam. As experience with lovastatin grows, it has not been linked with any increased risk for cataracts. A slit lamp eye exam is only necessary for lovastatin patients who have cataracts or are prone to develop them, such as diabetics and users of steroid medications.

At the time of this writing, very few interactions are known between lovastatin and other drugs. If the blood thinner warfarin (Coumadin) is used concurrently with lovastatin, its dose may need to be decreased. Lovastatin has been combined with other lipid drugs such as niacin and the bile acid drugs, augmenting their effect on cholesterol and triglycerides.

Dosage is started at 20 mg once daily with the evening meal. (The body makes most of its cholesterol at night.) If needed, the dose may be increased after 4 weeks up to a maximum of 40 mg twice daily. The cost is about $1.50 per pill, or $45 to $180 per month, depending on the dosage required.

Combination Therapy. Drugs from different categories can be combined if necessary to lower cholesterol to an acceptable range. The bile acid sequestrants in particular have been shown to safely augment the benefits of niacin or lovastatin (124). A lovastatin-colestipol regimen was shown to reduce LDL by almost 50% and to raise HDL by 17% (126, 127). Similar results were obtained from combining cholestyramine with lovastatin in the 1988 Lovastatin Study Group III (122). The combination of colestipol and niacin resulted in a 43% decrease in LDL and a 37% increase in HDL in a 1987 study led by Blankenhorn (113). Evidence that atherosclerotic plaque regressed was present in 16% of their patients.

Drugs to Lower Triglycerides. Triglyceride levels of 150 to 250 mg/dl (1.7-2.8 mmol/L) can be controlled by lifestyle, especially regular exercise;

attaining ideal weight; and minimizing sugar and alcohol intake. Also beneficial is eating certain cold-water fish such as salmon and mackerel, which are rich sources of omega-3 oils. In rare cases, the treating physician may advise cautious use of commercially prepared fish-oil capsules.

Medications are sometimes used for moderate triglyceride elevations (250 to 500 mg/dl or 2.8 to 5.6 mmol/L) if the patient has familial combined hyperlipidemia. A family history of heart attacks occurring before age 55 deserves investigation into the presence of this or other genetic disorders.

Triglyceride levels that persist higher than 500 mg/dl are definitely elevated and in need of treatment (128). Drugs such as niacin or gemfibrozil may be indicated after 6 months of an adequate dietary trial. Treatment is more urgent for triglyceride elevations greater than 1,000 mg/dl (11.3 mmol/L), which tend to cause pancreatitis. Again, the bile acid sequestrants tend to elevate triglycerides and should be avoided in people with hypertriglyceridemia. (See Table 3.4 for a comparison of the major cholesterol-lowering drugs.)

In summary, the drugs with proven long-term safety records and proven effectiveness in decreasing CHD are the bile acid drugs, nicotinic acid, and gemfibrozil. Except for gemfibrozil, they require considerable patient education and a meticulous dosage schedule to avoid side effects. As with many medications, taking lipid-lowering agents consistently and regularly makes them safer and more effective.

Gemfibrozil and niacin have two advantages over the bile acid powders: They frequently lower triglycerides and raise HDL. Gemfibrozil is convenient and has a good safety record, but it is somewhat expensive. Niacin is by far the least expensive of these medications but has annoying and sometimes dangerous side effects.

Lovastatin is the most powerful lipid drug known to date. It dramatically lowers LDL and triglycerides while boosting HDL. Though convenient to use, it is expensive and its long-term safety is only now being established. If no serious side effects arise in the future, however, lovastatin and other drugs in its class may become the most frequent first-line medications for hypercholesterolemia.

Recent advances in pharmaceutical research allow control of virtually any cholesterol elevation. As an adjunct to heart-healthy diets, proper use of these agents can save thousands of lives each year. No longer can we accept a laissez-faire attitude toward plasma cholesterol: Control of our major health problem is now within our grasp.

Medical and Surgical Intervention

Impressive medical and surgical advances have been developed to treat CHD, including coronary bypass surgery, balloon dilation, and

Table 3.4 Summary of Cholesterol-Lowering Drugs[a]

Drug	Dose per day	LDL-cholesterol lowering	Side effects	Monitoring required	Reduce CHD risk?	Long-term safety record?	Effect on HDL	Mechanism of action
Colestipol and Cholestyramine	12-30 gm	15%-30%	Constipation, bloating, may increase triglycerides	Other drug levels, triglycerides	Yes	Yes	Minimal	Increases excretion of bile acids in stool and increases LDL-receptor activity
Nicotinic acid	2-6 gm	15%-30%	Skin flushing, stomach upset, liver inflammation	Uric acid, liver function, glucose, ulcer	Yes	Yes	Increases	Decreases liver's synthesis of VLDL and possibly cholesterol
Gemfibrozil	1200 mg	5%-15%	Gallstones, nausea	Liver function	Yes	Preliminary evidence	Increases	Reduces incorporation of free fatty acids into triglycerides

	Dose	%	Side effects	Monitoring				Mechanism
Probucol	1 gm	10%-15%	Nausea, diarrhea, flatulence, prolonged QT interval on ECG	HDL ECG	Unproven	Unproven	Increases	May inhibit oxidation of LDL
Lovastatin	20-80 mg	25%-45%	Liver, muscle enzymes elevated	Liver function, eye exams (?)	Unproven	Unproven	Increases	Decreases cholesterol synthesis by inhibiting the enzyme HMG CoA reductase

aResults are based on average performance in groups of people.

clot-dissolving drugs. These interventions have become the standard of medical care and pillars of hope for people with CHD. However, none of these techniques cures atherosclerosis or even delays its progression. All of them incur certain risks, and many patients do not benefit from them. A brief summary of the newer treatments and some of their problems and limitations follows.

Coronary Artery Bypass Surgery

More than 350,000 coronary bypass surgeries are performed each year in the United States at a cost of billions of dollars. In this procedure, a new conduit from the aorta or internal mammary artery is connected to one of the heart's coronary arteries at a point beyond its blockage (see Figure 3.8).

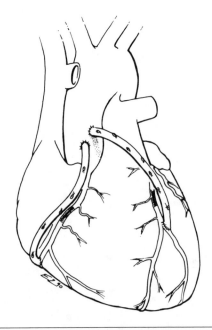

Figure 3.8   Coronary artery bypass surgery using a vein graft to detour plaque obstruction to the right coronary artery and the left anterior descending artery.

Although bypass surgery was first performed in 1964, it was not until 1977 that a study to assess its benefit was reported (129). The study showed that bypass surgery did not prolong life any more than medical therapy did. However, this study was severely criticized, especially by surgeons, for its small size and design. The results were generally disregarded, and the number of operations escalated each year.

Results from another larger study, the Coronary Artery Surgery Study (CASS), were first released in 1983 (130, 131). It found that bypass grafting did not extend life expectancy except for a small subgroup of patients.[5] The European Coronary Surgery Study Group (132) was somewhat more successful in demonstrating a benefit from bypass surgery. After 12 years, the surgically treated group had a 4% lower death rate than those treated medically (132).

Though little evidence exists that bypass grafting prolongs life, it does temporarily relieve angina pectoris. It should be considered for patients with severely limiting pain that has been unresponsive to diet and drug therapy. Nonetheless, the procedure should be postponed for as long as possible. Two thirds of bypass patients have angina chest pain again 5 years after their operations (133).

Many of these discouraging statistics stem from the fact that instead of halting the underlying process, bypass surgery actually accelerates atherosclerosis (134-138). Atherosclerotic changes become prominent in the vein graft only 3 years after bypass surgery and reach dangerous levels in 7 to 10 years. Up to 70% of vein grafts become completely occluded within 12 years. These same microscopic changes would take 35 to 40 years to peak in normal arteries.

Research at UCLA's Atherosclerosis Research Institute showed that plaque buildup (defined as further loss of 25% of the passageway) proceeded 10 times more frequently in vessels that had been operated on than in comparable arteries not bypassed (139). Some of the new conduits rapidly and completely closed due to clotting. In the bypass grafts that were still open 5 years after surgery, Kroncke and colleagues found that 74% had plaque progression and in the majority of these (78%), the artery had become totally occluded (140).

Given these problems, is bypass surgery performed too often or too early? A 1988 review of 386 bypass procedures found that slightly more than half were done for appropriate reasons, whereas the remainder were performed on questionable or inappropriate grounds. The rates of inappropriate surgery varied from 37% to 78% in the hospitals surveyed (141).

In spite of technique improvements, operative deaths and complication rates from bypass surgery have quadrupled over the past 15 years, possibly reflecting more patients returning for subsequent surgery (142). Nevertheless, the number of coronary bypass surgeries has continued to soar. It has now become the most common operation of all time, outstripping even the tonsillectomy in its heyday (143).

---

[5]These were people who had severe blockage in the first (proximal) part of the left main coronary artery. Surgery may also be indicated when all three major coronary arteries are severely affected and/or there is abnormal heart muscle contraction (ventricular dyskinesis). The operation is futile when plaque is distributed all along the artery, even in the tiny branches, or arterioles.

More than 2 million Americans today have had this procedure performed, yet only a minority of them are being treated aggressively with diet or drug therapy to lower their cholesterol. Very few are given adequate instruction on a heart-healthy diet or smoking cessation. Sometimes changes in health habits are suggested, but only rarely are they emphasized to a sufficient degree. Detailed education and vigorous support and follow-up are necessary to change health habits. Experience has shown that a perfunctory admonition to "give up cigarettes" or "eat less fat" is heeded by only a small minority.

Balloon Dilation: The Plaque Busters

Since its first application in 1977, balloon angioplasty, or PTCA,[6] has attracted considerable media coverage and public interest. Using a thin wire with an inflatable tip would seem the perfect alternative to bypass surgery. Indeed, in only 10 years, the use of PTCA has expanded to over 200,000 patients per year (143). However, convincing evidence is lacking for any long-term benefit from it.

The public's expectations of PTCA have grown inappropriately. Like surgery, it does not cure atherosclerosis but is a stopgap measure that may temporarily reduce symptoms for patients in serious trouble. Cequier noted that one third of PTCA patients had developed re-stenosis (repeat closure) of the treated segments when evaluated again 6 months after treatment (144). The blockage averaged 73% of the artery's diameter. Another third had significant progression of atherosclerosis after an average period of 3 years. PTCA benefits only a minority of patients and seems to increase the likelihood of later bypass surgery (145).

As with bypass surgery, the risks of PTCA must not be taken lightly. Intuitively, it is easy to imagine that a tiny balloon threaded through an artery could squash the plaque and allow normal blood flow to resume. Expanding the catheter tip usually does increase the arterial opening, but not simply because the plaque has been flattened. Arterial plaque is a solid tumor and frequently contains scar tissue and calcium. Plaque is rarely compressible by the balloon pressures used in PTCA, so two dire consequences frequently result: plaque rupture or overstretching of the artery wall (146).

Although it is not desirable, sometimes the only way to open the artery is to rupture the plaque. In the words of a leading PTCA specialist, "Although it might initially seem to indicate a failed procedure, plaque rupture may often be the key to a clinically successful treatment" (147, p. 13).

---

[6]PTCA stands for percutaneous (through the skin) transluminal (down the lumen, or arterial passageway) coronary (heart artery) angioplasty ("repairing" the artery).

Another tactic in balloon angioplasty is to severely dilate the artery beyond its ability to recoil into its original shape. This overstretching literally rips the cells and fibers within the artery's wall (the media and adventitia layers). The outer diameter is permanently dilated, forming what is known as an aneurysm (see Figure 3.9). Sometimes a particularly solid plaque retains its shape and is pushed (herniated) through the

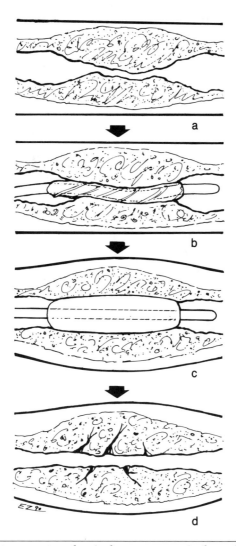

Figure 3.9   Percutaneous transluminal coronary angioplasty (PTCA). Through the narrowed segment of artery (a), a thin catheter tip directed by X-ray fluoroscopy is positioned (b) and inflated (c). Plaque fissure (d), aneurysm formation, or both, are dangerous and common results of the procedure.

artery's middle layer. "For long-lasting favorable results, angioplasty must produce major damage to the wall structures" (147, p. 14).

In addition to the desired and expected results of PTCA, life-threatening complications may also occur, though generally only in about 5% or less of cases. Sometimes the balloon completely rips through the arterial wall. Or a blood clot may form suddenly, completely blocking the artery. In either case emergency surgery is necessary to save the patient from bleeding to death or sustaining a heart attack.

A new alternative is *atherectomy*, a procedure in which a specialized catheter is used to shave off plaque while an attempt is made to retrieve the particles into a rotating chamber. Unfortunately, this procedure severely damages the endothelium layer before the bulk of the plaque's mass underneath is reached. Also, as the arterial rotator breaks off particles of the plaque, some are dispersed downstream as emboli.

Laser treatments have been in an experimental stage for several years. Early lasers had the unfortunate side effect of heating the tissue to 600 degrees Fahrenheit. Newer lasers are being developed that are much cooler. However, the danger persists that a hole will be burned completely through the arterial wall during the attempt to vaporize dense, calcified plaque.

Anti-Clotting Drugs

Drugs to counteract the body's clotting mechanism have been used as an emergency measure in recent years to attempt to dissolve clots forming within arteries. Starting in the early 1980s, streptokinase and urokinase were used with marginal success, causing toxicity and complications from bleeding. Tissue plasminogen activator (TPA) was introduced in 1988 and has shown slightly greater effectiveness with fewer side effects (148).

Although they represent a great step forward in treating heart attacks, the anticlotting drugs are not without their drawbacks and limitations. In the majority of patients (80%), treatment opens only 30% or less of the artery's original diameter, and the rest remains occluded by dense plaque (149). The drugs must be given within the first 6 hours of the heart attack, necessitating rapid access to a hospital. The cost is more than $2,000 per injection, and several injections per patient have become fairly routine in modern cardiac care units.

The availability of bypass surgery, PTCA, and anticlotting drugs does not suggest that someone can simply check into a hospital and have his or her arteries "cleaned out." By the time an individual experiences the symptoms of atherosclerosis, plaque has covered most of the surface area of medium and large arteries throughout the body. Completely cleaning out the arteries of the average middle-aged American using PTCA or laser treatment is clearly impossible.

None of these medical or surgical procedures can cure atherosclerosis and in fact are much more likely to fuel the underlying process by further damaging the arteries. At best they can buy time for those in dire straits. An individual who has had one of these treatments needs to exercise even tighter control of cholesterol and the other CHD risk factors. Health professionals must not fail to stress this critically important point to their patients.

References

1. Leibowitz, J.O. (1970). *The history of coronary heart disease*. London: Wellcome Institute of the History of Medicine.
2. Vogel, J. (1847). *The pathological anatomy of the human body*. Philadelphia: Lea and Blanchard.
3. Anitschkow, N. (1933). Experimental arteriosclerosis in animals. In E.V. Cowdry (Ed.), *Arteriosclerosis*. New York: Macmillan.
4. Anitschkow, N., & Chalatow, S. (1913). Ueber experimentelle cholesterinsteatose und ihre Bedentung fur die Entstehung einiger Pathologischer Prozesse [Centralblatt fuer Allyemeine, Pathologie, und Pathologische Anatomie]. *Centralbl Allg Pathol, 24,* 1.
5. Keys, A. (1980). *Seven countries. A multivariate analysis of death and coronary heart disease*. Cambridge, MA: Harvard Univ Press.
6. Keys, A. (1970). Coronary heart disease in seven countries. *Circulation, 41*(4, Suppl. 1), 1-211.
7. Rose, G. (1982). Incubation period of coronary heart disease. *British Medical Journal, 284,* 1600-1601.
8. McGill, H.C., Jr. (1968). *Geographic pathology of atherosclerosis*. Baltimore: Williams and Wilkins.
9. Keys, A. (1969). Serum cholesterol and the question of normal. In Benson, E.S., & Strandjord, P.E. (Eds.), *Multiple laboratory screenings* (p. 1). Orlando: Academic Press.
10. White, N.K., & Edwards. J.E. (1950). Correlations in coronary artery disease. *Circulation, 1,* 645.
11. Hegsted, D.M., McGandy, R.B., Myers, M.L., & Stare, F.J. (1965). Quantitative effects of dietary fat on serum cholesterol in man. *American Journal of Clinical Nutrition, 17,* 281.
12. Keys, A., Anderson, J.T., & Grande, F. (1965). Serum cholesterol response to changes in the diet. Part I, II, & III. *Metabolism, 14,* 747-787.
13. Connor, W.E., Stone, D.B., & Hodges, R.E. (1964). The interrelated effects of dietary cholesterol and fat upon human serum lipid levels. *Journal of Clinical Investigation, 43,* 1691.

14. Shekelle, R.B., & Stamler, J. (1989). Dietary cholesterol and ischaemic heart disease. *Lancet*, **I**, 1177-1179.
15. Kushi, L.H., Lew, R.A., Stare, F.J., & Ellison, C.R. (1985). Diet and 20-year mortality from coronary heart disease: The Ireland-Boston Diet-Heart Study. *New England Journal of Medicine*, **312**, 811-818.
16. Kahn, H.A., Phillips, R.L., Snowden, D.A., & Choi, W. (1984). Association between reported diet and all-cause mortality. Twenty-one year follow-up on 27,530 adult Seventh-Day Adventists. *American Journal of Epidemiology*, **119**, 775-787.
17. Thorogood, M., Carter, R., Benfield, L., McPherson, K., & Mann, J. (1987). Plasma lipids and lipoprotein cholesterol concentrations in people with different diets in Britain. *British Medical Journal*, **295**, 351-353.
18. Sacks, F.M., Castelli, W.P., Donner, A., & Kass, E.H. (1975). Plasma lipids and lipoproteins in vegetarians and controls. *New England Journal of Medicine*, **292**, 1148-1151.
19. Sacks, F.M., Rosner, B., & Kass, E.H. (1974). Blood pressure in vegetarians. *American Journal of Epidemiology*, **100**, 390-398.
20. Philips, R., Lemon, F., Kuzma, J., & Beeson, W.L. (1978). Coronary heart disease mortality among Seventh-Day Adventists with differing dietary habits. *American Journal of Clinical Nutrition*, 1915-1985.
21. Katz, L.N., Stamler, J. & Pick, R. (1958). *Nutrition and atherosclerosis.* Philadelphia: Lea and Febiger.
22. Robertson, T.L., Kato, H., Gordon, T., Kagan, A., Rhodes, G.G., Land, C.E., Worth, R., Belsky, J.L., Dock, D.S., Miyanishi, M., & Kawamoto, S. (1977). Epidemiological studies of coronary heart disease and stroke in Japanese men lining in Japan, Hawaii and California. *The American Journal of Cardiology*, **39**, 244-249.
23. Kagan, A., Harris, B.R., & Winkelstein, W., Jr. (1974). Epidemiologic studies of coronary heart disease and stroke in Japanese men living in Japan, Hawaii, and California: Demographic, physical, dietary, and biochemical characteristics. *Journal of Chronic Disease*, **27**, 345-364.
24. Worth, R.M., Kato, H., & Rhoads, G.G. (1975). Epidemiologic studies of coronary heart disease and stroke in Japanese men living in Japan, Hawaii, and California: Mortality. *American Journal of Epidemiology*, **102**, 481-490.
25. Kato, H., Tillotson, J., Nichaman, M.Z., Rhoads, G.G., & Hamilton, H.B. (1973). Epidemiologic studies of coronary heart disease and stroke in Japanese men living in Japan, Hawaii and California. Serum lipids and diet. *American Journal of Epidemiology*, **97**, 372-385.
26. Marmot, M.G., Syme, S.L., Kagan, A., Kato, H., Cohen, J.B., & Belsky, J. (1975). Epidemiologic studies of coronary heart disease and stroke in Japanese men living in Japan, Hawaii, and California:

Prevalence of coronary and hypertensive heart disease and associated risk factors. *American Journal of Epidemiology, 102,* 514.

27. National Diet-Heart Study Research Group. (1969). The national diet-heart study final report. *Circulation, 37*(Suppl. I), 1, 1-412.

28. Turpeinen, O., Karvonen, M.J., Pekkarinen, M., Miettinen, M., Elosuo, R., & Paavilainen, E. (1979). Dietary prevention of coronary heart disease: The Finnish Mental Hospital Study. *International Journal of Epidemiology, 8,* 99-118.

29. Dayton, S., Pearce, M.L., Hashimoto, S., Dixon, W.J., & Tomiyasu, U. (1969). A controlled clinical trial of a diet high in unsaturated fat in preventing complications of atherosclerosis. *Circulation, 40*(Suppl. II), 1-63.

30. Multiple Risk Factor Intervention Trial Research Group. (1982). Multiple Risk Factor Intervention Trial: Risk factor changes and mortality results. *Journal of the American Medical Association, 248,* 1465-1477.

31. Hjermann, I., Holme, I., & Leren, P. (1986). Oslo Study diet and antismoking trial. Results after 102 months. *American Journal of Medicine, 80*(2A), 7-11.

32. Hjermann, I., Byre, K.V., Holme, I., & Leren, P. (1981). Effect of diet and smoking intervention on the incidence of coronary heart disease: Report from the Oslo Study Group of a randomized trial in healthy men. *Lancet, 2,* 1303-1310.

33. Shekelle, R.B., Shryock, A.M., Paul, O., Lepper, M., Stamler, J., Liu, S., & Raynor, W.J., Jr. (1981). Diet, serum cholesterol and death from coronary heart disease. The Western Electric Study. *New England Journal of Medicine, 304,* 65-70.

34. Arntzenius, A.C., Kromhout, D., Barth, J.D., Reibor, J.H., Bruschke, A.V., Buis, B., van-Gent, C.M., Kempen-Voogd, N., Strikwerda, S., & Van-der Velde, E.A. (1985). Diet, lipoproteins, and the progression of coronary atherosclerosis. The Leiden Intervention Trial. *New England Journal of Medicine, 313,* 805-811.

35. Frick, M.H., Elo, O., Haapa, K., Heinonen, O.P., & Heinsalmi, P., Helo, P., Huttenen, J.K., Kaitaniemi, P., Koskinen, P., & Manninen, V. (1987). Helsinki Heart Study. Primary-prevention trial with gemfibrozil in middle-aged men with dyslipidemia: Safety of treatment, changes in risk factors, and incidence of coronary heart disease. *New England Journal of Medicine, 317,* 1237-1245.

36. Manninen, V., Elo, O., Frick, H., Haapa, K., Heinonen, O.P., Heinsalmi, P., Helo, P., Huttunen, J.K., Kaitaniemi, P., Koskinen, P. (1988). Lipid alterations and decline in the incidence of coronary heart disease in the Helsinki Heart Study. *Journal of the American Medical Association, 260,* 641-651.

37. Lipid Research Clinics Program. (1984). The Lipid Research Clinics

Coronary Primary Prevention Trial results I. Reduction in incidence of coronary heart disease. *Journal of the American Medical Association, 251,* 351-364.

38. Lipid Research Clinics Program. (1984). The Lipid Research Clinics Coronary Primary Prevention Trial results II. The relationship of reduction in incidence of coronary heart disease to cholesterol lowering. *Journal of the American Medical Association, 251,* 365-374.

39. Expert Panel of the National Cholesterol Education Program. (1988). Report of the National Cholesterol Education Program Expert Panel on detection, evaluation, and treatment of high blood cholesterol in adults. *Archives of Internal Medicine, 148,* 36-68. (Also available as NIH Publication No. 88-2925, January 1988)

40. American Heart Association Nutrition Committee. (1988). Dietary guidelines for healthy American adults. *Circulation, 77,* 721A.

41. U.S. Department of Health and Human Services, Public Health Service. (1988). *The Surgeon General's report on nutrition and health* (DHHS [PHS] Publication No. 88-50210). Washington, DC: Superintendent of Documents.

42. Committee on Diet and Health, Food and Nutrition Board, Commission on Life Sciences, National Research Council. (1989). *Diet and health. Implications for reducing chronic disease risk.* Washington, DC: National Academy Press.

43. National Institutes of Health, Office of Medical Applications of Research. (1985). Lowering blood cholesterol to prevent heart disease. Consensus development conference statement. *Journal of the American Medical Association, 251,* 2080.

44. Committee on Technological Options to Improve the Nutritional Attributes of Animal Products. Board on Agriculture, National Research Council. (1988). *Designing foods. Animal product options in the marketplace.* Washington, DC: National Academy Press.

45. U.S. Department of Health and Human Services, Department of Agriculture. (1986, December). *The relationship between dietary cholesterol and blood cholesterol and human health and nutrition. A report to the Congress, pursuant to the Food Security Act of 1985.* P.L. 99-198. Subtitle B, Section 1453.

46. American Heart Association. (1968). *Diet and heart disease.* Dallas: Author.

47. American Heart Association, Nutrition Committee and Council on Arteriosclerosis. Recommendations for Treatment of Hyperlipidemia in Adults. (1984). *Circulation, 69,* 1065A-1090A.

48. Anderson, J.W., & Tietyen-Clark, J. (1986). Dietary fiber: hyperlipidemia, hypertension, and coronary heart disease. *American Journal of Gastroenterology, 81,* 907-919.

49. Morris, J.N., Heady, J.A., & Raffle, P.A.B. (1956). Physique of London busmen. The epidemiology of uniforms. *Lancet, 2,* 569.

50. Morris, J.N., Heady, J.A., Raffle, P.A.B., Roberts, C.G., Parks, W.J. (1953). Coronary heart-disease and physical activity of work. *Lancet*, **2**, 1053.
51. Keys, A. (1976). Overweight and the risk of heart attack and sudden death. In G.A. Bray (Ed.), *Obesity in perspective, Part 2* (Vol. 2, p. 215). Washington, DC: U.S. Department of Health, Education, and Welfare. (DHEW Publication No. NIH 75-708)
52. Hopkins, P.N., & Williams, R.R. (1986). Identification and relative weight of cardiovascular risk factors. *Cardiology Clinics*, **4**(1), 3-32.
53. Paffenbarger, R.S., Hyde, R.T., Wing, A.L., & Hsieh, C.C. (1986). Physical activity, all-cause mortality and longevity of college alumni. *New England Journal of Medicine*, **314**, 605-613.
54. Paffenbarger, R.S., Wing, A.L., & Hyde, R.T. (1978). Physical activity as an index of heart attack risk in college alumni. *American Journal of Epidemiology*, **108**, 161.
55. Powell, K.E., Thompson, P.D., Caspersen, C.J., & Kendrick, J.S. (1987). Physical activity and the incidence of coronary heart disease. *Annual Review of Public Health*, **8**, 253-287.
56. Wood, P.D., Stefanick, M.L., & Dreon, D.M. (1988). Changes in plasma lipids and lipoproteins in overweight men during weight loss through dieting as compared with exercise. *New England Journal of Medicine*, **319**, 1173-1179.
57. Garcia-Palmieri, M.R., Costas, R., Cruz-Vidal, M., Sorlie, P.D., & Havlik, R.J. (1982). Increased physical activity: A protective factor against heart attacks in Puerto Rico. *American Journal of Cardiology*, **50**, 749.
58. Kannel, W.B., & Sorlie, P. (1979). Some health benefits of physical activity. The Framingham Study. *Archives of Internal Medicine*, **139**, 857.
59. Magnus, K., Matroos, A., & Strackee, J. (1979). Walking, cycling, or gardening, with or without seasonal interruption, in relation to acute coronary events. *American Journal of Epidemiology*, **110**, 724.
60. Leon, A.S., Connett, J., Jacobs, D.R., & Rauramaa, R. (1987). Leisure-time physical activity and risk of coronary heart disease and death: The Multiple Risk Factor Intervention Trial. *Journal of the American Medical Association*, **258**, 2388-2395.
61. Thomas, G.S., Lee, P.R., Franks, P. (1981). *Exercise and health: The evidence and the implications*. Cambridge, MA: Oelgeschlager, Gunn & Hain.
62. Bray, G.A. (1985). Complications of obesity. *Annals of Internal Medicine*, **103**(Suppl.), 1052-1062.
63. Nestel, P.J., Schreibman, P.H., & Ahrens, E.H. (1973). Cholesterol metabolism in human obesity. *Journal of Clinical Investigation*, **52**, 2389-2397.
64. Ballantyne, D., Clark, R.S., & Ballantyne, R.C. (1981). The effect of

physical training on plasma lipids and lipoproteins. *Clinical Cardiology,* **4**, 1-4.

65. Multiple Risk Factor Intervention Trial Research Group. (1977). Contributions of weight reduction to lowering serum cholesterol. *Circulation,* **56**(Suppl. III), 113.

66. Haskell, W.L. (1984). Exercise-induced changes in plasma lipids and lipoproteins. *Preventive Medicine,* **13**, 23-36.

67. Castelli, W.P., & Anderson, K., (1986). A population at risk. Prevalence of high cholesterol levels in hypertensive patients in the Framingham Study. *American Journal of Medicine,* **80**(Suppl. 2A), 23-32.

68. Wood, P.D., Haskell, W., Klein, H., Lewis, S., Stein, M., & Farquhar, J. (1976). The distribution of plasma lipoproteins in middle-aged male runners. *Metabolism,* **25**, 1249-1257.

69. Johannessen, S., Holly, R.G., Lui, H., & Amsterdam, E.A. (1986). High-frequency, moderate-intensity training in sedentary middle-aged women. *Sports Medicine,* **14**, 99-102.

70. Joseph, J.J., & Bena, L.L. (1977). Cholesterol reduction: A long term intense exercise program. *Journal of Sports Medicine and Physical Fitness,* **17**, 163-168.

71. Hespel, P., Lijnen, P., Fagard, R., Van Hoof, R., Rosseneu, M., & Amery, A. (1988). Changes in plasma lipids and apoproteins associated with physical training in middle-aged sedentary men. *American Heart Journal,* **115**, 786-792.

72. Christie, R.J., Bloore, H.G., & Logan, R.L. (1980). High-density lipoprotein (HDL) cholesterol in middle-aged joggers. *New Zealand Medical Journal,* **91**, 39-40.

73. Lopez, S.A., Vial, R., & Balart, L. (1974). Effect of exercise and physical fitness on serum lipids and lipoproteins. *Atherosclerosis,* **20**, 1-9.

74. Wood, P.D., Haskell, W.L., Blair, S.N., Williams, P.T., Krauss, R.M., Lindgren, F.T., Albers, J.J., Ho, P.H., & Farquhar, J.W. (1983). Increased exercise level and plasma lipoprotein concentrations: A 1 year randomized, controlled study in sedentary middle-aged men. *Metabolism,* **32**, 31-39.

75. Williams, P.T., Wood, P.D., Stefanick, M.L., Dreon, D.M. (1988). Changes in plasma lipids and lipoproteins in overweight men during weight loss through dieting as compared with exercise. *New England Journal of Medicine,* **319**, 1173-1179.

76. Brownell, K.D., Bachorik, P.S., & Ayerle, R.S. (1982). Changes in plasma lipid and lipoprotein levels in men and women after a program of moderate exercise. *Circulation,* **65**, 477.

77. Zimmerman, J., Kaufman, N.A., & Fainaru, M. (1984). Effect of weight loss in moderate obesity on plasma lipoprotein and apolipoprotein levels and on high density lipoprotein composition. *Arteriosclerosis,* **4**, 115-123.

78. Streja, D., & Mymin, D. (1979). Moderate exercise and high-density lipoprotein-cholesterol: Observations during a cardiac rehabilitation program. *Journal of the American Medical Association, 242,* 2190-2192.

79. Tran, Z.V., & Weltman, A. (1985). Differential effects of exercise on serum lipid and lipoprotein levels seen with changes in body weight. A meta-analysis. *Journal of the American Medical Association, 254,* 919-924.

80. Blackburn, H. (1986). Physical activity and hypertension. *Journal of Clinical Hypertension, 2,* 154-162.

81. Tuck, M.L., Sowers, J., Dornfeld, L., Kledzik, G., & Maxwell, M. (1981). The effect of weight reduction on blood pressure, plasma renin activity, and plasma aldosterone levels in obese patients. *New England Journal of Medicine, 304,* 930-933.

82. Stamler, J., Farinaro, E., Mojonnier, L.M., Hall, Y., Moss, D., & Stamler, R. (1980). Prevention and control of hypertension by nutritional-hygienic means: Long-term experience of the Chicago Coronary Prevention Evaluation Program. *Journal of the American Medical Association, 243,* 1819-1823.

83. Boyer, J.L., & Kasch, R.W. (1970). Exercise therapy in hypertensive men. *Journal of the American Medical Association, 211,* 1668.

84. Rauramaa, R. (1984). Relationship of physical activity, glucose tolerance, and weight management. *Preventive Medicine, 13,* 37.

85. Richter, E.A., Ruderman, N.B., & Schneider, S.H. (1981). Diabetes and exercise. *American Journal of Medicine, 247,* 2674-2679.

86. Pederson, O., Beck-Nielsen, J., & Jeding, L. (1980). Increased insulin receptors after exercise in patients with insulin-dependent diabetes mellitus. *New England Journal of Medicine, 302,* 886.

87. Bennett, P.N. (1972). Effect of physical exercise on platelet adhesiveness. *Scandinavian Journal of Haematology, 9,* 138.

88. Stephens, T. (1988). Physical activity and mental health in the United States and Canada: Evidence from four population surveys. *Preventive Medicine, 17,* 35-47.

89. Greist, J.H., Klein, M.H., Eischens, R.R., Foris, J., Gurman, A.S., & Morgan, W.P. (1979). Running as a treatment for depression. *Comprehensive Psychiatry, 20,* 41-54.

90. Dishman, R.K. (1985). Medical psychology in exercise and sport. *Medical Clinics of North America, 69,* 123-143.

91. Stern, M.J., & Cleary, P. (1981). National exercise and heart disease project: Psychosocial changes observed during a low-level exercise program. *Archives of Internal Medicine, 141,* 1463.

92. Brownell, K.D., Marlatt, G.A., Lichtenstein, E., & Wilson, G.T. (1986). Understanding and preventing relapse. *American Psychology, 41,* 765-782.

93. Fox, S.M. (1972). Physical activity in cardiovascular health: III The exercise prescription, frequency and type of activity. *Modern Concepts of Cardiovascular Health, 41,* 25-30.

94. Barr, S.I. (1987). Women, nutrition, and exercise: a review of athletes' intakes and a discussion of energy balance in active women. *Progress in Food and Nutrition Science*, 11, 307-361.

95. Donato, K.A. (1988). Efficiency and utilization of various energy sources for growth. *American Journal of Clinical Nutrition*, 45(Suppl.), 164.

96. Dreon, D.M., Frey-Hewitt, B., Ellsworth, N., Williams, P.T., Terry, R.B., & Wood, P.D. (1988). Dietary fat: Carbohydrate ratio and obesity in middle-aged men. *American Journal of Clinical Nutrition*, 47, 995.

97. Lissner, L., Levitsky, D.A., Strupp, B.J., Kalkwarf, H.T., & Roe, D.A. (1987). Dietary fat and the regulation of energy intake in human subjects. *American Journal of Clinical Nutrition*, 46, 886.

98. Pariza, M.W., & Boutwell, R.K. (1987). Historical perspective: Calories and energy expenditure in carcinogenesis. *American Journal of Clinical Nutrition*, 45(Suppl.), 151.

99. Björntorp, P., Vahouny, G.V., & Kritchevshy, P. (Eds.) (1985). *Dietary fiber and obesity*. New York: Alan P. Liss.

100. Brownell, K.D. (1985). Behavioral treatment for obesity. *Female Patient*, 9, 85-95.

101. Romanczyk, R.G. (1974). Self-monitoring in the treatment of obesity: Parameters of reactivity. *Behavioral Therapy*, 5, 531.

102. Haskell, W.L. (1978). Cardiovascular complications during exercise training of cardiac patients. *Circulation*, 57, 920.

103. Bruce, R.A. (1974). The benefits of physical training for patients with coronary heart disease. In F.J. Ingelfinger, R.V. Ebert, M. Finland, & A.S. Relman (Eds.), *Controversy in internal medicine II* (pp. 145-161). Philadephia: W.B. Saunders.

104. Schuler, G., Schlierf, G., Wirth, A., Mautner, H.P., Scheurlen, H., Thumm, M., Roth, H., Schwarz, F., Kohlmeier, M., & Mehmel, H.C. (1988). Low-fat diet and regular, supervised physical exercise in patients with symptomatic coronary artery disease: Reduction of stress-induced myocardial ischemia. *Circulation*, 77, 172-181.

105. Oldridge, N.B., Guyatt, G.H., Fischer, M.E., & Rimm, A.A. (1988). Cardiac rehabilitation after myocardial infarction. *Journal of the American Medical Association*, 260, 945-950.

106. Van Camp, S.P., & Peterson, R.A. (1986). Cardiovascular complications of outpatient cardiac rehabilitation programs. *Journal of the American Medical Association*, 256, 1160-1163.

107. Hoeg, J.M., Maher, M.B., Bailey, K.R., & Brewer, J.B. (1987). Comparison of six pharmacologic regimens for hypercholesterolemia. *American Journal of Cardiology*, 59, 812-815.

108. Weintraub, M.S., Eisenberg, S., & Breslow, J.L. (1987). Different patterns of postprandial lipoprotein metabolism in normal, type IIa, type III, and type IV hyperlipoproteinemic individuals: Effects of

treatment with cholestyramine and gemfibrozil. *Journal of Clinical Investigation*, **79**, 1110-1119.

109. Levy, R.I., Brensike, J.F., Epstein, S.E., Fisher, M.L., Friedman, L., Friedewald, W., & Detre, K.M. (1984). The influence of changes in lipid values induced by cholestyramine and diet on progression of coronary artery disease: Results of the NHLBI Type II Coronary Intervention Study. *Circulation*, **69**(2), 325-337.

110. Glueck, C. (1983). Influence of clofibrate, bile-sequestering agents and probucol on high-density lipoprotein levels. *American Journal of Cardiology*, **52**, 28B.

111. Schaeffer, E.J., & Levy, R.I. (1985). Pathogenesis and management of lipoprotein disorders. *New England Journal of Medicine*, **312**, 1300-1310.

112. Canner, P.L., Berge, K.G., Wenger, N.K., Stamler, J., Friedman, L., Prineas, R.J., & Friedewald, W. (1986). Fifteen year mortality in Coronary Drug Project patients: Long-term benefit with niacin. *Journal of the American College of Cardiology*, **8**, 1245-1255.

113. Blankenhorn, D.H., Nessim, S.A., Johnson, R.L., Sanmarco, M.E., Azen, S.P., & Cashin-Hemphill, L. (1987). Beneficial effects of combined Colestipol-Niacin therapy in coronary atherosclerosis and coronary venous bypass grafts. *Journal of the American Medical Association*, **257**, 3233-3240.

114. Hoeg, J.M., Gregg, R.E., & Brewer, H.B. (1986). An approach to the management of hypercholesterolemia. *Journal of the American Medical Association*, **255**, 512-521.

115. Hunninghake, D.B., & Peters, J.R. (1987). Effects of fibric acid derivatives on blood lipid and lipoprotein levels. *American Journal of Medicine*, **83**(Suppl. 5B), 44-49.

116. WHO Cooperative Trial. (1980). Committee of principal investigators: WHO cooperative trial on primary prevention of ischemic heart disease using clofibrate to lower serum cholesterol: Mortality follow-up. *Lancet*, **2**, 379.

117. Steinberg, D., Parthasorathy, S., Corew, T.E., Khoo, J., & Witztum, J.L. (1989). Beyond cholesterol: Modifications of low-density lipoprotein that increase its atherogenicity. *New England Journal of Medicine*, **320**, 915-924.

118. Grundy, S.M. (1988). HMG-CoA reductase inhibitors for treatment of hypercholesterolemia. *New England Journal of Medicine*, **319**, 24-32.

119. Illingworth, D.R., & Sexton, G.J. (1984). Hypocholesterolemic effects of mevinolin in patients with heterozygous familial hypercholesterolemia. *Journal of Clinical Investigation*, **74**, 1972-1978.

120. Tobert, J.A., Hitzenberger, G., Kukovetz, W.R., Holmes, I.B., & Jones, K.H. (1982). Rapid and substantial lowering of human serum cholesterol by mevinolin, an inhibitor of hydroxymethyl glutaryl-coenzyme A reductase. *Atherosclerosis*, **41**, 61-65.

121. The Lovastatin Study Group II. (1986). Therapeutic response to

Lovastatin (Mevinolin) in nonfamilial hypercholesterolemia. *Journal of the American Medical Association*, **256**, 2829-2834.

122. The Lovastatin Study Group III. (1988). A multi-center comparison of lovastatin and cholestyramine therapy for severe primary hypercholesterolemia. *Journal of the American Medical Association*, **260**, 359-366.

123. Illingworth, D.R. (1986). Comparative efficacy of once versus twice daily mevinolin in the therapy of familial hypercholesterolemia. *Clinical Pharmacological Therapy*, **40**, 338-343.

124. Coronary Drug Project Research Group. (1975). Clofibrate and niacin in coronary heart disease. *Journal of the American Medical Association*, **231**, 360-381.

125. Tobert, J.A. (1988). Rhabdomyolysis in patients receiving lovastatin after cardiac transplantation. *New England Journal of Medicine*, **318**, 48.

126. Vega, L.G., & Grundy, S.M. (1987). Treatment of primary moderate hypercholesterolemia with lovastatin and colestipol. *Journal of the American Medical Association*, **257**, 33-38.

127. Illingworth, D.R. (1984). Mevinolin plus colestipol in therapy for severe heterozygous familial hypercholesterolemia. *Annals of Internal Medicine*, **101**, 598-604.

128. National Institutes of Health Consensus Development Conference. (1984). Treatment of hypertriglyceridemia. *Journal of the American Medical Association*, **251**, 1196-1200.

129. Murphy, M.L., Hultgren, H.N., Detre, K., Thomsen, J., Takaro, T., and participants of the Veterans Administration Cooperative Study. (1977). Treatment of chronic stable angina: A preliminary report of survival data. *New England Journal of Medicine*, **297**, 621-627.

130. CASS Principal Investigators. (1984). Myocardial infarction and mortality in the Coronary Artery Surgery Study (CASS): Randomized trial. *New England Journal of Medicine*, **310**, 750-758.

131. CASS Principal Investigators. (1983). Coronary Artery Surgery Study (CASS): A randomized trial of coronary artery bypass surgery: survival data. *Circulation*, **68**, 939-50.

132. Varnauskas, E. and the European Coronary Surgery Study Group. (1988). Twelve-year follow-up of survival in the randomized European Coronary Surgery Study. *New England Journal of Medicine*, **319**, 332-337.

133. Seides, S.F., Borer, J.S., Kent, K.M., Rosing, D.R., McIntosh, C.L., & Epstein, S.E. (1978). Long-term anatomic fate of coronary-artery bypass grafts and functional status of patients 5 years after operation. *New England Journal of Medicine*, **298**, 1213-1217.

134. Campeau, L., Enjalbert, M., Lesperance, J., Bourassa, M.G., Kwiterovich, P., Wacholder, S., & Sniderman, A. (1984). The relation of risk factors to the development of atherosclerosis in saphenous-vein bypass grafts and the progression of disease in the native

circulation: A study 10 years after aortocoronary bypass surgery. *New England Journal of Medicine,* **311,** 1329-1332.

135. Levine, J.A., Bechtel, D.J., & Gorlin, R., et al. (1975). Coronary artery anatomy before and after direct revascularization surgery: Clinical and cinearteriographic studies in 67 selected patients. *American Heart Journal,* **89,** 561-70.

136. Maurer, B.J., Oberman, A., & Holt, J.H., Jr., et al. (1974). Changes in grafted and nongrafted coronary arteries following saphenous vein bypass grafting. *Circulation,* **50,** 293-300.

137. Griffith, L.S.C., Achuff, S.C., & Conti, C.R. (1973). Changes in intrinsic coronary circulation and segmental ventricular motion after saphenous-vein coronary bypass graft surgery. *New England Journal of Medicine,* **288,** 589-95.

138. Kakos, G.S., Oldham, H.N. Jr., & Dixon, S.H., Jr. (1972). Coronary artery hemodynamics after aorto-coronary artery vein bypass: An experimental evaluation. *Journal of Thorasic and Cardiovascular Surgery,* **63,** 49-53.

139. Cashin, W.L., Sanmarco, M.E., Nessim, S.A., Blankenthorn, D.H. (1984). Accelerated progression of atherosclerosis in coronary vessels with minimal lesions that are bypassed. *New England Journal of Medicine,* **311,** 824-8.

140. Kroncke, G.M., Kosolcharoen, P., Claymen, J.A., Peduzzi, P.N., Detre, K., & Takaro, T. (1988). Five-year changes in coronary arteries of medical and surgical patients of the veterans administration randomized study of bypass surgery. *Circulation,* **78**(Suppl. I), 144-150.

141. Winslow, C.M., Kosecoff, J.B., Chassin, M., Kanouse, D., & Brook, R.H. (1988). The appropriateness of performing coronary artery bypass surgery. *Journal of the American Medical Association,* **260,** 505-509.

142. Naunheim, K.S., Fiore, A.C., Wadley, J.J., McBride, L.R., Kanter, K.R., Pennington, D.G., Borner, H.B., Kaiser, G.C., & Willman, V.L. (1988). The changing profile of the patient undergoing coronary artery bypass surgery. *Journal of the American College of Cardiology,* **11,** 494-8.

143. National Center for Health Statistics 1987. 1986 summary: National Hospital Discharge Survey. Advance data from vital and health statistics. No. 145. DHHS Publ No (PHS) 87-1250. Public Health Service. Hyattsville, MD.

144. Cequier, A., Bonan, R., Crepeau, J., Coté, G., DeGuise, P., Joly, P., Lespérance, J., & Waters, D.D. (1988). Restenosis and progression of coronary atherosclerosis after coronary angioplasty. *Journal of the American College of Cardiology,* **12,** 49-55.

145. Ellis, S.G., Fisher, L., Dishman-Ellis, S. (1989). Comparison of coronary angioplasty with medical treatment for single- and double-vessel

coronary disease with left anterior descending artery involvement. Long-term outcome based on an Emory-CASS registry study. *American Heart Journal,* **118**, 208.

146. Waller, B.F. (1989). PCTA: Mechanisms of dilation and causes of acute and late closures. *Cardiovascular Review and Reports,* **April**, 35-47.

147. Angelini, Paolo. (1987). *Balloon catheter coronary angioplasty.* Mt. Kisco, NY: Futuro Publ Co.

148. Yusef, S., Wittes, J., & Friedman, L. (1988). Overview of results of randomized clinical trials in heart disease. I. Treatment following myocardial infarction. *Journal of the American Medical Association,* **260**, 2088-2093.

149. Satler, L.F., et al. (1987). Assessment of residual coronary arterial stenosis after thrombolytic therapy during acute myocardial infarction. *American Journal of Cardiology,* **59**, 1231-1233.

Suggested Readings

Diet

Grundy, S.M, Bilheimer, D., Blackburn, H., Brown, W.V., Kwiterovich, P.O., Jr., Matterson, F., Schonfeld, G., & Weidman, W.H. (1982). Rationale of the diet-heart statement of the American Heart Association. Report of the Nutrition Committee. *Circulation,* **65**, 839A-854A.

Lewis, B., Hammett, F., Katan, M., Kay, R.M., Merkx, I., Nobels, A., Miller, N.E., & Swan, A.V. (1981). Towards an improved lipid-lowering diet: Additive effects of changes in nutrient intake. *Lancet,* **2**, 1310-1313, 8259.

Exercise and Weight Control

Blair, S.N., & Oberman, A. (1987). Epidemiologic analysis of coronary heart disease and exercise. *Cardiology Clinics,* **5**, 271-83.

Exercise testing and training of apparently healthy individuals: A handbook for physicians. (1972). The Committee on Exercise, American Heart Association.

Katch, F.I., & McArdle, W.D. (1983). *Nutrition, weight control, and exercise* (2nd ed.). Philadelphia: Lea & Febiger.

Morgan, W.P., & Goldston, S.E. (Eds.) (1987). *Exercise and mental health.* Washington, DC: Hemisphere.

National Institutes of Health Consensus Development Conference Statement. (1985). Health implications of obesity. *Annals of Internal Medicine,* **103**, 1073-1077.

Newman, D. (1986). *The sports medicine fitness course*. Palo Alto, CA: Bull.

Pollock, M., Wilmore, J., & Fox, S. (1984). *Exercise in health and disease*. Philadelphia: W.B. Saunders.

U.S. Department of Health and Human Services, Public Health Service. (1985). *Health implications of obesity. National Institutes of Health Consensus Development Conference statement* (Vol. 5, No. 9).

II

THE OTHER RISK FACTORS FOR ATHEROSCLEROSIS

☐

A high blood level of cholesterol, in and of itself, can cause plaque to form in arteries. Smoking and high blood pressure, however, greatly accelerate this dangerous process. Together with cholesterol they make up the three major risk factors and atherosclerosis. Minor risk factors are diabetes, stress, heredity, low HDL levels, and being male, sedentary, or seriously overweight (≥30% above ideal weight).

When more than one risk factor is present, the consequences are compounded. In particular, high cholesterol, smoking, and high blood pressure act synergistically to promote atherosclerosis and to undermine health. When two of these risk factors are present, the risk of athero-sclerosis is not simply doubled, but quadrupled. With all three present, the risk is eight times higher (see Figure II) (1). Thus, a 55-year-old man with most of the major and minor risk factors will stand greater than a 50-50 chance of having a heart attack within 8 years. This is like playing Russian roulette with a half-loaded gun, yet many of us live with these incredibly high risks—and many suffer bad consequences.

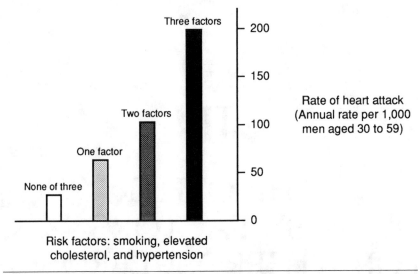

Risk factors: smoking, elevated cholesterol, and hypertension

Figure II   The major risk factors for CHD—hypercholesterolemia, hypertension, and smoking—have a synergistic effect when present in combination. If an individual has two of these, the risk for CHD is three to four times as great as if neither were present. The presence of all three risk factors incurs a risk almost eight times higher. (Source: NHLBI *Facts at Your Fingertips*.)

Is Cholesterol the Most Important Risk Factor?

Some of the recent statistical studies that have evaluated risk factors independently judge elevated cholesterol to be the most critical risk factor for CHD. Data from the World Health Organization indicates that nearly half of the variance in CHD rates between countries is due to differences in average blood cholesterol levels (2). Elevated blood pressure is the most powerful risk factor for stroke, and smoking has the greatest relative impact on peripheral vascular disease, but these are much less common causes of death and disability than CHD. In the Multiple Risk Factor Intervention Trial (MRFIT), which involved 365,000 men, 46% of the total number of preventable deaths were attributed to cholesterol levels over 180 mg/dl (4.7 mmol/L) (3).

In an extensive review of the literature, Hopkins and Williams (4) calculated that CHD rates would decrease by

- 44% if serum cholesterol levels averaged 160 mg/dl (4.1 mmol/L),
- 43% in a tobacco-free society,
- 36% if average diastolic blood pressures were under 80 mmHg,

• 33% with ideal stress management, and
• 15% with prevention of diabetes.

A concerted societal effort to target cholesterol as our major health issue is justified for several reasons. First, cholesterol is the substance that becomes impregnated in the artery walls. If cholesterol levels are normal—below 160 mg/dl (4.1 mmol/L)—serious atherosclerosis rarely occurs. The Japanese have only one tenth the rate of heart attack found among Americans in spite of very high rates of hypertension and smoking. Their average cholesterol level is approximately 160 mg/dl (4.1 mmol/L), compared with 215 mg/dl (5.6 mmol/L) for Americans.

Second, hypercholesterolemia is the most common of the three major risk factors for atherosclerosis. About three quarters of American adults have blood cholesterol concentrations over 180 mg/dl (4.7 mmol/L), levels that are too high for optimal health. Over half of U.S. adults have borderline-high or definitely high-risk cholesterol levels. In contrast, only a third of American adults have borderline or high-risk blood pressure, with slightly less being smokers and only 4% being diabetic.

Next, cholesterol levels generally begin to rise as early as the 20s and 30s, allowing more time for this factor to wreak havoc on our cardio-vascular systems. Blood pressure does not increase, on the average, until the 30s and 40s. Moreover, some blood pressure problems may well result from the stiffness and hardening of arteries from atherosclerotic plaque. Autopsy studies show a higher correlation between coronary athero-sclerosis and blood cholesterol levels than with any other risk factor (5).

The cholesterol problem also frequently goes unrecognized, allowing the lethal process of arterial sludging to continue unchecked. Fully half of American adults are unaware that they have elevated cholesterol. As late as 1985, only 38% of respondents to a government survey ever recalled having had a cholesterol test. Fewer than 3% knew the actual results, and only a small percentage of these were receiving treatment. In contrast, nearly all those surveyed could recall having had a blood pressure measurement; more than half had been measured in the past year. Unlike most hypercholesterolemic people, most hypertensives are now aware of their problem, know their usual blood pressure measurements, and are receiving treatment.

Though hypercholesterolemia may be the preeminent cause of CHD in our population, heavy smoking or severe hypertension may be an even more critical factor for a given individual. The bottom line in CHD preven-tion is to keep cholesterol from entering the arterial walls, not just to control its level in the bloodstream. Thus, the other risk factors must be recognized and controlled for optimal health.

Part II of this book contains background information about and tools for controlling these other cardiovascular risk factors. Chapter 4 addresses high blood pressure and chapter 5 deals with stress, two important risk factors with considerable overlap. Chapter 6 includes important material on smoking, diabetes, and heredity. Because an in-depth treatment of each topic is clearly beyond the scope of this book, Part II attempts to clarify the salient points and provide answers to commonly asked questions. A review of this material will assist health professionals in motivating their clients to change unhealthy lifestyle habits.

Chapter

4

High Blood Pressure

High blood pressure, or hypertension, is one of the three most powerful contributors to atherosclerosis. Along with hypercholesterolemia and smoking, it is considered one of the three major risk factors for CHD (6). An estimated one third of American adults, or 60 million, have border-line or high blood pressure (7, 8).

The principal reason to control hypertension is to block its tendency to promote atherosclerosis, and thus heart attack and stroke. Studies show that hypertension is hazardous for males and females of all ages and races. It is a particularly potent risk factor for stroke, especially in blacks.

Definitions of Hypertension

Blood pressure is represented by two numerical values, such as 120/80, and is measured in millimeters of mercury (mmHg). Systolic pressure (the higher value) is the force inside the arteries at the moment the heart muscle contracts, pumping blood into the body. This can be thought of as the pumping pressure. Diastolic pressure (the lower value) is the pressure that remains inside the arteries as the heart relaxes between beats. This represents the resting pressure.

Mild & Borderline. Diastolic pressures between 90 and 104 mmHg are defined as mild, whereas systolic pressures between 140 and 159 mmHg are referred to as borderline (8). But, as with cholesterol levels, these terms are misnomers. There is nothing borderline or mild about the danger of a blood pressure in these ranges. More than 70% of all hypertensives in the United States fall under the borderline classification, and 60% of coronary deaths attributed to blood pressure occur to people with so-called "mild" hypertension (9).

Systolic or Diastolic. Some individuals have an elevation in only one of the two blood pressure values and thus have either systolic or diastolic hypertension. Elevation of either measurement is detrimental to a person's health. Such conditions affect about one third of U.S. adults. Diastolic hypertension usually develops earlier in life whereas systolic is more prevalent in the elderly.

Labile or Fixed. Many individuals find that their blood pressure fluctuates considerably from day to day, sometimes by as much as 30 to 40 points (mmHg). This condition is frequently the result of psychological stress. Often disregarded and untreated, labile hypertension also predisposes a person to heart attack and stroke (10). Fixed hypertension has traditionally referred to blood pressure that continuously remains elevated. Since blood pressure fluctuates in nearly everyone, however, the distinction between labile and fixed is seldom considered useful today (11). The average of several blood pressure values, not just the lowest recordings, should be used to determine the need for and effectiveness of treatment.

Table 4.1 classifies blood pressure into five categories, with "ideal" being the suggested value for optimal health (8). For every 10 mmHg rise in systolic pressure over the ideal 120, there is a 30% increase in the rate of cardiovascular disease (12). Even though a diastolic blood pressure of 85 is generally considered normal, the risk of CHD at that level is twice that at 60 mmHg (13). The health risks are even greater if hypertension is accompanied by other risk factors, especially hypercholesterolemia or smoking.

Cutoff points, although somewhat arbitrary, have been designated to help physicians make uniform and rational decisions about blood pressure treatment. Usually, the diagnosis of hypertension is made when readings repeatedly exceed 150/90 mmHg. Medications are then considered as well as dietary measures. If drugs are needed to control blood pressure, the goal should *not* be to lower it as much as possible. Using drugs to lower blood pressure below 140/80 is not warranted and may actually increase the risk of CHD. This may be due to adverse drug effects or some other unknown mechanism (14).

Analogous to the situation of cholesterol levels described in chapter 1, the health hazard of rising blood pressure is not an all-or-none phenomenon. Instead, the risk gradually increases as blood pressure rises above 120 systolic or 80 diastolic. In the higher ranges, the risk rapidly mounts so that people with very high pressures are six times more likely to suffer from CHD than people with healthy pressures (6, 15). The continuous and graded nature of the blood pressure hazard is illustrated in Figure

Table 4.1 Classification of Blood Pressure

Range, mmHg	Category
	Diastolic
<85	Normal blood pressure
85-89	High normal blood pressure
90-104	Mild hypertension
105-114	Moderate hypertension
≥115	Severe hypertension
	Systolic (when diastolic blood pressure is <90)
<140	Normal blood pressure
140-159	Borderline isolated systolic hypertension
≥160	Isolated systolic hypertension

This blood pressure classification is based on the average of two or more readings on two or more occasions in adults age 18 or older. A classification of borderline isolated systolic hypertension (SBP 140 to 159 mmHg) or isolated systolic hypertension (SBP ≥160 mmHg) takes precedence over high normal blood pressure (diastolic blood pressure, 85 to 89 mmHg) when both occur in the same person. High normal blood pressure (DBP 85 to 89 mmHg) takes precedence over a classification of normal blood pressure (SBP <140 mmHg) when both occur in the same person.

Note. From ''The 1988 Report of the Joint National Committee on the Detection, Evaluation, and Treatment of High Blood Pressure.'' (1988). NIH Publication No. 88-1088 (p. 3).

4.1 (16). As this graph shows, 30% of 65-year-olds with blood pressures higher than 180/105 are expected to die from cardiovascular disease in 8 years compared to 10% with pressures of 126/60 mmHg.

From the standpoint of optimal health, the lower blood pressure can be maintained through diet and exercise, the better.[1] Health professionals and their clients should not wait until the blood pressure reaches the definitive hypertension range before instituting lifestyle changes.

---

[1]The obvious exceptions are states of serious disease such as shock and treatment using medication. Also, persons with quite low blood pressure may experience occasional light-headedness when in warm temperatures or when standing up suddenly but need not be concerned if they are otherwise healthy.

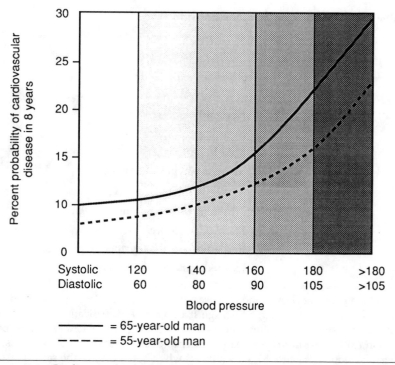

Figure 4.1   Cardiovasuclar problems do not suddenly appear at a particular blood pressure threshold, but instead gradually increase over a broad range of values. The risks of higher blood pressure rise more steeply for older persons.

Note. From "Blood Pressure and the Development of Cardiovascular Disease in the Aged" by W.B. Kannel. In *Cardiology in Old Age* (p. 59), 1976, New York: Plenum Publishing Corporation. Adapted by permission.

The Cholesterol Connection

Cholesterol and blood pressure contribute independently and in concert to the formation of arterial plaque. Neither risk factor causes symptoms until the terminal stages. Both can usually be prevented if intervention is begun early (17).

The lifestyle-related causes for blood pressure and cholesterol elevation are very similar. As a group, hypertensives have above-average cholesterol levels (19). People with systolic blood pressure values over 150 mmHg have cholesterol levels that average 237 mg/dl in men and 223 mg/dl in women. Those with systolic pressures under 106 mmHg have below-average cholesterol levels: 192 mg/dl for men and 198 mg/dl for women (13). This is due in part to similar dietary factors that elevate both cholesterol and blood pressure. In addition, many of the antihypertensive medications can have deleterious effects on blood lipids. (This will be discussed later in the chapter.)

The lifestyle measures to control hypertension parallel those for cholesterol management. These focus on eating fresh foods that contain less fat, particularly saturated fat, and salt. The diet should also contain more potassium, fiber, and polyunsaturated oils (19-21). Exercise, weight loss, and stress management also benefit blood pressure as they do blood cholesterol (22-24). The effect of these lifestyle measures on blood pressure varies considerably from one individual to another but is generally significant (25-27).

Causes of Hypertension

In only 5% of cases, hypertension can be traced to drugs[2] or an internal disease such as kidney failure or excessive thyroid or adrenal hormones. The cause remains medically undetermined in the other 95%; these hypertensives are diagnosed with essential (or primary) hypertension. Hypertensive patients are often told, "We do not know the cause for your blood pressure elevation." This is not entirely true, as decades of research confirm that certain lifestyle characteristics promote hypertension (28).

Age and Heredity

Advancing age and heredity are often mistakenly thought to be direct causes of hypertension. It is true that in societies plagued with hypertension, blood pressure tends to increase with age. But members of most primitive societies do not develop higher blood pressures as they mature. The Carajas Indians of Brazil, for example, have an average systolic blood pressure of only 109 mmHg even when they are 60 to 70 years old; Americans in their 60s average 145 mmHg. The Indians are thin; exercise frequently; consume a low-salt, low-fat, high-fiber diet; and seem to have little psychological tension.

The rarity of hypertension in certain populations does not signify a genetic protection from the condition. When primitive groups adopt the foods of advanced societies, their rates of hypertension escalate. An example is the Xhosa tribe of South Africa. Blood pressures of Xhosa living in cities is higher than their fellow tribe members living in villages. The urban dwellers are heavier and less active and consume more salt

---

[2]These include over-the-counter cold medications and appetite suppressants, steroids, amphetamines, cocaine, and, in a small minority of women, birth control pills.

and fat than the villagers. Other examples are the Indians of Easter Island who migrated to Chile (29) and Eskimos who moved to Denmark. In these cases, the indigenous people quickly develop "modern" blood pressures with changes in lifestyle (30).

A comparison of two genetically similar Polynesian groups provides another example. Figure 4.2 illustrates the relative stability of blood pressure with advancing age in those members who remained in the traditional culture (31). Polynesian men and women who moved to cities had a much more pronounced rise in blood pressure than those living in the traditional society.

Thus, blood pressure does not normally or inevitably increase with advancing age. Rather, people in affected societies just tend to be older by the time their arteries stiffen from decades of cholesterol infiltration. More so than genetic inheritance, unhealthy dietary and lifestyle habits are passed on to younger generations. Most people who consume more than 4,500 mg of sodium a day will eventually develop hypertension regardless of their genetic endowment.

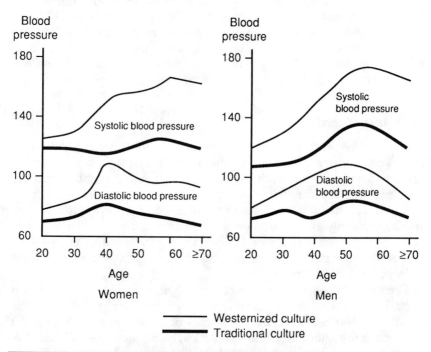

Figure 4.2 Polynesians who remain in their traditional culture (represented by heavy lines) have much less systolic and diastolic blood pressure rise with age than those who have adopted modern diets (thin lines).

Note. From "Studies of Hypertension in Migrants" by J.H. Cassel. In *Epidemiology and Control of Hypertension* by O. Paul (Ed.) (p. 43), 1975, New York: Stratton Intercontinental.

Fortunately, because of the relation of lifestyle to blood pressure most hypertension can be prevented. In addition, many of those who already have elevated pressures can reduce their blood pressure by improved health habits enough so they can minimize or even discontinue medications (17, 32). The strategies primarily involve diet—reducing salt, saturated fat, alcohol, and excess calories while increasing intake of fish, fiber, and potassium. Stress management, another important tool, is discussed in chapter 5.

Dietary Factors

Eating a wide variety of natural foods will promote a healthy blood pressure by supplying ample amounts of potassium, calcium, magnesium, and fiber. These foods also tend to be low in sodium and saturated fat, all of which help maintain a healthy blood pressure.

Sodium. Many studies support the theory that excessive sodium[3] is a common cause for hypertension (33). Sodium accumulation forces the body to retain water, which then increases blood volume, cardiac output, and blood pressure. No populations have been described that have high sodium intake and yet little hypertension.

In contrast, several diverse populations with low sodium intakes—less than 1,500 mg a day—have been studied. Their members do not gain weight with age and have essentially no hypertension. Examples include the Eskimos, Polynesians, Pygmies, Central and South American Indians, African Bushmen and nomads, and the aborigines in Australia, New Guinea, and China (34).

Even members of traditional societies, though, may have relatively high blood pressures if they consume considerable amounts of sodium. Japanese in the rural Akila prefecture average a whopping 25,000 to 35,000 mg of sodium a day, primarily from soy sauce and salted fish. As a result, 85% of the adult males have systolic blood pressure over 140 mmHg. In Akila, as in Japan as a whole, stroke is the most common cause of death (35).

The inhabitants of the South Pacific Solomon Islands present another fascinating illustration. Tribes on different islands were compared as to their diets, cooking methods, and average blood pressures. Nine percent of one group, the Lau, were noted to have hypertension. Though closely related genetically to the other tribes, the Lau used seawater for cooking,

---

[3]Sodium atoms make up about a third of table salt (by weight), and chloride atoms make up the remainder. One teaspoon of table salt weighs 5,500 mg and contains about 2,132 mg of sodium. Or approximately 1 gm of sodium is found in 2.5 gm of salt. "Sodium" and "salt" are generally used interchangeably because chloride is unrelated to blood pressure. But to avoid confusion, the sodium content rather than salt will be used here for specific quantities and recommendations, as is generally done elsewhere.

and thus had a much higher sodium intake. The other tribes had virtually no hypertension, their rates ranging from 0% to 3% (36).

Since the early 1900s it has been known that sodium restriction is generally effective in lowering blood pressure in hypertensive persons (37). This received little attention at the time, because hypertension was somewhat unusual and generally not detected. Numerous studies since then have verified that many hypertensives benefit from sodium restriction, some dramatically (38-41).

Sodium restriction will decrease systolic and diastolic blood pressure on the average by about 10 mmHg, but individual variation is considerable. Approximately half of all hypertensives are salt-sensitive, meaning they will significantly benefit from cutting back on salt (42). Avoiding salty foods early in life may prevent or delay the development of hypertension (39).

The average American consumes 10 to 50 times the necessary amount of sodium. Many use 10 to 15 gm each day when they could live quite well on 0.2 gm per day (43). As a result, the 1988 report of the Joint National Committee on Detection, Evaluation, and Treatment of Hypertension recommended restricting sodium to no more than 2,500 mg a day (8). The National Research Council reports that 500 mg of sodium a day is adequate for practically all adults (44).

An estimated two thirds of U.S. salt intake is hidden in prepared foods, with the remaining third added during cooking and at the table. Replacing heavily salted foods with natural, unprocessed foods will alleviate the bulk of this sodium overload. Fresh or frozen vegetables, for example, usually have less than 35 mg of sodium in a half-cup serving. Canned vegetables, however, have up to 500 mg, and canned vegetable juice has over 300 mg per half cup. Canned and luncheon meats are also particularly high in sodium. Even ready-to-eat grain products, such as pancake mixes and macaroni and cheese, are heavily salted, though these same grain products are naturally very low in sodium. (Table 4.2 lists the sodium content of some common foods.)

In reading food labels, "low sodium" means the product contains 140 milligrams (mg) of sodium or less per serving. "Very low sodium" foods contain 35 mg of sodium or less per serving. "Sodium-free" or "salt-free" foods contain less than 5 mg of sodium per serving. "Unsalted" and "no salt added" mean the product is processed without the salt normally added to such products. It is not necessarily "sodium free" because other sodium-based compounds may be added. A "reduced sodium" listing simply means that the manufacturer has eliminated at least 75% of the sodium. It may still be too high in sodium, however.

Some foods are so high in sodium that they should be avoided completely or used only in small quantities. Examples include pickles and olives, which are soaked in brine during the preserving process. Antacids, too, can contain more than 1,000 mg of sodium in only two tablets.

Table 4.2 Sodium and Potassium Content of Foods

Food	Sodium (mg/100 g)	Potassium (mg/100 g)
Almonds, shelled	4	773
Apples, raw	1	110
Apricots, dried	26	979
Avocados	4	604
Bacon, Canadian	2,555	432
Bananas	1	370
Beans, frozen, cooked	1	152
Beef, lean, cooked	60	370
Breads, whole wheat, regular	527	273
unsalted	30	230
Broccoli, frozen	13	244
Butter, salted	987	23
unsalted	10	23
Cantaloupe or honeydew	12	251
Carrots, raw	47	341
Cashew nuts	15	464
Cereals, cornflakes	1,005	120
oatmeal, cooked	218	61
wheat, shredded, unsalted	3	348
Cheese, cheddar	700	82
cottage	229	85
Chicken, cooked, white meat	64	441
dark meat	86	321
Corn, frozen, cooked	1	184
canned	236	97
Crackers, graham	670	384
soda	1,100	120
Cucumbers	6	160
Dates, natural and dry	1	648
Egg, whole	122	129
Figs, dried	34	640
Fish, halibut, broiled	134	525
salmon, broiled	116	443
Honey, strained	5	51

(Cont.)

Table 4.2 Continued

Food	Sodium (mg/100 g)	Potassium (mg/100 g)
Margarine, regular	987	23
unsalted	10	10
Milk, whole or skim	50	144
Mushrooms, canned	400	197
fresh	15	414
Olives, green	2,400	55
Oranges or orange juice	1	200
Peanuts, roasted, unsalted	5	701
Peanut butter	606	652
Peas, canned, regular	236	96
canned, low sodium	3	96
Pickles, dill	1,428	200
Pork, ham, cured	930	326
sausage, cooked	958	269
Potatoes, peeled, boiled, unsalted	2	285
chips	1,000	1,130
Prunes, uncooked	8	694
Raisins, uncooked	27	763
Rice, cooked, unsalted	2	28
Salad dressing, Italian	2,097	15
Soybean curd (tofu)	7	42
Tomatoes, raw	3	244
Tomato catsup, regular	1,338	370
low sodium	5-35	370
Yams	—	600
Yogurt	51	143

Note. Adapted from *Cooper's Nutrition in Health and Disease* (pp. 592-594) by H.S. Mitchell, H.J. Rynbergen, L. Anderson, and M.V. Dibble (Eds.), 1968, Philadelphia: Lippincott. Adapted by permission.

Health professionals should emphasize to clients that humans are not born with a craving for salt. It is learned over years of eating high-salt foods and can thus be unlearned. In one year's time, a person can gradually adjust to much less sodium in food and gain an appreciation of the more subtle flavors of foods prepared with herbs and spices. Those who reflexively grab the salt shaker should taste the food first, then add only enough salt to suffice, one shake at a time.

Potassium. In addition to reducing the amount of sodium in the diet, it is beneficial to increase potassium intake (45-47). A practical way to do so is by eating healthy foods high in potassium, including the following: apricots, avocados, bananas, beans (including red, white, lima, and soy) bran, broccoli, dates, cucumbers, lentils, melons, mushrooms, orange juice, peaches, potatoes (both the white and the sweet varieties), peas, prunes, prune juice, salmon, sardines, tomatoes, and winter squash. Table 4.2 also lists the potassium content of some common foods (48).

Reducing sodium and increasing potassium can be achieved simultaneously by using one of the commercially available salt substitutes. Some of these are half sodium chloride and half potassium chloride (such as Lite Salt, by Morton). This combination provides an appreciable seasoning effect and is an easy initial adjustment for the hard-core "salt-a-holic." (Note: Potassium supplementation is not recommended for people with kidney disease.)

Other Minerals. Although deficiencies in calcium or magnesium intake are not as clearly established as for potassium, they may have a small effect on blood pressure (49). Communities with hard water and thus more calcium and magnesium intake have slightly lower rates of hypertension (50, 51). In one experiment, supplementing the diet of 48 hypertensive persons with 1 gm per day of calcium had a modest lowering effect of 4 mmHg on their systolic blood pressure. There was no change in subjects who had normal blood pressure (52).

Fats and Fiber. Excessive amounts of fat in the diet, particularly saturated fat, tend to increase blood pressure as well as cholesterol. Replacing these with polyunsaturated fat tends to lower blood pressure to a similar extent as does sodium restriction (19, 20, 53, 54). The highly unsaturated omega-3 fats found in certain cold-water fish are at least partially responsible for the very low incidence of hypertension in Eskimos (55). Similarly, the low incidence of hypertension in Mediterranean populations may be related to their relatively high intake of monounsaturated olive oil.

To study the relationship of fats to blood pressure, 57 Finnish couples were placed on a low-fat diet (23% of total calories) containing as much polyunsaturated fat as saturated fat (56). After 6 weeks their average systolic blood pressure dropped 10 points and diastolic blood pressure nearly 8. This effect could not be explained by weight loss or sodium restriction. Their blood pressures quickly rose again once they reverted to their usual diet, high in saturated fat. The investigators also noted a "pronounced reduction" in serum cholesterol during the trial.

Fiber also seems to be beneficial for lowering blood pressure, perhaps by slowing the absorption of fat, reducing the body's insulin requirement, or both. Vegetarians, who consume at least twice as much fiber as non-vegetarians, consistently have lower average blood pressures than other groups of comparable age, sex, and weight (57). Their lower fat consumption and body fat also contribute to their blood pressure control.

Alcohol. Excessive alcohol intake bears a strong relationship to hypertension. Heavy drinking is responsible for an estimated 10% of the hypertension in American men (58, 59). Drinking more than 2 ounces of alcohol a day tends to elevate blood pressure (60, 61). Two ounces of alcohol corresponds to 4 ounces of 100-proof whiskey, 16 ounces of wine, or 48 ounces of beer. Paradoxically, a lower level of alcohol consumption, two drinks a day or less, tends to lower blood pressure (62).

Weight and Activity Level

Obesity is another major promoter of hypertension. This was suspected for decades and confirmed by a survey of a million Americans (63). Half of the hypertensive men and 40% of the hypertensive women in America are overweight. Obesity was determined to be responsible for 70% of the new-onset hypertension in the Framingham Heart Study (64). Obesity is responsible for 50% to 70% of all hypertension in whites and 30% in blacks. In contrast, hypertension is rare in primitive populations without obesity (34).

Although blood pressure is clearly elevated in overweight people in general, the effects of obesity on different individuals vary considerably. Just as some heavy persons have normal cholesterol, some may have normal blood pressure. All obese persons have large blood volumes, but those with normal blood pressure seem to keep their arteries relaxed and dilated, allowing blood to traverse under lower pressures (34).

Obese individuals have increased blood levels of hormones, such as aldosterone, and adrenaline-like hormones, that affect the kidney. These substances raise blood pressure by constricting small arteries (23, 65). Obesity also requires the pancreas to secrete extra amounts of insulin, which causes sodium retention by the kidneys. The expansion in blood volume and cardiac output is another proposed mechanism for increasing blood pressure (66).

Recent evidence shows that not all forms of obesity carry the same health risks. Particularly likely to become hypertensive are those individuals with most of their fat on the torso or around the waistline—so-called central or male-pattern obesity. This pattern also predisposes an individual to diabetes and hypercholesterolemia. Fat accumulation on the buttocks, hips, and legs—the female pattern—is less likely to create hypertension and these other problems (67-70).

Exercise and weight loss, in turn, lower blood pressure (71). In the Harvard Alumni Study, the men participating in vigorous activity were half as likely to have developed hypertension (72). The change in blood pressure with exercise is variable, usually being greater in those with the highest initial pressures. The average drop in both systolic and diastolic blood pressure is about 10 mmHg and requires a 10% to 30% reduction in body weight (23).

Those who lose weight are found to have reduced blood volume and cardiac output. Regular exercise also reduces adrenaline-like substances in the bloodstream, thus relaxing the blood vessels and enlarging their diameter (73-75). This effect reduces the blood pressure and the heart's work load.

The major effect of exercise on blood pressure is in reducing weight. Independent of weight loss, exercise has a modest blood pressure-lowering effect. Weight training is a much poorer blood pressure–reducer than isotonic or aerobic exercises such as running, cycling, rowing, swimming, and cross-country skiing.

Reisin and co-workers reported that they helped moderately overweight subjects achieve a 26/20 mmHg (systolic/diastolic) blood pressure drop simply by weight loss, which averaged 20 pounds (76). Salt intake was not restricted during the 4 months of the trial.

In 1981, Tuck and colleagues demonstrated that weight loss reduces blood pressure independently of sodium restriction (23). Figure 4.3 demonstrates the effect of weight reduction on blood pressure over the course of 12 weeks. Sodium intake was restricted only in the subjects with higher initial blood pressure values, but pressures fell similarly in both groups with weight loss.

Another study compared weight loss averaging 16 pounds to the use of a blood pressure drug (beta blocker), Metoprolol, in 56 overweight, hypertensive patients (77). From average diastolic blood pressures of 101 mmHg, the Metoprolol group reduced their blood pressure 7 mmHg, whereas the weight loss group attained a 10–mmHg drop. The drug group had an unfavorable increase in total cholesterol as well as a 10% decrease in beneficial HDL. In contrast, the weight loss group averaged a 6% decrease in total cholesterol combined with a 6% increase in HDL. Triglycerides increased 56% in the drug group and decreased 8% in the diet group.

Several studies suggest that maintaining ideal weight during the ages of 30 to 50 may be more effective in curbing hypertension from its inception (primary prevention) than reducing weight once hypertension is established (secondary prevention). In the Framingham Heart Study, obese young adults were eight times more likely to develop hypertension later in life. Improvement in pressures with weight loss in older persons is less consistent (78).

In Florida, Cade and co-workers put 105 hypertensive patients on an exercise program (79). Nearly all received a significant benefit from jogging two miles (3.3 km) 3 to 5 times a week. Half of those initially on drug therapy were able to discontinue all medications. The 58 patients who

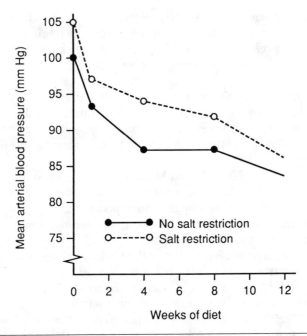

Figure 4.3 Mean arterial pressure fell equally in two groups of individuals on weight-reducing diets. Salt intake was restricted only in those with higher initial values (upper curve). Mean blood pressure is a composite of both systolic and diastolic blood pressures, calculated from the diastolic blood pressure plus one third of the difference between the systolic and diastolic values.

Note. Adapted from information appearing in *New England Journal of Medicine.* "The Effect of Weight Reduction on Blood Pressure, Plasma Serum Activity, and Plasma Aldosterone Levels in Obese Patients" by M. Tuck, J. Sowers, L. Dornfeld, G. Kladzik, and M. Maxwell, 1981, *New England Journal of Medicine,* **304**, p. 932.

had been on medication attained an average mean blood pressure reduction of 15 mmHg as a result of the exercise program.[4]

As with hypercholesterolemia, blood pressure responses are most dramatic in response to a comprehensive approach. Stamler and associates helped 115 hypertensives lower their blood pressure through a healthy diet, smoking cessation, and exercise (17). The subjects were taught how to reduce their dietary calories as well as their fat, cholesterol, alcohol, and sodium intakes. The average blood pressure reduction was a respectable 10/13 mmHg, and the participants who made the most changes

---

[4]Mean BP is the diastolic value plus one third of the difference between the systolic and diastolic pressures. Warning: In cases of severe uncontrolled hypertension, the exercise program should be closely supervised by a physician. Also, salt tablets are not needed unless the amount of sweat lost per day exceeds 1 gallon (equivalent to a 7-pound weight loss).

achieved even greater success. In 1989, the Stamlers reported that this approach was also successful in preventing definite hypertension from developing in over 90% of their subjects who had borderline pressures (80). For an in-depth review of non-drug treatments for hypertension, see Frumkin et al., 1978 (24).

Blood Pressure Medications

Although high blood pressure has been repeatedly shown to be a major risk factor for predicting CHD, only one study has demonstrated that reducing blood pressure prevents subsequent heart attacks: the Hypertension Detection and Follow-up Program (15). In contrast, large studies in the United States (3, 84, 85), England (81), Norway (82), and Australia (83) have consistently shown that antihypertensive medications help prevent stroke.

One explanation for this apparent inconsistency is that blood pressure is not as important in causing CHD as stroke. Another reason is that many of the drugs used to treat hypertension have unfortunate side effects that militate against CHD protection; they frequently cause an elevation in LDL and triglycerides or a drop in HDL (42, 86, 87). As a result, 50% of treated hypertensives have high-risk cholesterol levels, whereas only 40% of nontreated hypertensives and 30% of those with normal blood pressure fall into this category (88). These untoward effects are found in the drugs used most commonly for hypertension: the diuretics and beta blockers.

The most commonly prescribed diuretics fall into the thiazide group. These elevate blood cholesterol an average of 12 to 19 mg/dl (.3 to .5 mmol/L) and triglycerides an average of 23 to 29 mg/dl (.26 to .3 mmol/L) (12, 42, 88). The rise in serum cholesterol and triglycerides is generally blunted if the individual maintains a low-fat diet (89).

At least some adverse effect on cholesterol and triglycerides occurs to nearly anyone taking the thiazide diuretics, and it persists as long as they are used. Lasix (furosemide) is a less common diuretic that lowers beneficial HDL cholesterol, leaving LDL and triglycerides unaffected (90).

Thiazides also cause the body to excrete potassium as well as sodium. If an individual does not increase intake of dietary or commercially prepared potassium, the level in the blood may fall too low. This makes the heart tend to beat in an abnormal and lethal rhythm called ventricular fibrillation (91).

If a diuretic is required, as in congestive heart failure, indapamide (Lozol) may be used even in those with hypercholesterolemia. It has not been shown to affect LDL cholesterol and may actually increase HDL.

Beta blockers are another standard class of blood pressure medications for which more than 30 million prescriptions were written in 1988. Most of these drugs have the unfortunate consequence of increasing blood triglycerides by up to 65% (92). Some of these also decrease beneficial HDL cholesterol (82, 93). Particularly troublesome are propanolol, atenolol, and metoprolol.

Newer beta blockers may not affect HDL cholesterol if they have the property of ISA (intrinsic sympathomimetic activity). Examples are acebutolol (Sectral), oxprenolol (Trasicor, Iset), and pindolol (Visken). Pindolol may even raise HDL and lower total cholesterol (92). Labetalol is a related drug (with both alpha- and beta-blocking properties) that has no effect on blood lipids. Table 4.3 summarizes antihypertensive medications that affect lipids. If these drugs are used, blood tests should be done 1 to 2 months after initiating therapy to determine if any detrimental changes have occurred to lipids or potassium. This is especially important because the duration of therapy may extend over decades.

Over 100 million prescriptions are filled each year in the United States for blood pressure medications, making them the most widely used of

Table 4.3   Effect of Blood Pressure Drugs on Lipids

| Generic name (trade name) | Possible effect on | | | |
	Total cholesterol	LDL	HDL	Triglycerides
Beta blockers				
Propranolol (Inderol)	i, 0, d	0	dd	ii
Atenolol (Tenormin)	i	0	d	ii
Metoprolol (Lopressor)	i, 0, d	0, d	d	ii
Nadolol (Corgard)	0	0	0, d	d
Diuretics				
Thiazides (Diuril, Esidrix)	i	i	0	ii
Chlorthalidone (Hygroton)	i	i	0	ii
Furosemide (Lasix)	i	0	d	i
Other				
Reserpine (in Ser-Ap-Es)	0	0	d	d
Methyldopa (Aldomet) variable effect	0, d	0	0, d	0, i

Key i = increases; ii = greatly increases; 0 = no change; d = decreases; dd = greatly decreases; LDL = low-density lipoproteins; HDL = high-density lipoproteins.

Note. If these antihypertensive drugs must be used, blood tests should be done to note any detrimental lipid (and electrolyte) changes, especially because therapy may extend over several decades.

all drugs. The cost of these drugs exceeds $3 billion a year by the most conservative estimates. As late as 1985, Dyazide, a thiazide diuretic, and Inderol, a beta blocker, were the two most frequently prescribed of all drugs. Because of their adverse effects on lipids and the availability of alternative drugs, their use in blood pressure management should be minimized.

Cholesterol-Lowering Effects

Lowering blood pressure alone without control of cholesterol does not reduce CHD risk (6). Half of all hypertensive patients also have high blood levels of cholesterol or triglycerides. Thus, the clinician must not lose sight of cholesterol and other cardiovascular risk factors when treating hypertension. Prazosin (Minipress), a vasodilator, has been available for many years, and studies have shown that it tends to decrease total cholesterol 7 to 8 mg/dl while raising HDL 2 to 3 mg/dl. It usually lowers triglycerides. A newer and closely related drug, Terazocin (Hytrin) offers these same lipid benefits combined with one-a-day dosage convenience (94). Other advantages are that neither drug raises blood sugar or causes impotence, problems common with thiazide diuretics and beta blockers, respectively. They do tend to cause light-headedness, however, for the first week or two of use.

In addition to the drugs discussed previously, two new classes of agents that lower blood pressure without adversely affecting lipids are the calcium antagonists and angiotensin converting enzyme (ACE) inhibitors. One of the latter group, captopril, may even have a beneficial effect on HDL if given for longer than 6 months. In addition to improving blood pressure, ACE inhibitors can alleviate the excess fluid accumulation of congestive heart failure, and with calcium antagonists can alleviate angina chest pain. These new drug classes are generally safe and effective medications but are expensive. Other blood pressure medications that do not affect lipids include clonidine (Catapress), guanabenz (Wytensin), and hydralazine (Apresoline).

In summary high blood pressure is a common and powerful contributor to atherosclerosis in men and women of all ages and races. All but the lowest pressures are associated with increased risk for cardiovascular diseases. It is not natural or acceptable for blood pressure to rise with age. Only when primitive groups become acculturated do their blood pressures increase. On the other hand, if modern cultures adopt the dietary and lifestyle habits of those more traditional, average blood pressures would probably remain low into old age.

Nature has simplified things for us—lifestyle approaches for cholesterol control will also help contain blood pressure. Eating healthy amounts of sodium, fat, and calories; managing stress; and engaging in regular physical activity are effective in reducing blood pressure as well as cholesterol level. These health habits reduce or eliminate the need for medication and provide many other health benefits as well. If drugs are needed to control hypertension, they are frequently continued for life. They should be taken in a regular, consistent fashion, never stopped by a patient's own volition. A patient should discuss any troublesome side effects with the treating physician. It is essential that the patient maintain healthy lifestyle habits to maximize the effect and minimize the dosages of the medications.

References

1. National Heart, Lung, and Blood Institute. (1990). Facts at your fingertips. In: NHLBI Kit 1990.
2. Simons, L.I. (1986). Interrelations of lipids and lipoproteins with coronary artery disease in 19 countries. *American Journal of Cardiology*, 57, 5G-10G.
3. Multiple Risk Factor Intervention Trial Research Group. (1982). Multiple Risk Factor Intervention Trial. *Journal of the American Medical Association*, 248, 1465-1477.
4. Hopkins, P.N., & Williams, R.R. (1986). Identification and relative weights of cardiovascular risk factors. *Cardiology Clinics*, 4, 3-32.
5. Holme, I., Enger, S.C., Helgeland, A., Hjermann, I., Leren, P., Lund-Larsen, P.G., Solberg, L.A., & Strong, I.P. (1981). Risk factors and raised atherosclerotic lesions in coronary and cerebral arteries. *Arteriosclerosis*, 1, 250-256.
6. Kannel, W.B. (1989). Impact of risk factors. *Consultant*, 29, 104-114.
7. National Heart, Lung, and Blood Institute. (1986, September). *A guide to heart and lung health at the workplace* (NIH Publication No. 86-2210). Bethesda, MD.
8. Joint National Committee on Hypertension. (1988). The 1988 report of the Joint National Committee on detection, evaluation, and treatment of high blood pressure. *Archives of Internal Medicine*, 148, 1023-1038.
9. Rehman, A.S. (1980). Mild hypertension: No more benign neglect. *New England Journal of Medicine*, 302, 293.
10. Kannel, W.B., Sorlie, P., & Gordon, T. (1980). Labile hypertension: A faulty concept? The Framingham Study. *Circulation*, 61, 1183-1187.
11. Kaplan, N.M. (1990 4/7/90). Personal communication.
12. Castelli, W.P. (1987). Dyslipidemia and the effect of antihypertensive therapy on lipids. *Practical Cardiology*, 13 (Suppl. Mar.), 8-14.
13. Pooling Project Research Group. (1978). Relationship of blood pressure, serum cholesterol, smoking habit, relative weight and ECG ab-

normalities to incidence of major coronary events. *Journal of Chronic Disorders,* **31,** 201.

14. Alderman, M.H., Ooi, W.L., Madhavan, S., & Cohen, H. (1989). Treatment-induced blood pressure reduction and the risk of myocardial infarction. *Journal of the American Medical Association,* **262,** 920-924.

15. Hypertension Detection and Follow-Up Program Cooperative Group. (1982). The effect of treatment on mortality in "mild" hypertension. *New England Journal of Medicine,* **307,** 976-980.

16. Kannel, W.B. (1976). Blood pressure and the development of cardiovascular disease in the aged. In Caird, F.I., Dall, J.L., & Kennedy, R.D. (Eds.), *Cardiology in old age,* pp. 143-175. NY: Plenum Press.

17. Stamler, R., Stamler, J., Grimm, R., Dyer, A., Gosch, F.C., Benman, R., Elmen, P., Fishman, J., Van-Heel, N., & Civinelli, J. (1985). Nonpharmacologic control of hypertension. *Preventive Medicine,* **14,** 336-345.

18. Castelli, W.P., & Anderson, K. (1986). A population at risk: Prevalence of high cholesterol levels in hypertensive patients in the Framingham study. *American Journal of Medicine,* **80**(Suppl. 2A), 23-32.

19. Smith-Barbaro, P.A., & Pucak, G.J. (1983). Dietary fat and blood pressure. *Annals of Internal Medicine,* **98,** 828-831.

20. Rouse, I.L., Beilin, L.J., Armstrong, B.K., & Vandonger, R. (1983). Blood-pressure-lowering effect of a vegetarian diet: Controlled trial in normotensive subjects. *Lancet,* **1,** 5-10.

21. McCarron, D.A., Filer, L.J., & Van Itallie, T. (Eds.) (1982). Current perspectives in hypertension: A symposium on food, nutrition, and health. *Hypertension,* **2**(5), 4.

22. Wilcox, R.G., Bennett, T., Brown, A.M., & Macdonald, I.A. (1982). Is exercise good for high blood pressure? *British Medical Journal,* **285,** 767-769.

23. Tuck, M.L., Sowers, J., Dornfeld, L., Kledzik, G., & Maxwell, M. (1981). The effect of weight reduction on blood pressure, plasma renin activity, and plasma aldosterone levels in obese patients. *New England Journal of Medicine,* **304,** 930-933.

24. Frumkin, K., Nathan, R.J., Prout, M.F., & Cohen, M.C. (1978). Nonpharmacologic control of essential hypertension in man: A critical review of the experimental literature. *Psychosomatic Medicine,* **40,** 294-320.

25. McCarron, D.A., & Kotchen, T.A. (Eds.) (1983). Nutrition and blood pressure control. Current status of dietary factors and hypertension. *Annals of Internal Medicine,* **98,** 5.

26. Dustan, H.P. (1987, February). Controlling dietary causes of hypertension. *Primary Cardiology,* **13,** 35-42.

27. Grundy, S.M., Bilheimer, D., Blackburn, H., Brown, W.V.,

Kwitenovich, P.O., Jr., Mattson, F., Schonfeld, G., & Weidman, W.H. (1982). Rationale of the diet-heart statement of the American Heart Association. Report of the Nutritional Committee. *Circulation*, **65**, 839-854A.

28. Trowell, H. (1981). Hypertension, obesity, diabetes mellitus, and coronary heart disease. In H.C. Trowell & D.P. Burkitt (Eds.), *Western diseases: Their emergence and prevention* (pp. 3-32). London: Edward Arnold.

29. Cruz-Coke, R., Elcheverry, R., & Nagel, R. (1964). Influence of migration on blood-pressure of Easter Islanders. *Lancet*, **1**, 697-699.

30. Beaglehole, R., Salmond, C.E., Hooper, A., Huntsman, J., Stanhope, J.M., Cassel, J.C., & Prior, I.A. (1977). Blood pressure and social interaction in Tokelauan migrants in New Zealand. *Journal of Chronic Disorders*, **30**, 803.

31. Cassel, J.H. (1975). Studies of hypertension in migrants. In Paul, O. (Ed.), *Epidemiology and control of hypertension*, p. 43. New York: Stratton Intercontinental.

32. Dodson, P.M., Pacy, P.J., & Cox, E.V. (1985). Long-term follow-up of the treatment of essential hypertension with a high-fibre, low-fat and low-sodium dietary regimen. *Human Nutrition Clinical Nutrition*, **39C**, 213-220.

33. Freis, E.D. (1976). Salt, volume, and the prevention of hypertension. *Circulation*, **53**, 589.

34. Dustan, H.P. (1985). Obesity and hypertension. *Annals of Internal Medicine*, **103**, 1047-1049.

35. Takahashi, E., Sasaki, N., Takeda, J., & Ho, H. (1957). The geographic distribution of cerebral hemorrhage and hypertension in Japan. *Human Biology*, **29**, 139.

36. Page, L.B., Damon, A., & Moellering, R.C. (1974). Antecedents of cardiovascular disease in six Solomon Islands societies. *Circulation*, **49**, 1132.

37. Ambard, L., & Beaujard, E. (1904). Causes de l'hypertension arterielle [The etiology of arterial hypertension]. *Archives of General Medicine*, **1**, 520.

38. Australian National Health and Medical Research Council Dietary Salt Study Management committee. (1989). Fall in blood pressure with modest reduction in dietary salt intake in mild hypertension. *Lancet*, **I**, 399-402.

39. Kaplan, N.M. (1985). Non-drug treatment of hypertension. *Annals of Internal Medicine*, **102**, 359-373.

40. MacGregor, G.A., Markandu, N.D., Best, F.E., Elder, D.M., Cam, J.M., Sagnella, G.A., & Squires, M. (1982). Double-blind randomized crossover trial of moderate sodium restriction in essential hypertension. *Lancet*, **1**, 351-355.

41. Morgan, T., Adam, W., Gillies, A., Wilson, M., Morgan, G., &

Carney, S. (1978). Hypertension treated by salt restriction. *Lancet*, **1**, 227.

42. Weinberger, M. (1986). Antihypertensive therapy and lipids: Paradoxical influences on cardiovascular disease risk. *American Journal of Medicine*, **80**(Suppl. 2A), 64-70.

43. Meneely, G., & Battarbee, H.D. (1976). Sodium and potassium. In Hegsted, D.M., Chichester, C.O., Darby, W.S., McNutt, K.W., Stalvey, R.M., & Stotz, E.H. (Eds.), *Present knowledge in nutrition*, pp. 259-280. (4th ed.). Washington, DC: National Academy of Sciences.

44. National Research Council Subcommittee on the Recommended Dietary Allowances. (1989). Washington, D.C.: Academic Press.

45. Siani, A., Strazzullo, P., Russo, L., Guglielmi, S., Iacoviella, L., Ferrara, L.A., & Mancini, M. (1987). Controlled trial of long term oral potassium supplementation in patients with mild hypertension. *British Medical Journal*, **294**, 1453-1456.

46. Langford, H. (1983). Dietary potassium and hypertension: Epidemiologic data. *Annals of Internal Medicine*, **98**(Part 2), 770-772.

47. MacGregor, G.A., Smith, S.J., Markandu, N.D., Banks, R.A., & Sagnella, G.A. (1982). Moderate potassium supplementation in essential hypertension. *Lancet*, **2**, 567-570.

48. Mitchell, H.S., Rynbergen, H.J., Anderson, L., & Dibble, M.V. (Eds.) (1968). *Cooper's Nutrition in Health and Disease*. Philadelphia: Lippincott, pp. 592-594.

49. McCarron, D.A. (1983). Calcium and magnesium nutrition in human hypertension. *Annals of Internal Medicine*, **98**(Part 2), 800-805.

50. Neri, L.C., & Johansen, H.L. (1978). Water hardness and cardiovascular mortality. *Annals of the New York Academy of Sciences*, **304**, 203-219.

51. Schroeder, H.A. (1960). Relation between mortality from cardiovascular disease and treated water supplies: Variations in states and 163 largest municipalities. *Journal of the American Medical Association*, **172**, 1902-1908.

52. McCarron, D.A., & Morris, C.D. (1985). Blood pressure response to oral calcium in persons with mild to moderate hypertension. *Annals of Internal Medicine*, **103**, 825-831.

53. Ehnholm, C., Huttunen, J., & Pietenen, P. (1982). Effect of a low fat, high P/S diet on serum lipoproteins in a free-living population with high incidence of coronary heart disease. *New England Journal of Medicine*, **307**, 850-855.

54. Rao, R.H., Rao, U.B., & Srikantia, S.G. (1981). Effect of polyunsaturated rich vegetable oils on blood pressure in essential hypertension. *Clinical and Experimental Hypertension*, **3**, 27-38.

55. Sanders, T.A.B., Vickers, M., & Haines, A.P. (1981). Effect on blood lipids and haemostasis of a supplement of cod-liver oil, rich in

eicosapentanoic and docosahexaenoic acids, in healthy young men. *Clinical Science, 61,* 317-324.

56. Puska, P., Iacona, J.M., Nissinen, A., Korhonen, H.J., Vartianinen, E., Pietinen, P., Dougherty, R., Leino, U., Mutanen, M., Moisio, S., & Huttunen, J. (1983). Controlled, randomized trial of the effect of dietary fat on blood pressure. *Lancet, 1,* 1-5.

57. Armstrong, B., Van Merwyk, A.J., & Coates, J. (1977). Blood pressure in Seventh-Day Adventist vegetarians. *American Journal of Epidemiology, 105,* 444-449.

58. Jackson, R., Stewart, A., Beaglehole, R., Scragg, R. (1985). Alcohol consumption and blood pressure. *American Journal of Epidemiology, 122,* 1037-1044.

59. Friedman, G.D., Klatsky, A.L., & Siegelaub A.B. (1983). Alcohol intake and hypertension. *Annals of Internal Medicine, 98*(Part 2), 846-849.

60. MacMahon, S.W. (1987). Alcohol consumption and hypertension. *Hypertension, 9,* 111-121.

61. Klatsky, A.L., Friedman, G.D., & Armstrong, M.A. (1986). The relationships between alcoholic beverage use and other traits to blood pressure: A new Kaiser Permanente study. *Circulation, 73,* 628-636.

62. Heinsimer, J.A., & Irwin, J.M. (1986). Alcohol and the cardiovascular system. *Cardiovascular Review Reports, 7,* 848-860.

63. Stamler, R., Stamler, J., Riedlinger, W.F., Algena, G., & Roberts, R.H. (1978). Weight and blood pressure: Findings in hypertension screening of 1 million Americans. *Journal of the American Medical Association, 240,* 1607-1610.

64. Garrison, R.J., Kannel, W.B., Stokes, J., III, & Castelli, W.P. (1987). Incidence and prevalence of hypertension in young adults: The Framingham Offspring Study. *Preventive Medicine, 16,* 235-251.

65. Fagerberg, B., Andersson, O.K., Persson, B., & Hedner, T. (1985). Reactivity to norepinephrine and effect of sodium on blood pressure during weight loss. *Hypertension, 7,* 586-592.

66. Anderson, J.W. (1983). Plant fiber and blood pressure. *Annals of Internal Medicine, 98*(Part 2), 842-846.

67. Williams, P.T., Fortmann, S.P., Terry, R.B., Garay, S.C., Vranizan, K.M., Ellsworth, N., & Wood, P.D. (1987). Associations of dietary fat, regional adiposity, and blood pressure in men. *Journal of the American Medical Association, 257,* 3251-3256.

68. Weinsier, R.L., Norris, D.J., Birch, R., Bernstein, R.S., Wang, J., Yang, M.U., Pierson, R.N., Jr., & Van-Itallie, T.B. (1985). The relative contribution of body fat and fat pattern to blood pressure level. *Hypertension, 7,* 578-585.

69. Blair, D., Habicht, J.P., Sims, E.A., Sylwester, D., & Abraham, S. (1984). Evidence for increased risk for hypertension with centrally

located body fat and the effect of race and sex on this risk. *American Journal of Epidemiology*, **119**, 526-540.

70. Stallones, L., Mueller, W.H., & Christensen, B.L. (1982). Blood pressure, fatness and fat patterning among USA adolescents from two ethnic groups. *Hypertension*, **4**, 483-486.

71. Stamler, J., Farino, E., Mojonnier, L.M., Hall, Y., Moss, D., & Stamler, R. (1980). Prevention and control of hypertension by nutritional-hygienic means. *Journal of the American Medical Association*, **243**, 1819-1823.

72. Paffenbarger, R.S., Hyde, R.T., Wing, A.L., & Hsieh, C.C. (1986). Physical activity, all-cause mortality and longevity of college alumni. *New England Journal of Medicine*, **314**, 605-613.

73. Jennings, G., Nelson, L., Nestel, P., Esler, M., Korner, P., Burton, D., & Bazelmans, J. (1986). The effects of changes in physical activity on major cardiovascular risk factors, hemodynamics, sympathetic function, and glucose utilization in man. *Circulation*, **73**, 30-40.

74. Duncan, J.J., Farr, J.E., Upton, S.J., Hagan, R.D., Oglesby, M.E., & Blair, S.N. (1985). The effects of aerobic exercise on plasma catecholamines and blood pressure in patients with mild essential hypertension. *Journal of the American Medical Association*, **254**, 2609-2613.

75. Martin, J.E., Dubbert, P.M., & Cushman, W.C. (1985). Controlled trial of aerobic exercise in hypertension [abstract]. *Circulation*, **72**(Suppl. 3), 13.

76. Reisen, E., Abel, R., Modan, M., Silverberg, D.S., Eliahou, H.E., & Modan, B. (1978). Effect of weight loss without salt restriction on the reduction of blood pressure in overweight hypertensive patients. *New England Journal of Medicine*, **298**, 1-6.

77. MacMahon, S.W., MacDonald, G.J., Bernstein, L., Andrews, G., & Blacket, R.B. (1985). Comparison of weight reduction with metoprolol in treatment of hypertension in young overweight patients. *Lancet*, **1**, 1233-1236.

78. Page, L.B. (1981). Nutritional determinants of hypertension. In Winick, M. (Ed.), *Nutrition and the killer diseases* (pp. 113-126). New York: John Wiley.

79. Cade, R., Mars, D., Wagemaker, H., Zauner, C., Packer, D., Privette, M., Cade, M., Peterson, J., & Hood-Lewis, D. (1984). Effect of aerobic exercise training on patients with systemic arterial hypertension. *American Journal of Medicine*, **77**, 785-790.

80. Stamler, R., Stamler, J., Gosch, F.C., Civinelli, J., Fishman, F., McKeever, P., McDonald, A., & Dyer, A.R. (1989). Primary prevention of hypertension by nutritional-hygenic means. *Journal of the American Medical Association*, **262**, 1801-1807.

81. Medical Research Council Working Party. (1985). The Medical

Research Council Trial of treatment of mild hypertension: Principal results. *British Medical Journal, 291,* 87-104.

82. Helgeland, A., Hjermann, I., & Leren, P. (1978). High-density lipoprotein cholesterol and antihypertensive drugs: The Oslo study. *British Medical Journal, 2,* 403.

83. Australian National Blood Pressure Study Management Committee. (1980). Report by the Management Committee. The Australian Therapeutic Trial in mild hypertension. *Lancet, 1,* 1261-1267.

84. Veterans Administration Cooperative Study on Antihypertensive Agents. (1970). Effects of treatment on morbidity in hypertension. II. *Journal of the American Medical Association, 213,* 1143-1152.

85. Veterans Administration Cooperative Study on Antihypertensive Agents. (1967). Effects of treatment on morbidity in hypertension. I. *Journal of the American Medical Association, 202,* 1028-1034.

86. Leren, P., Helgeland, A., Holme, I. (1986). Coronary heart disease and treatment of hypertension. Some Oslo Study data. *American Journal of Medicine, 80*(Suppl. 2A), 3-6.

87. Ames, R.P., & Hill, P. (1982). Antihypertensive therapy and the risk of coronary heart disease. *Journal of Cardiovascular Pharmacology, 4*(Suppl. 2), S206-S212.

88. MacMahon, S.W., & MacDonald, G.J. (1986). Antihypertensive treatment and plasma lipoprotein levels. *American Journal of Medicine, 80*(Suppl. 2A), 40-47.

89. Grimm, R.H., Jr., Lean, A.S., Hunninghake, D.B., Lenz, K., Hannan, P., & Blackburn, H. (1981). Effects of thiazide diuretics on plasma lipids and lipoproteins in mildly hypertensive patients: A double-blind controlled trial. *Annals of Internal Medicine, 94,* 7-11.

90. Cutler, R. (1983). Effect of antihypertensive agents on lipid metabolism. *American Journal of Cardiology, 51,* 628-631.

91. Holland, O.B., Nixon, J.V., & Kuhnert, L. (1981). Diuretic-induced ventricular ectopic activity. *American Journal of Medicine, 70,* 762-768.

92. Lehtonen, A. (1985). Effect of beta-blockers on blood lipid profile. *American Heart Journal, 109,* 1192-1196.

93. Leren, P., Helgeland, A., Holme, I. (1986). Effect of propranolol and prazosin in blood lipids: The Oslo study. *Lancet, 2,* 4-6.

94. Deger, G. (1986). Effect of terazosin on serum lipids. *American Journal of Medicine, 80*(Suppl. 5B), 82-85.

Chapter

5

Stress

The traditional risk factors for heart disease—high cholesterol, blood pressure, smoking, and diabetes—leave a considerable number of CHD cases unaccounted for. What influences the remainder is subject to speculation, but many researchers are convinced that stress accounts for a sizable part of it. This may explain why Americans have twice as many heart attacks as Europeans with similar cholesterol levels, blood pressures, and smoking histories (1).

The mind-body relationship is exceedingly complex, however, and research in this vital area is still in its infancy. Stress is inherently a difficult factor to objectively quantify; something eminently distressful to one person may be a welcome challenge to another. Even the same individual may consider something mildly aggravating at one time but may later find it to be intolerable. As a result, stress research eludes the clean analytic scrutiny of double-blind, prospective, placebo-controlled cross-over studies. We will probably never know just how much CHD is due to stress. Nevertheless, we must not discount the importance of mental tension to health just because it requires an intuitive approach.

Defining Stress As a Process

Some researchers consider stress to be a situation or event (the stressor) or emphasize the body's physiological or psychological reaction to the stressor. Other groups study the result of stress—that is, the change in health or perceived level of distress. A workable definition for stress, though, requires a holistic approach to the entire stress process.

Events and situations that force us to adapt are called stressors. Each person has his or her own unique set of stressors in the home, workplace, and community. But the stressor itself cannot be considered "stress," because a dreadful situation for one person, such as an in-law visit, may be a celebration for another. Or, on a particularly trying day, a major upset may result from something that is usually not very troublesome, such as misplacing one's keys. Thus, it is not the stressor alone—the in-law visit or the search for the keys—that determines stress, but rather how an individual perceives and responds to it. People who do not become upset over difficult circumstances enjoy better health and freedom from disease, according to a concept known as "hardiness" (2).

A useful concept here is the distinction between good and bad stress. Hans Selye has termed these *eustress* and *distress*, respectively (3). Eustress comes from the Greek root "eu" meaning "good," as in euphoria. Examples of eustress include enjoyable exercise, humor, music, love, and sex. The mental and physical response to the sensation is pleasant and can have healing properties (4, 5). Eustress is the spice of life; it turns us on rather than wearing us out.

Or a stressor can lead to an entirely different experience, one of distress. Sometimes a situation that really poses no threat causes anxiety. We battle trivial problems, anguish over unfounded fears, or assume social tensions instead of relying on facts (thinking, for example, "He must be angry at me; he didn't even speak to me.").

Very seldom do we encounter truly urgent, menacing situations. Sometimes our perception and mind-set alone create stressors out of thin air. An example is a tense reaction to hearing a police siren and seeing flashing lights in the rearview mirror. We may immediately become alarmed and defensive, even though the squad car could be responding to an emergency across town.

Much of what we experience as stress stems from our attitudes toward or perceptions of the event. This is a product of many factors, including our expectations, temperament, upbringing, experience, mood at the time, habitual ways of thinking and behaving, and outlook on life in general. When confronted with a (potentially) stressful situation, we consciously or unconsciously make an immediate judgment about it. When this judgment is affected by a lack of knowledge, understanding, or patience, we find we have painted an unnecessarily gloomy picture.

Hundreds of times a day we encounter events or sensations to which we must react. These stressors pass through our perceptual filtering system, which either enjoys them, ignores them, or creates concern about them. If we choose to perceive them as unpleasant and react negatively, the result is distress. Over a period of days, weeks, or years, distress eventually results in disease. Figure 5.1 illustrates the stress process.

The stress process, then, involves a real or imagined event to which an individual reacts in a positive or negative manner. Or to paraphrase Selye, stress is the response of the body to any demands made upon it (6). To avoid confusion, when the word "stress" is used in this book, it refers to distress.

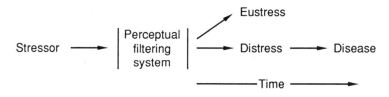

Figure 5.1 The experience of stress is a process. Whenever we encounter an external stimulus, or stressor, we make an instantaneous judgment and emotional response. This "perceptual filtering" is affected by our experiences, expectations, outlook on life, and mood at the time. The event may or may not be pleasant, depending on how it is perceived.

Psychosocial pressures contribute to at least half of the illnesses seen by family physicians, with the cardiovascular system being particularly susceptible. Blood pressure, cholesterol, triglycerides, and clotting tendencies can all be increased by mental tension (7-9). The stressors in our society that have been most closely linked to cardiovascular disease are disturbing emotions, job strain, lack of social support, and the Type A behavior pattern. These are discussed in the following sections.

Disturbing Emotions

Occasionally we hear a dramatic account of someone dropping dead during an emotionally charged incident such as hearing that a spouse has had a fatal accident. Although emotionally induced sudden deaths do occur, they are uncommon (10). Like the other cardiovascular risk factors, stress generally kills over decades, not in one fell swoop. Chronic, unrelenting, poorly identified, and unresolved stressors are the most deadly (11). The most commonly cited emotions linked to hypercholesterolemia and CHD are hostility, depression, and lack of control over one's life.

In a study by Blumenthal et al., hostility correlated with the degree of atherosclerosis seen during angiography, a special X-ray evaluation of arteries (12). The worst arterial blockage was seen in hostile men, and the least was noted in nonhostile women.

Hostility tends to raise both serum cholesterol levels and the risk of CHD (13-16). An individual thus afflicted has "free-floating" hostility brewing just under the emotional surface. Trivial occurrences can then trigger a sudden and inappropriate burst of anger. Repressed anger may also breed an attitude of self-righteousness or resentment. Hostility has been shown to be a risk factor for premature death in general, not only for CHD (17).

Depression is a common and devastating source of distress and ill health. It has been strongly implicated in raising serum cholesterol (18).

It may be manifested as a perception of defeat, loss of self-esteem, loss of identity, or dissatisfaction with personal life (19).

Lack of control over one's life is another source of emotional turmoil (20). Examples include forced retirement, prejudice, unemployment, poverty, and lack of education or authority. Deep-seated fears and insecurities often surface in situations of inadequate control. Some people, such as the Type As described in a later section, are particularly distressed by a lack of control.

Job Strain

As many as one in four workers suffers from a work-related stress disorder (21). The total cost of stress to business and industry has been estimated to range from $75 billion to $150 billion (22, 23). Job overload and dissatisfaction can and does increase blood pressure, serum triglycerides, and cholesterol. If the stress continues, blood pressure and lipids remain high (8, 24).

Having an occasional hectic day is not as dangerous as working steadily under conditions of unrelenting agitation. This is especially perilous when a failure to remain vigilant could lead to drastic consequences involving money or lives. A well-documented example of this process has been noted with air traffic controllers (25).

Contrary to popular thought, so-called "workaholics" may not be at a higher risk for heart attack. If a person truly enjoys and receives satisfaction from his or her work, putting in long hours is not necessarily unhealthy for that individual. Excessive work hours may disrupt the family unit, however. Executives do not corner the market on job stress, either. Many blue-collar workers experience high stress due to shift work, physical danger, or having little control over their jobs or careers (26).

Key stressors at work include the following:

1. Responsibility without authority
2. Too much to do in the time available, excessive deadlines, and insufficient control over job demands
3. Unresolved conflict, especially with the supervisor
4. Worry about quality
5. Ambiguity in role or task
6. Conflict in role or task; double binds
7. Lack of fulfillment or achievement through the job, leading to dissatisfaction
8. Poor interpersonal relationships with the supervisor and co-workers
9. Excessive changes in the company or work environment; frequent changes in position, policies, or responsibilities
10. Rivalry for status or success

11. Insufficient compensation
12. Losing, or fear of losing, employment

A worker who can control the pressure or pace at work is much less likely to develop disease than a worker who is controlled by a clock, machine, payment mechanism, or competition (20, 26, 27). Another perilous situation occurs when job stress affects family life, a valuable source of social support and defusing.

Lack of Social Support

The Japanese are known for their tradition of strong family support. The extended family frequently shares the same house, and decisions are made by consensus. Syme and Marmot studied the effect of westernization on 3,809 Japanese who had migrated to California (28). They found that those who retained strong ties to the Japanese language, diet, and culture had the same low rate of CHD as found in native Japanese.

In contrast, the Japanese-Americans who adopted the American life of high mobility and little family support had CHD rates three to five times higher. The authors concluded that it was primarily the loss of social support that explained the increase in heart attack rate in the more Americanized immigrants. Differences in diet, smoking, or blood pressure could not account for all of the detrimental change in their cardiovascular health.

Another indicator of the importance of social support comes from statistics on marital status. Heart attacks occur more frequently in single persons and those in marriages in which spouses frequently disagree. Widowers die from heart attacks 67% more often than expected (29, 30).

Type A Behavior Pattern

Type A behavior is a set of personality traits that is thought to predispose an individual to CHD. The pattern encompasses impatience, aggressiveness, hard-driving competitiveness, and a sense of urgency about time. These people strive to achieve more and more in less and less time. Their unbridled ambition compels them not only to compete, but to dominate. They are caught in a ceaseless struggle against time and circumstance, fighting against themselves and others (31-33).

Type A persons do not constantly display their coronary-prone behavior; rather, it is triggered by circumstances in their environment (8). Situations likely to evoke Type A behavior are those requiring vigilance, deadlines, competition, or lack of control.

Type A's reveal their impatience and suppressed hostility by their body language and speech mannerisms. These telltale psychomotor characteristics include hurried movements, doing two or more things simultaneously (polyphasic activities), speaking rapidly and loudly, using obscenities, interrupting others who speak slower, pounding with the fists, clenching the jaw, tapping fingers and legs, and a loud, jarring laugh. Type A's are fixated on numbers rather than concepts, quantity rather than quality. They frequently lack appreciation of emotions and the arts. Emotional consequences of Type A behavior include depression, personal struggles leading to the perception of defeat, free-floating hostility, insecurity, loss of identity, and loss of self-esteem (34).

Individuals without any of these traits are considered to possess the Type B behavior pattern. They do not harbor free-floating hostility and feel little need to display or discuss their achievements unless the situation demands they do so. Unlike Type A persons, they are able to do the following:

- Accept delays without impatience and let others do things at their own pace
- Enjoy other people and let other people help them
- Play for pleasure and relaxation and enjoy games and sports just for fun, not to compete or to exhibit superiority
- Relax without guilt
- Leave some tasks uncompleted while they relax and enjoy themselves

Type A men and women have been shown in some studies to have twice the number of heart attacks than their Type B counterparts, even after adjusting for the other risk factors (32, 35). Although more common in men, Type A behavior has the same deleterious effects in women (36). Among women employed outside of the home, Type A's have four times the amount of CHD as Type B women. Even Type A homemakers have higher heart attack rates (31).

The Type A hypothesis has several problems, however, that limit its usefulness. The determination of Type A status, either by interview or by questionnaire, is fairly subjective and imprecise. Several large studies failed to show any correlation between the pattern and future incidence of CHD (37). And a study by Ragland and Brand indicated that Type A's may have a better rate of long-term survival after a heart attack than do Type B's (38).

Much of the risk associated with Type A behavior could be due to its contribution to other risk factors, such as elevations in blood pressure and cholesterol (13, 39). Type A's have less social support and are more prone to disturbing emotions such as hostility and depression. Type A's report (perceive) greater job stress than Type B's who work at the same exact job (36). Type A's also manage stress differently. They tend to work alone under periods of stress, possibly contributing to their sense of work overload (40).

Most importantly, perhaps, the Type A concept suffers from a lack of specificity. Fully half to three quarters of urban men possess Type A behavior, but not all of them are having heart attacks. Type A or B classification is thus too general and not very helpful in determining people at greatest risk. A Type A person who remains in control of his or her environment, is not in a position to compete, and is not depressed or hostile may not be at any increased risk whatsoever (41).

Thus, a more specific test for stress is needed, one that measures an individual's physical reaction to stressors. Questionnaires for stress can only roughly classify people as more or less susceptible to CHD. Future research must focus on objective physiological measures of the stress response. Blood pressure response appears to be a promising avenue because it changes rapidly in response to stress, is a well-known risk factor, and can be accurately measured by externally placed monitors (26). The blood pressure–stress relationship will be preceded here by a review of the body's overall response to stress.

The Stress Response

Human physiology describes a "fight-or-flight" response that served a vital purpose in centuries past (42). When confronted by a savage animal, a cave dweller needed all the mental and physical alertness that could be mustered. By an outflow of nerve impulses from the brain, heart rate, blood pressure, breathing, and muscle tone were quickly activated.

Though physical dangers such as this are rare today, stress still activates our sympathetic nervous system. We respond to a traffic jam in the same manner as the cave dweller who faced near-certain death. Cholesterol levels and blood pressure may soar to dangerous heights in response to trivial problems, brief delays, and minor frustrations. By not filtering out or properly managing the stressors of daily life, our bodies become perpetually vigilant.

The fight-or-flight response is not usually under our conscious control but rather is mediated through the autonomic nervous system. Via the sympathetic division of autonomic nerves, catecholamine hormones such as epinephrine (formerly called adrenaline), norepinephrine, and cortisol are released into the bloodstream to charge up the entire body.[1] The cardiovascular system is particularly vulnerable to activation of the sympathetic nervous system and the subsequent release of catecholamines. Type A's have higher levels of catecholamines and cortisol in their bloodstreams (13, 19).

---

[1]These substances are discharged into the circulation by the tips of sympathetic nerves and, to a lesser extent, by the adrenal glands resting atop the kidneys.

The major stress chemical of the autonomic nervous system seems to be norepinephrine. It affects cholesterol metabolism by mobilizing triglycerides out of fat cells as VLDL, very low–density lipoproteins. Some of these become transformed in the circulation into atherogenic LDL particles. Norepinephrine and related hormones also raise blood pressure and heart rate, promote clotting, and predispose the heart to beat in an irregular rhythm.

Stress and Cholesterol

Animal experiments have shown that stress can raise blood cholesterol and induce narrowing of the arteries with plaque. For obvious ethical reasons we cannot plan a similar experiment in humans. However, in natural experiments in which people subject themselves to stress, the changes in cholesterol are illustrative.

It was noted that the serum levels of accountants peaked just prior to the April 15 income tax deadline. Corporate accountants experienced another peak in January, when they were completing annual financial reports (43). The cholesterol differences between periods of high and low

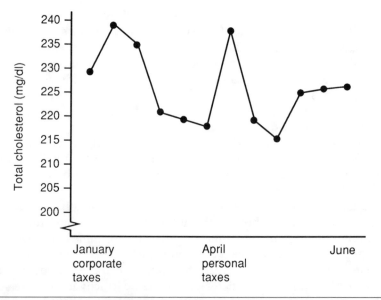

Figure 5.2 Blood cholesterol levels of accountants were noted to have two distinct seasonal peaks, both of which coincided with heavy work demands: corporate and personal tax deadlines.

Note. From "Changes in the Serum Cholesterol and Blood Clotting Time in Men Subjected to Cyclic Variation of Occupational Stress" by R.H. Rosenman and V. Carroll, 1958, *Circulation,* **17,** p. 852. Copyright 1958 by the American Heart Association. Adapted by permission of the American Heart Association, Inc.

stress averaged 42 mg/dl (1.1 mmol/L). The lowest values were noted during the periods of the least amount of job pressure (see Figure 5.2). In general, persons reporting mental tension have higher blood cholesterol levels (7). This is particularly true for Type A's (39) and ''hot reactors'' described in the next section (44).

In more than 60 studies, people responded to stress with blood cholesterol elevations of 8% to 65% above their baseline levels (9, 45, 46). The stressors varied from examinations, films, life changes, surgery, race-car driving, flying, and military training to immersing a hand in cold water. Cholesterol levels in subjects who were asked very personal, emotional questions increased 70 mg/dl (1.8 mmol/L) within an hour after the interview (47). The changes that result from stress occur in the dangerous LDL cholesterol, not the HDL.

Some persons have much more labile, or fluctuating, cholesterol levels than others. Grundy and Griffin found that 10% of student subjects averaged 90 mg/dl (2.3 mmol/L) increases in their cholesterol levels during exams (48). In another study, just anticipating the discomfort of immersing a hand in cold water caused cholesterol levels to rise (49). In some subjects the cholesterol went up well over 100 mg/dl (2.6 mmol/L) in just a few hours.

Stress and Hypertension

Although stress is by no means the sole cause of hypertension, evidence is steadily accumulating in support of a cause-and-effect relationship between psychological stress and high blood pressure. Mind-body inter-actions are known that could explain a role for stress in hypertension (26, 50-52). Although intuitively this link seems obvious, it has been very diffi-cult to design a study that either proves or explains the association for the general population. In some individuals, such as the air traffic controllers studied by Rose and co-workers, stress clearly elevated pressures (25).

A major contributor to hypertension is the narrowing of the diameter of small arteries by the smooth muscle cells in a process called vaso-constriction. Pressure increases because the blood is forced through smaller caliber arteries. This is analogous to the pressure that builds up in a garden hose when the nozzle opening is narrowed. Though excessive cardiac output (increased pumping of blood) is more characteristic of younger hypertensives, vasoconstriction is the hallmark of hypertension in persons over age 40.

Though it is difficult to determine the precise cause of vasoconstriction, stress is frequently implicated—especially hostility, loss of control, or chronic vigilance (25). A likely mechanism is the release of norepinephrine and cortisol as described previously (53). Arteries afflicted with athero-sclerosis have exaggerated vasoconstriction in response to these chemicals, an effect that frequently contributes to heart attack (54).

Over the past decade, investigators have developed methods to study cardiovascular responses to various stressors. Pressure changes in the stress lab correlate very well with an individual's average daily blood pressure (55). Sophisticated electronic monitors evaluate the subject's cardiovascular response to competitive video games, mental arithmetic, and immersion of a hand in cold water.

According to Robert Eliot of Denver's Institute of Stress Medicine, vasoconstriction from stress hormones plays a pivotal role in the blood pressure of people he calls "hot reactors." They exhibit no symptoms or observable behaviors as clues to their blood pressure reaction yet have as many as 30 to 40 blood pressure surges a day (50). As many as 20% of apparently healthy Americans are hot reactors and are thought to be at increased risk for heart attack or stroke. Blood pressure changes in the classic hot reactor are mediated via vasoconstriction, though other hot reactors develop increased pulse rate, cardiac output, or both as manifestations of their hyperreactivity.

Figure 5.3 demonstrates the striking degree of vasoconstriction in a hot reactor as compared with a cool reactor (56). The two male subjects were outwardly very similar—both were hard-driving, Type A bank presidents.

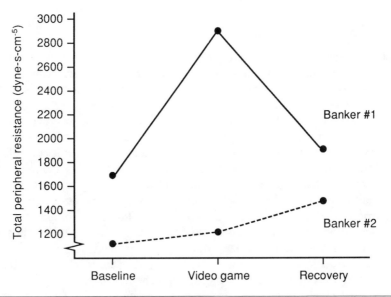

Figure 5.3 Blood pressure surges can be dramatic in hot reactors, as demonstrated by the response of Banker #1 to a competitive video game. In contrast, Banker #2 had minimal blood pressure change in response to the same challenge.

Note. From "Predicting Workplace Blood Pressure" by R. Eliot, 1987, *Practical Cardiology* (special supplement), p. 5. Copyright 1987 by *Practical Cardiology*. Adapted by permission.

Their inner physiological responses were entirely different, however. Banker 2's blood pressure remained stable during the competitive video game. Banker 1's blood pressure sykrocketed to 240/140, and the test was canceled for fear he would have a stroke. (Somewhat annoyed, he protested, "I was just getting into it!") (57).

Stress-induced hypertension can be missed during a physical examination unless the patient is quite anxious at the time of the office visit. Unless the blood pressure elevation is always present, the individual may be diagnosed as a labile hypertensive and left untreated. But the stress-induced blood pressure fluctuations may well herald future fixed hypertension (58). The hot reactor is predisposed to CHD even if pressures remain normal under relaxed conditions (56).

Evidence is accumulating that the dangers of hypertension can be averted if hot reactors change their physiological responses to stress through counseling and behavior modification (59). Drug therapy may be necessary, especially until behavior changes have become established. Calcium channel blockers, a newer class of antihypertensive drugs, work particularly well for vasoconstrictive hot reactors (60).

Blood Clotting and Sudden Cardiac Death

Another effect of catecholamines is more rapid blood clotting. Friedman and others also found that the accountants had accelerated clotting times during their periods of high stress (43). This is illustrated in Figure 5.4. Increased clotting tendency is hazardous for the bulk of middle-aged and older Americans, whose inner arterial surfaces are roughened by atherosclerotic plaque.

Numerous reports suggest an association between psychological stress, norepinephrine, and sudden cardiac death (61). The mechanism seems to be via microscopic tears in the heart muscle fibers called contractile bands. The hormonally flogged heart literally tears itself apart, bit by bit, at sites of contractile bands (50). The resultant scar tissue cannot properly conduct electrical impulses from the heart's pacemaker, setting the stage for an abnormal heart rhythm and sudden cardiac death.

Steps in Personal Stress Management

In describing the counterpart of the stress response, Benson coined the term "relaxation response" for what he and others discovered about the physiology of relaxation (62). Not surprisingly, it entails the opposite of the stress response: Alerting messages from the brain and norepinephrine secretion diminish, quickly followed by a drop in heart rate, blood pressure, and muscle tone. Research done since the 1960s has demonstrated

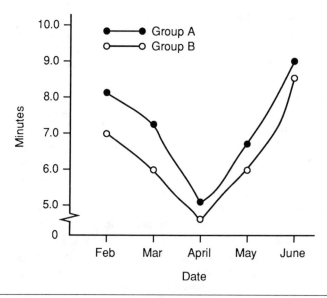

Figure 5.4 Blood clotting time decreased dramatically in accountants during months of high work load and stress. This tendency could precipitate a heart attack in persons with arteries damaged by atherosclerosis. Testing was performed at approximately the mid-point of each month.
Note. From "Behavior Pattern and CHD" by M. Friedman and R. Rosenman,1958, *Circulation,* **17**, p. 852. Copyright 1958 by the American Heart Association. Adapted by permission of the American Heart Association, Inc.

that relaxation exercises also can have a modest cholesterol-lowering effect.

We all encounter stress, but due to our different perceptions of and responses to the situation, only some of us suffer from it. A stressor becomes problematic when it is perceived in a negative sense and is out of our control. Much of stress management involves simply changing one's perspective—that is, modifying one's reaction to the stressor. Otherwise, effective problem solving is thwarted by reflexive anxiety, dread, and catastrophic expectations.

No single method of stress management is best for everyone. Each individual has a unique set of stressors as well as a unique filtering mechanism for determining whether the stressor results in eustress or distress. Each of us has a personal collection of strengths, weaknesses, experiences, coping mechanisms, and support bases. The best approach to stress management is thus an eclectic one: Identify those situations that elicit the alarm reaction ("fight-or-flight"), and modify the mental and physical response to them.

The first step, then, is to know one's own stressors: psychological, interpersonal, sociocultural, physical, financial, and others. Next, avoid coping techniques that are ineffective, such as acting out, regressing, abusing drugs, denial, overworking, or blaming others. The third step is to use techniques that do work. These include a healthy diet, adequate exercise, and one or more relaxation techniques. Ultimately, stress management parallels self-care—maintaining healthy lifestyle habits and living in a clean and psychologically enriching environment.

A healthy diet is crucial to the control of obesity, diabetes, and high levels of cholesterol and blood pressure—conditions that only add another source of stress to life. It may also act as a buffer to stress. Unsaturated fats, especially the omega-3 oils in fish, inhibit blood clotting and resist the vasoconstrictive response to norepinephrine (63). Someone who is angry should never eat a meal high in saturated fat because these fats and stress both increase blood pressure and clotting.

Most of us have noticed that "letting off steam" through exercise has a relaxing effect. Fit persons do not seem to perceive as much distress as unfit persons do from the same stressors (64, 65). Regular exercise also helps improve self-esteem and decrease depression and anxiety (66, 67). Decreased norepinephrine together with lower cholesterol, blood pressure, and blood glucose has also been noted as a result of an exercise program (68).

Recent evidence extols aerobic exercise in particular. Researchers in Montreal studied a group of 45 men in a YMCA fitness program. Compared with unfit men, the aerobically trained men recovered faster from experimentally induced stress. Furthermore, when the unfit men became physically conditioned, they too were able to recover more quickly from the stressor (69). Aerobically fit individuals have also been found to be more resilient to major life changes (70).

Relaxation Techniques

Meditation and other relaxation techniques are not only effective in relaxation and stress management, but also have a limited role in control of hypertension and cholesterol (71, 72). Ornish and co-workers have been using meditation and a low-fat diet to help patients already stricken with severe coronary heart disease (73, 74). The results have been striking, not only in relieving angina chest pain (a 90% decrease), but also in slowing the progression of the disease. Using sophisticated diagnostic equipment, Ornish has documented plaque regression in one quarter of his patients' coronary arteries within one year (73).

Cooper and Aygen used meditation to decrease the cholesterol in their subjects by 30 mg/dl (75). The initial training involved only four consecutive lessons of transcendental meditation. The subjects meditated twice daily for approximately 20 minutes. In England, Patel used yoga and biofeedback to help control cholesterol levels and blood pressure (51, 76).

The improvement in blood pressure was particularly impressive, averaging 25/10 mmHg.

Other valuable relaxation techniques include breathing exercises, visualization, biofeedback (77), progressive relaxation (78), and autogenic training (46). The Health and Public Policy Committee of the American College of Physicians in its 1985 review of the literature credited biofeedback with lowering blood pressures by an average of 7.8/5.6 (systolic/diastolic) (79). Relaxation studies indicated an average 11/7.1 blood pressure decrease. Using data from the Hypertension Detection and Follow-Up Program this degree of blood pressure control translates into a 20% reduction in CHD risk (80).

Major concepts in behavioral approaches include the following (81):

- Using positive "self-talk" and positive reinforcement
- Looking for win/win solutions in resolving conflicts rather than proving someone wrong
- Listening in a nonjudgmental way
- Being flexible and trusting
- Expressing feelings and emotions; asking for support from family and friends
- Developing healthy diversions such as music or hobbies
- Seeking counseling if needed, either for psychological problems or for communication skills, assertiveness training, or time management

Because a thorough discussion of stress management techniques is beyond the scope of this book, readers wishing to explore this subject further are directed to the Suggested Readings list at the end of this chapter.

In summary, stress is the body's response, positive or negative, to any demand made on it. Each person has his or her own unique set of stressors as well as a personal collection of strengths and weaknesses in dealing with them.

Perhaps the most important factor in determining the impact of stress is our perceptual filtering mechanism. This is heavily influenced by our attitudes, perspectives, experiences, and moods. Our stress filter determines whether the stressor results in eustress or distress. Eustress, or positive stress, is exciting and challenging and motivates us to change. Distress wears us out and promotes disease.

If left unchecked, disturbing emotions, overload, and lack of control maintain us inappropriately in a high state of arousal. Chronic and excessive amounts of hormones raise blood pressure, glucose, and cholesterol; increase clotting tendencies; and may even induce dangerous heart arrhythmias.

Because stress cannot be completely avoided, it needs to be managed at an optimal level. This is best accomplished by first knowing the sources of stress and what effect they have on our bodies. Stressors are best managed by a well-rounded repertoire of stress management techniques. These include relaxation exercises, time management and interpersonal skills, and changing habitual thoughts and behaviors.

References

1. Keys, A. (1970). Coronary heart disease in seven countries: XIII. Multiple variables. *Circulation,* **41**(Suppl.), 138-144.
2. Kobasa, S.C. (1979). Stressful life events, personality, and health: An inquiry into hardiness. *Journal of Personality and Social Psychology,* **37**, 2-3.
3. Selye, H. (1983). The stress concept: Past, present, and future. In C.L. Cooper (Ed.), *Stress research: Issues for the eighties* (pp. 1-20). Chinchester, Eng: Wiley.
4. Siegel, B.J. (1986). *Love, Medicine, & Miracles.* New York: Harper & Row.
5. Cousins, N. (1983). *The Healing Heart: Antidotes to Panic and Helplessness.* New York: W.W. Norton.
6. Selye, H. (1974). *Stress without distress.* Scarborough, NY: New American Library.
7. Trevisan, M., Tsong, Y., Stamler, J., Tokich, T., Mojonnier, L., Hall, Y., Cooper, R., & Moss, D. (1983). Nervous tension and serum cholesterol: Findings from the Chicago Coronary Prevention Evaluation Program. *Journal of Human Stress,* **9**, 12-16.
8. Jenkins, C.D. (1982). Psychosocial risk factors for coronary heart disease. *Acta Medica Scandinavica,* **660**(Suppl.), 123-136.
9. vanDoornen, L.J.P., & Orlebeke, K.F. (1982). Stress, personality and serum-cholesterol level. *Journal of Human Stress,* **8**, 24-29.
10. Brackett, C.D., & Powell, L.H. (1988). Psychosocial and physiological predictors of sudden cardiac death after healing of acute myocardial infarction. *American Journal of Cardiology,* **61**, 979-983.
11. Pelletier, K.R. (1977). *Mind as healer, mind as slayer: A holistic approach to preventing stress disorders.* New York: Delacorte and Delta.
12. Blumenthal, J.A., Williams, R., Kong, Y., Schanberg, S.M., & Thompson, L.W. (1978). Type A behavior and angiographically documented coronary disease. *Circulation,* **58**, 634-639.
13. Weidner, G., Sexton, G., McLellarm, R., Connor, S.L., & Matarazzo, J.D. (1987). The role of Type A behavior and hostility in an elevation of plasma lipids in adult women and men. *Psychosomatic Medicine,* **49**, 136-145.
14. Williams, R.B. (1987). Refining the Type-A hypothesis: Emergence of the hostility complex. *American Journal of Cardiology,* **60**, 27J.

15. Barefoot, J.C., Dahlstrom, W.G., & Williams, R.B. (1983). Hostility, CHD incidence, and total mortality: A 25-year follow-up study of 255 physicians. *Psychosomatic Medicine*, 45, 59-63.
16. Matthews, K.A., Glass, D.C., Rosenman, R.H., & Bortner, R.W. (1977). Competitive drive, pattern A, and coronary heart disease: A further analysis of some data from the Western Collaborative Group Study. *Journal of Chronic Disorders*, 30, 489-498.
17. Shekelle, R.B., Gale, M., Ostfeld, A.M., & Paul, O. (1983). Hostility, risk of coronary heart disease, and mortality. *Psychosomatic Medicine*, 45, 109-114.
18. Rahe, R.H., Rubin, R.T., Gunderson, E.K.E., & Arthur, R.J. (1971). Psychological correlates of serum cholesterol in men. *Psychosomatic Medicine*, 33, 399-410.
19. Eliot, R.S. (1988a). *Stress and the heart*. Mount Kisco, NY: Futura.
20. Karasek, R.A., Jr., Baker, D., Marxer, F., & Ahlbom, A. (1981). Job decision latitude, job demands, and cardiovascular disease: A prospective study of Swedish men. *American Journal of Public Health*, 71, 694-705.
21. Gallup Poll. (1989). Stress, anxiety and depression in the workplace. New York Business Group.
22. Fielding, J.E. (1989). Work site stress management: National survey results. *Journal of Occupational Medicine*, 31, 990-995.
23. Rosch, P. (1984). The health effects of job stress. *Business and Health*, 1, 5-8.
24. Sales, S.M. (1969). Organizational role as a risk factor in coronary disease. *Administrative Science Quarterly*, 14, 325-336.
25. Rose, R.M., Jenkins, C.D., & Hurst, M.W. (1978, June). *Air traffic controller health change study: A prospective investigation of physical, psychological, and work-related changes* (FAA-AM-78-39). Springfield, VA: National Technical Information Service.
26. Schnall, P.L., Pieper, C., Schwartz, J.E., Karasek, R.A., Schlussel, Y., Devereux, R.B., Ganau, A., Alderman, M., Warren, K., & Pickering, T. (1990). The relationship between 'job strain,' workplace diastolic blood pressure, and left ventricular mass index. *Journal of the American Medical Association*, 263, 1929-1935.
27. Kasl, S.V. (1984). Stress and health. *Annual Review of Public Health*, 5, 319-341.
28. Syme, L., & Marmot, M. (1976). Acculturation and coronary heart disease in Japanese Americans. *American Journal of Epidemiology*, 104, 225-247.
29. Weidner, G., Hollis, J.F., Carmody, R.P., Connor, W.E., & Matarazzo, J.D. (1984). The relationship of life events and Type A behavior to standard coronary risk factors in women and men. *Psychosomatic Medicine*, 46, 79-80.
30. Berkman, L.F., & Syme, S.L. (1979). Social networks, host resistance,

and mortality: A nine-year follow-up study of Alameda County residents. *American Journal of Epidemiology*, **109**, 186-204.

31. Haynes, S.G., Feinleib, M., & Kannel, W. (1980). The relationship of psychosocial factors to coronary heart disease in the Framingham study. III. Eight-year incidence of coronary heart disease. *American Journal of Epidemiology*, **111**, 37-58.

32. Rosenman, R.H., Brand, R.J., Scholtz, R.I., & Friedman, M. (1976). Multivariate prediction of coronary heart disease during 8.5 years follow-up in the Western Collaborative Group Study. *American Journal of Cardiology*, **37**, 903-910.

33. Friedman, M., & Rosenman, R.H. (1971). Type A behavior pattern: Its association with coronary heart disease. *Annals of Clinical Research*, **3**, 300-312.

34. Jenkins, C.D. (1976). Psychologic and social risk factors for coronary disease. *New England Journal of Medicine*, **294**, 987, 1033.

35. Brand, R.J. (1978). Coronary-prone behavior as an independent risk factor for coronary heart disease. In T.M. Dembroski, S.M. Weiss, J.L. Sheilds, (Eds.), *Coronary-prone behavior*. New York: Springer-Verlag.

36. Waldron, J. (1978). The coronary-prone behavior pattern, blood pressure, employment and socioeconomic status in women. *Journal of Psychosomatic Research*, **22**, 79-87.

37. Shekelle, R.B., Hully, S.B., Neaton, J.D., Billings, J.H., Borhani, N.O., Grace, T.A., Jacobs, D.R., Lasser, N.L., Mittlemark, M.B., & Stamler, J. (1985). The MRFIT behavior pattern study: II. Type A behavior and incidence of coronary heart disease. *American Journal of Epidemiology*, **122**, 559-570.

38. Ragland, D.R., & Brand, R.J. (1988). Type A behavior and mortality from coronary heart disease. *New England Journal of Medicine*, **318**, 65-69.

39. Friedman, M. (1977). Type A behavior pattern: Some of its pathophysiological components. *Bulletin of the New York Academy of Medicine*, **53**, 593-604.

40. Siegel, J.M. (1984). Type A behavior. *Annual Review of Public Health*, **5**, 357-358.

41. Review Panel on Coronary Prone Behavior and Coronary Heart Disease. (1981). Coronary-prone behavior and coronary heart disease: A critical review. *Circulation*, **63**, 1199-1215.

42. Cannon, W.B. (1941). The emergency function of the adrenal medulla in pain and the major emotions. *American Journal of Physiology*, **33**, 356-372.

43. Friedman, M., Rosenman, R.H., & Carroll, V. (1958). Changes in the serum cholesterol and blood clotting time in men subjected to cyclic variation of occupational stress. *Circulation*, **17**, 852.

44. Dembroski, T.M., MacDougall, J.M., Slaats, S., Eliot, R.S., & Buell,

J.C. (1981). Challenge-induced cardiovascular response as a predictor of minor illnesses. *Journal of Human Stress, 7*, 2-5.

45. O'Donnell, L., O'Meara, N., Owens, D., Johnson, A., Collins, P., & Tomkin, G. (1987). Plasma catecholamines and lipoproteins in chronic psychological stress. *Journal Royal Society of Medicine, 80*, 339-342.

46. Luthe, W. (1972). Autogenic therapy: Excerpts on applications to cardiovascular disorders and hypercholesterolemia. *Biofeedback and self-control, 1971.* Chicago: Aldine-Atherton.

47. Dimsdale, J.E., & Herd, J.A. (1982). Variability of plasma lipids in response to emotional arousal. *Psychosomatic Medicine, 44*, 413-430.

48. Grundy, S., & Griffin, A. (1959). Effects of periodic mental stress on serum cholesterol levels. *Circulation, 19*, 496-498.

49. Peterson, J., Keith, R., & Wilcox, A. (1962). Hourly changes in serum cholesterol concentration. *Circulation, 25*, 798-803.

50. Eliot, R.S. (1988b). The dynamics of hypertension—an overview. *American Heart Journal, 116*, 583.

51. Patel, C., Marmot, M.G., Terry, D.J., Carruthers, M., Hunt, B., & Patel, M. (1985). Trials of relaxation in reducing coronary risk: Four-year follow-up. *British Medical Journal of Clinical Research, 290*, 1103-1106.

52. Engel, B.T., Glasgow, M.S., & Gaarder, K.R. (1983). Behavioral treatment of high blood pressure. III. *Psychosomatic Medicine, 45*, 23-29.

53. Glass, D.S., & Contrada, R.J. (1982). Type A behavior and catecholamines: A critical review. In C.R. Lake & M. Ziegler (Eds.), *Norepinephrine: Clinical aspects.* Baltimore: Williams & Wilkins.

54. Forstermann, U., Mugge, A., Alheid, U., Haverich, A., Frolich, J. (1988). Selective attenuation of endothelium-mediated vasodilation in atherosclerotic human coronary arteries. *Circulation Research, 62*, 185-190.

55. Morales-Ballejo, H.M., Eliot, R.S., Boone, J.L., & Hughes, J.S. (1988). Psychophysiologic stress testing as a predictor of mean daily blood pressure. *American Heart Journal, 116*, 673-681.

56. Eliot, R.S. (1987). Predicting workplace blood pressure. *Practical Cardiology, 13* (Special Suppl., March), 3-7.

57. Personal communication, R. Eliot, 5/89.

58. Light, K.C., & Obrist, P.A. (1980). Cardiovascular reactivity to behavioral stress in young males with and without marginally elevated casual systolic pressures. *Hypertension, 2*, 802-808.

59. Lee, D.D., DeQuattro, V., Allen, J., Kimura, S., Aleman, E., Konugres, G., Davison, G. (1988). Behavioral vs beta blocker therapy in patients with primary hypertension: Effects of blood pressure, left ventricular function and mass, and the pressor surge of social anger. *American Heart Journal, 116*, 637-644.

60. Ruddel, H., Langewitz, W., Schachinger, H., Schmieder, R., &

Schulte, W. (1988). Hemodynamic response patterns to mental stress: Diagnostic and therapeutic implications. *American Heart Journal,* **116,** 617-627.

61. Brodsky, M.A., Sato, D.A., Iseri, L.T., Wolff, L.J., & Allen, B.J. (1987). Ventricular tachyrhythmia associated with psychological stress. *Journal of the American Medical Association,* **257,** 2064-2067.

62. Benson, H., Beary, J.F., & Carol, M.P. (1974). The relaxation response. *Psychiatry,* **37,** 37-46.

63. Lockette, W.E., Webb, R.C., Culp, B.R., & Pitt, B. (1982). Vascular reactivity and high dietary eicosapentaenoic acid. *Prostaglandins,* **24,** 631-639.

64. DeBenedette, V. (1988). Getting fit for life: Can exercise reduce stress? *Physician and Sportsmedicine,* **16,** 185-200.

65. Crews, D.J., & Landers, D.M. (1987). A meta-analytic review of aerobic fitness and reactivity to psychosocial stressors. *Medicine and Science in Sports and Exercise,* **19**(Suppl. 2), S114-S120.

66. Morgan, W.P., & Goldston, S.E. (Eds.) (1987). *Exercise and Mental Health,* Washington, DC: Hemisphere Publications.

67. Greist, J.H., Klein, M.H., Eischens, R.R., Faris, J., Gurman, A.S., & Morgan, W.P. (1979). Running as a treatment for depression. *Comprehensive Psychiatry,* **20,** 41-54.

68. Jennings, G., Nelson, L., Nestel, P., Esler, M., Korner, P., Burton, D., & Brazelmans, J. (1986). The effects of changes in physical activity on major cardiovascular risk factors, hemodynamics, sympathetic function, and glucose utilization in man: A controlled study of four levels of activity. *Circulation,* **73,** 30-40.

69. Keller, S., & Seraganian, P. (1984). Physical fitness level and autonomic reactivity to psychosocial stress. *Journal of Psychosomatic Research,* **28,** 279-287.

70. Roth, D.L., & Holmes, D.S. (1985). Influence of physical fitness in determining the impact of stressful life events on physical and psychological health. *Psychosomatic Medicine,* **47,** 164-173.

71. Jacob, R.G., Kraemer, H.C., & Agras, W.S. (1977). Relaxation therapy in the treatment of hypertension: A review. *Archives of General Psychiatry,* **34,** 1417-1427.

72. Benson, H., & Wallace, R.K. (1972). Decreased blood pressure in hypertensive subjects who practiced meditation. *Circulation,* **46,** 131.

73. Ornish, D., Scherwitz, L.W., Brown, S.E., Billings, J.H., Armstrong, W.T., Ports, T.A., McLanahan, S.M., Kirkeeide, R.L., Brand, R.J., & Gould, K.L. (1988). Can lifestyle changes reverse atherosclerosis? *Circulation,* **78**(Suppl. II), 11.

74. Ornish, D., Scherwitz, L.W., Doody, R.S., Kesten, D., McLanahan, S.M., Brown, S.E., DePuey, G., Sonnemaker, R., Haynes, C., Lester, J., McAllister, G.K., Hall, R.J., Burdine, J.A., & Gotto, A.M. (1983). Effects of stress management training and dietary changes in treating

ischemic heart disease. *Journal of the American Medical Association,* **249,** 54-59.

75. Cooper, M.J., & Aygen, M.M. (1979). A relaxation technique in the management of hypercholesterolemia. *Journal of Human Stress,* **5,** 24-27.

76. Patel, C., & Marmot, M. (1988). Can general practitioners use training in relaxation and management of stress to reduce mild hypertension? *British Medical Journal,* **296,** 21-24.

77. Brown, B.B. (1977). *Stress and the art of biofeedback.* New York: Bantam.

78. Jacobson, E. (1974). *Progressive relaxation.* Chicago: University of Chicago Press, Midway Reprint.

79. Health and Public Policy Committee, American College of Physicians. (1985). Biofeedback for hypertension. *Annals of Internal Medicine,* **102,** 709-715.

80. Hypertension Detection and Follow-Up Program Cooperative Group. (1979). Five-year finding of the Hypertension Detection and Follow-Up Program. 1. Reduction in mortality of persons with high blood pressure, including mild hypertension. *Journal of the American Medical Association,* **242,** 2562-2571.

81. Ellis, A., & Dryden, W. (1987). *The practice of rational emotive therapy.* New York: Springer Publ.

Suggested Readings

Alberti, R.E., & Emmons, M.L. (1975). *Stand up speak out talk back!* New York: Pocket.

Ardell, D.B. (1977). *High level wellness.* New York: Bantam.

Bach, G.R., & Wyden, P. (1968). *The intimate enemy. How to fight fair in love and marriage.* New York: Avon.

Benson, H. (1975). *The relaxation response.* New York: Avon.

Charlsworth, E.A., & Nathan, R.G. (1982). *Stress management.* New York: Ballantine.

Dyer, W.W. (1978). *Pulling your own strings.* New York: Avon.

Eliot, R.S., & Breo, D.L. (1984). *Is it worth dying for?* New York: Bantam.

Fromm, E. (1956). *The art of loving.* New York: Harper & Row.

Gordon, T. (1977). *Leader effectiveness training.* New York: Bantam.

Koestenbaum, P. (1974). *Managing anxiety.* Millbrae, CA: Celestial Arts.

Lakein, A. (1973). *How to get control of your time and your life.* New York: New American Library.

McKay, M., Davis, M., & Fanning, P. (1980). *The relaxation and stress reduction workbook.* Richmond, CA: New Harbinger.

McKay, M., Davis, M., & Fanning, P. (1981). *Thoughts and feelings.* Richmond, CA: New Harbinger.

McKay, M., Davis, M., & Fanning, P. (1983). *Messages. The communication book.* Oakland, CA: New Harbinger.

Pelletier, K. (1977). *Mind as healer, mind as slayer.* New York: Delta.

Reynolds, H., & Tramel, M.A. (1979). *Executive time management.* Englewood Cliffs, NJ: Prentice-Hall.

Rogers, C.R., & Stevens, B. (1971). *Person to person.* New York: Pocket.

Sehnert, K.W. (1981). *Stress/Unstress.* Minneapolis: Augsburg.

Simon, S. *Meeting yourself halfway. 31 value clarification strategies for daily living.* Niles, IL: Argus.

Stevens, J.O. (1971). *Awareness: Exploring, experimenting, experiencing.* New York: Bantam.

Surwit, R.S., Williams, R.B., & Shapiro, D. (1982). *Behavioral approaches to cardiovascular disease.* New York: Academic Press.

Tubesing, N.L., & Tubesing, D.A. (1984). *Structured exercises in stress management* (Vol. I & II). Duluth: Whole Person Press.

Chapter

6

Smoking, Heredity, and Diabetes

Tobacco use, inherited cholesterol problems, and diabetes mellitus also contribute to our nation's alarmingly high rate of atherosclerosis. Smoking is considered a major risk factor for heart disease, and the other two are minor risk factors. This designation is weighted in terms of populations, however, and does not always reflect the unique health profile of an individual. Smoking and diabetes will be of no concern if not present, whereas an inherited cholesterol problem will be a major contributor to CHD if the person is stricken with it. Health professionals must be familiar with all the common CHD risk factors to appropriately counsel clients interested in avoiding heart attack and stroke.

Smoking

Tobacco kills 350,000 Americans every year, more than the total number of U.S. soldiers lost in World War I, Korea, and Vietnam together. Cigarettes cause more premature deaths than all of the following combined: automobile accidents, cocaine, heroin, alcohol, AIDS, fire, homicide, and suicide. One third of smokers eventually die from their habit, losing an average 15 years of life (1, 2).

Most of these unnecessary deaths are due to CHD. Tobacco is estimated to contribute to as many as one third of all heart attacks in the United States—170,000 each year. Smokers have two to four times the risk of dying from a heart attack as nonsmokers (3-5). Women smokers who use contraceptive pills have up to a 10-fold increase in CHD (6). Various estimates show that as many as two out of three heart attacks suffered by women of reproductive age may be attributable to smoking.

Studies from various countries show that smokers also have about 50% more strokes than nonsmokers (7, 8).Cigarette smoking is a strong contributor to peripheral vascular disease (PVD), the narrowing of the blood vessels that supply the arms and legs. More than 90% of PVD victims are smokers (9).

Tobacco has several adverse effects that accelerate atherosclerosis. Smoking elevates LDL while lowering HDL cholesterol (10). The impact on HDL is especially pronounced and portentous. Exercise, which is usually effective in raising HDL, has no such effect in smokers. Smoking also incurs adverse effects to blood pressure, platelets, and the arterial lining that are equivalent in risk to an increase of 50 to 100 mg/dl (1.3 to 2.6 mmol/L) in total cholesterol.

Tobacco transiently increases both systolic and diastolic blood pressure, probably by an increase in the stress chemical norepinephrine and the resultant vasoconstriction and increased pulse rate (11, 12).[1] This forces the heart to work faster against greater resistance, increasing its need for oxygen. But simultaneously, the carbon monoxide that enters the circulation withholds oxygen from reaching the struggling heart muscle. Carbon monoxide is also directly toxic to the endothelial cells lining the arteries, which fosters more rapid cholesterol influx (13).

Both nicotine and carbon monoxide predispose the heart to beat in abnormal and potentially fatal rhythms (14, 15). They also promote blood clotting by making platelets more sticky (16-19). Smoking also escalates the production of fibrinogen, the precursor molecule to the fibrin strands that unite platelets into a formed clot. Thus, smoking not only initiates and hastens plaque formation, but it can also precipitate the final infarcting clot.

Besides the huge toll it takes on cardiovascular health, smoking also causes 80% to 85% of lung cancer, 30% of all cancers (20), and 80% to 90% of chronic bronchitis and emphysema (21, 22). Cigarette smoke contains more than 4,000 chemicals, including heavy metals, radioactive products, poisons such as hydrogen cyanide, and at least 48 known cancer-producing substances (23).

Smoking-related illnesses cost our country more than $50 billion in 1985. This includes $16 billion in medical care and $37 billion in lost productivity, premature death, and other indirect costs (1, 21). This does not include the $2 billion spent each year on tobacco advertising or the cost of purchasing cigarettes. Sadly, we spend more on tobacco than we do on public education (24).

Tobacco is easily the most addictive and physically dangerous drug in our society (25, 26). It is the only consumer product that is harmful when used as intended (27). Smoking more cigarettes daily, inhaling more

---

[1]When not smoking, however, smokers do not tend to have higher blood pressures than nonsmokers.

deeply, and starting at an earlier age all increase tobacco's danger. There is no safe cigarette—death rates of smokers who use low-tar and low-nicotine brands of cigarettes are still higher than those of nonsmokers. Although pipe and cigar smokers experience far less disease than cigarette smokers, switching to these forms of tobacco does not decrease the risk of atherosclerosis. Apparently, former cigarette users inhale pipe and cigar smoke much more than those who have never smoked cigarettes (28).

Tobacco's ill effects also act synergistically with high cholesterol and high blood pressure—the total health risk is more than the sum of each separate risk. If two of these risk factors are present, the risk is not twice as great, but four times higher. All three in combination result in a chance of disease eight times greater than if none was present.

Passive Smoking

Tobacco smoke in the environment arises from both mainstream smoke exhaled by the smoker and sidestream smoke from the burning end of the cigarette. Together they present a health hazard for nonsmokers, including an increased risk of CHD and cancer (29-31). Sidestream smoke from a smoldering cigarette has two to three times the carbon monoxide and nicotine concentration as the mainstream smoke received by the smoker (32). Passively inhaling another's smoke is sufficient to bring on the chest pain of angina pectoris in persons with CHD (33).

A particularly deplorable circumstance occurs when children and the unborn are exposed to passive smoke. Exposure to one or more smoking parent doubles most of the childhood respiratory infections, including bronchitis, pneumonia, tonsillitis, colds, and asthma. An estimated 5,000 stillborn deaths are attributed to smoking, as well as many thousands of birth defects. Passive smoke exposure also fosters an early start to atherosclerotic arteries.

Benefits of Smoking Cessation

The good news is that smoking cessation is a giant step toward a higher level of wellness. Cigarette smokers who quit have a lower incidence of heart attack, sudden death, stroke, peripheral vascular disease, and cancer than those who continue (8, 34-37).

As much as 90% of the excess risk for a heart attack is removed after a single smoke-free year (38, 39) and the risk is nearly that of nonsmokers after 2 to 3 years (40). Stroke risk also declines rapidly, reaching that of nonsmokers 5 years after cessation (34, 41). The damage to the lungs resolves in a more linear fashion.

In contrast to the recent proof about the benefits of lowering cholesterol, the merits of smoking cessation have been known for many years. Consequently, we have come much further in controlling this health hazard than we have with elevated blood cholesterol. As of 1990, fewer than 30% of American adults smoke, down from 50% three decades ago.

Heredity: Families With High Cholesterol

Coronary heart disease is known to cluster in certain families. The Western Collaborative Group Study determined family history in 3,154 men who were followed for more than 8 years (42). Men who had one or both parents afflicted with CHD were twice as likely to develop angina pectoris or heart attack. In the Framingham heart study, men whose brothers had CHD were half again as likely to develop coronary disease (43). Finally, a study of 117,156 women found that those who had a parent suffer a heart attack before age 60 were 2.8 times as likely to develop CHD as those without such a history (44).

Although family clustering of CHD does occur, it does not prove that heredity is responsible, because families share common environmental influences such as diet. For example, wives of heart attack victims as a group have higher-than-average cholesterol levels (45). All told, the family environment is a much stronger influence on cholesterol levels and atherosclerosis than is family inheritance (46, 47).

To complicate the environment/inheritance issue even further, some individuals inherit a predisposition to elevated cholesterol that is manifested only if they become obese, eat fatty foods, and so forth. Unfortunately, in America today these conditions are frequently realized. If these people maintained ideal weight, cholesterol levels, and blood pressure, they would incur little or no atherosclerosis.

Certainly no one inherits clogged arteries. At an early age, though, we learn eating and exercise habits that often lead to increases in weight, blood pressure, and cholesterol. Genetic changes cannot explain the relatively brisk rise or fall in atherosclerosis rates that occur when people emigrate and change their diets (48), or when food patterns change within a given locale (49). A natural experiment occurred in Scandinavia during the German occupation (50). Meats and dairy cream were sent to the military front lines, thus "leaning out" civilian diets. After a short interval, the incidence of atherosclerosis in the countries plummeted. The rates quickly climbed again after World War II, as depicted in Figure 6.1a, b, and c (50).

A true inherited cholesterol problem should be suspected when an individual has a very high cholesterol level, such as 300 mg/dl (7.8 mmol/L) and above. A positive or worrisome family history is defined throughout this book according to the guidelines of the National Cholesterol Education Program; namely, the occurrence of a heart attack or sudden cardiac death in at least one parent or sibling before the age of 55 (51).

Although they contribute to only a minority of the total CHD cases in this country, several clear-cut genetic abnormalities have been described. The classic situation is the inheritance of a chromosomal abnormality in the gene coding for the LDL receptors (52). The technical term for this condition is familial hypercholesterolemia, abbreviated FH.

A person with the heterozygous condition—that is, who has received one normal and one abnormal gene for cholesterol receptors—will have approximately half the normal number of receptors; twice normal blood cholesterol, in the range of 350 to 400 mg/dl (9.1 to 10.3 mmol/L); and

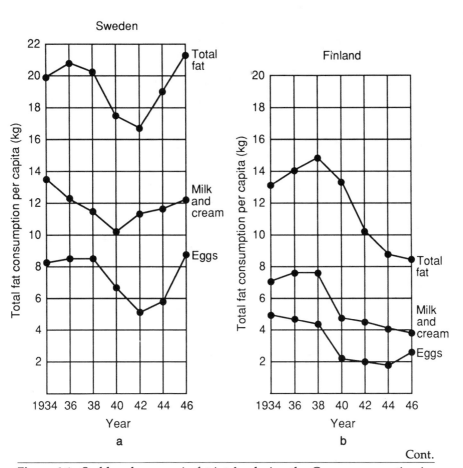

Figure 6.1 Sudden decreases in fat intake during the German occupation in Sweden (a) and Finland (b) coincided with a sharp temporary reduction of heart attacks (c).

Note. Figures 6.1a, b, and c are from ''The Relation of Nutrition to Health: A Statistical Study of the Effect of the War-Time on Arteriosclerosis'' by H. Malmros, 1950, *Acta Medica Scandinavica*, (suppl. 246), pp. 142, 144, 145. Copyright 1950 by *Acta Medica Scandinavica*. Adapted by permission.

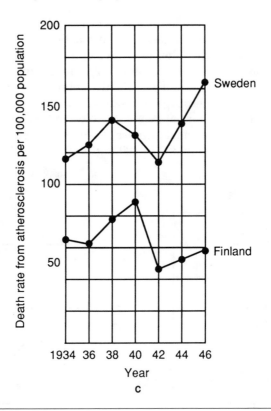

Figure 6.1 (Continued)

four times the average rate of heart attack. About one in every 500 persons has this form of familial hypercholesterolemia. Even in the absence of other risk factors, these unfortunate individuals are stricken with premature CHD. Approximately half of afflicted men die before reaching 50 years of age, and half the women die before age 60. Raised, yellow deposits of cholesterol, called xanthomas, occur over the achilles or hand tendons in about half of the FH cases by middle age. This clinical sign is virtually diagnostic of familial hypercholesterolemia.

Much less common is the homozygous condition—inheriting abnormal receptor genes from both parents, resulting in blood cholesterol elevation about four times normal (600 to 800 mg/dl or 15.5 to 20.6 mmol/L). Even with a strict diet these individuals are at extremely high risk, usually succumbing to CHD in their teens or early 20s. Fortunately this homozygous condition occurs only once in 1 million persons.

The most common inherited cholesterol problem is familial combined hyperlipidemia (FCHL), a condition in which the liver produces excessive amounts of LDL's apoprotein B-100 (53). This disorder is present in about 1% of our general population, but is present in perhaps 1 of 10 families of heart attack victims. One third of individuals with FCHL have cholesterol elevated into the range of 250 to 350 mg/dl (6.5 to 9 mmol/L). Another third have only increased triglyceride levels, and the final third have both conditions (54). Sometimes their lipid values vary considerably from one testing to another. Persons afflicted with FCHL who have average or only slightly elevated blood cholesterol are thought to produce particularly small, dense, and dangerous LDL particles. Helpful in pinning down the diagnosis is a determination of apoprotein B levels, which are often elevated in these cases.

Other inherited conditions occur when family members have particularly ineffective mechanisms to clear cholesterol from the circulation. In spite of a normal number of LDL receptors, they have one or more genetic factors that reduce the activity of the receptors (55). Such persons are overly sensitive to fatty foods and must develop excellent eating habits to stave off plaque. Some of these persons are diagnosed as having polygenic hypercholesterolemia, because multiple genes are probably interacting with the individual's diet to cause the cholesterol elevation.

Gender

Gender is a genetic factor that has a powerful influence on atherosclerosis. Before menopause, women have 1/10th the rate of CHD as men. Soon after menopause, when LDL levels and blood pressure climb rapidly, their risk becomes half that of men. Equality of the sexes in terms of CHD risk is approached in the ninth decade. In spite of the relative protection afforded by their gender, CHD has remained the leading overall cause of death in women since 1908.

Because hypercholesterolemia develops later in women, the majority of heart attacks occur at older ages in women than in men. Heart attack rates in white women are delayed 10 years behind men, and rates in non-white women are delayed 7 years. Heart disease becomes the leading cause of death in women over age 66, whereas it heads the list in men beyond age 39. Although most of the CHD prevention studies have used male subjects, a review of 9 studies that included women indicated that the NCEP guidelines also apply to women (56).

Much of women's CHD protection is presumably mediated through hormones. The estrogens released from the ovaries lower LDL and raise HDL (57). From puberty onward, females have HDL levels 10 points higher than those of males. Women's LDL levels are lower than men's until the early 50s, when their levels surpass men's. This is caused primarily by falling estrogen levels and parallels their rise in blood pressure after menopause (see Figure 6.2) (58, 59).

The effect of birth control pills on the cardiovascular system has been the topic of considerable research and discussion. Original formulations, which had higher concentrations of hormones, tended to cause blood

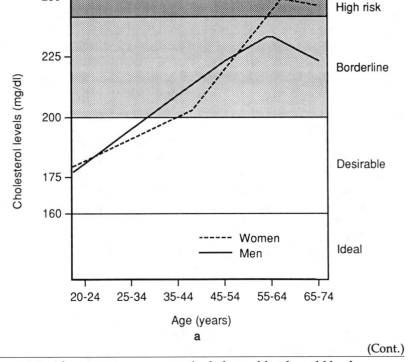

a

(Cont.)

Figure 6.2   After menopause, women's cholesterol levels and blood pressures climb and surpass men's (a and b); their rates of heart attack then climb significantly, also (c).
Note. Figures 6.2b and c are from "Symposium on Initial Antihypertensive Therapy" by W. Castelli and K. Anderson, 1986, *American Journal of Medicine, 80*, (suppl. 2A), pp. 28-29. Copyright 1986 by *American Journal of Medicine*. Reprinted by permission.

clots. But overall, the modern preparations do not seem to promote clotting or CHD in nonsmoking women. This was borne out in a long-term study of 120,000 nurses (60). In women who smoke, however, even low-dose contraceptive pills promote clotting and may also accelerate atherosclerosis (61).

Even today, some preparations are safer than others. Virtually all contraceptive pills today contain a combination of estrogens and progestins. The latter tend to offset some of the benefit of estrogens, generally resulting in a slight elevation of LDL and a reduction in HDL. Norgestrel has an especially deleterious impact on blood lipids, while that of ethynodiol diacetate is relatively weak (62). In addition, newer progestins, such as desogestrel and gestamine, seem to have no adverse effects on lipids. They have been studied and used extensively in Europe but are not yet approved in the United States (63).

A much-debated question has been whether or not estrogen replace-

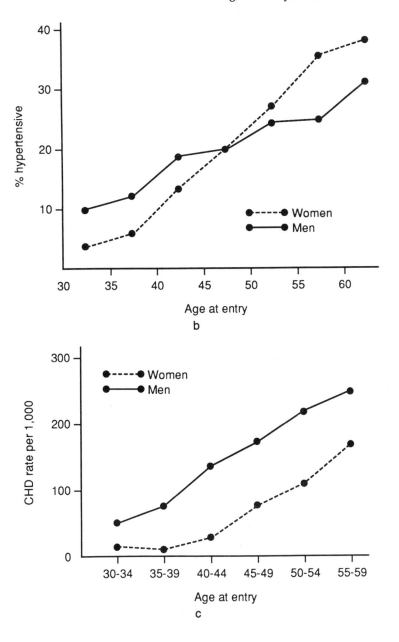

Figure 6.2 (Continued)

ment for the hot flushes of menopause would be safe. The major concern has been that when used without progestins, estrogens have a slight tendency to promote hyperplasia and cancer of the uterus. Opinions regarding this important topic have swayed in recent years toward noting an overall benefit to using combined estrogen and progesterone hormones after menopause. Not only does estrogen replacement therapy cut CHD rates by one third to one half in these women, but it may also be helpful in preventing stroke and osteoporosis (along with vitamin D, calcium, and exercise for the latter) (64-67).

Estrogens tend to elevate triglycerides though the effect is variable and generally small, especially with the estrogen skin patches. Nonetheless, a fasting lipid profile should be done before and three to six weeks after initiating estrogens. The decision to use oral contraceptives or estrogen replacement therapy ultimately rests with the individual and her physician. Clearly, estrogen-containing compounds should be used with extreme caution in smokers, if at all.

On a societal level, diet, rather than gender or heredity, is far and away the major promoter of hypercholesterolemia and CHD (68, 69). The major role of genetics is that we have not inherited from our ancestors the ability to process food that is permeated with saturated fat and cholesterol. We lack the appropriate genes for handling what our modern diet has become, a diet that was rare before this century. For 250,000 years, humans lived on wild grains, nuts, seeds, shoots, and lean game meat (70). How can we expect to eat the typical modern American diet and remain unscathed?

Sadly, we've become a race of hypercholesterolemics. Our modern eating patterns have created a cholesterol epidemic. On the other hand, if we were to resume diets for which we are genetically designed, atherosclerosis would once again be rare. In short, we inherit bad habits far more often than we inherit faulty genes.

Diabetes

Diabetes mellitus (sugar diabetes) has two basic categories, depending on whether the onset of the disease was in childhood or adolescence (Type I) or in adulthood (Type II). At least 80% of all diabetics in the United States have the adult-onset type and can usually control the disease by diet and oral medications. In contrast, nearly all Type I or juvenile-onset diabetics require insulin injections to control their blood sugar.

Overall, diabetics have two to three times the incidence of CHD, but much of the apparent risk of the disease is due to the frequent accompaniment of other cardiovascular risk factors. About 80% of the adult-onset diabetes is related to obesity. The risk of diabetes doubles for every 20% rise above ideal weight. Diabetics are also twice as likely as the general population to have hypertension and also tend to have elevated LDL and triglycerides, combined with low HDL levels.

Sorting out the independent relationship of diabetes and CHD with sophisticated statistical techniques revealed that symptomatic diabetes imparts a slight increase in CHD risk if weight, blood pressure, and lipids are normal (45). Asymptomatic high blood sugar (hyperglycemia) does not seem to promote atherosclerosis if these other risk factors are absent (71, 72).[2]

For unknown reasons, diabetes has a greater impact in women than men for all aspects of atherosclerosis—CHD, stroke, and peripheral vascular disease (73). Diabetic men in their 40s have a 20% higher risk of CHD than nondiabetic men the same age, but diabetic women in their 40s have four times the risk as their nondiabetic counterparts. After age 50 this sex differential is less pronounced (74).

As with the other cardiovascular risk factors, diabetes has much more impact if it occurs together with smoking, hypertension, hypercholesterolemia, or a combination of these. Along with smoking and hypercholesterolemia, diabetes is a particularly strong risk factor for peripheral vascular disease, increasing the risk five- to tenfold (75). It is a weaker contributor to stroke and CHD.

Treatment for diabetes involves most of the same principles discussed throughout this book for the prevention of atherosclerosis. Of primary importance is diet—low-fat, high-fiber, calorically balanced meals. Exercise and weight loss improve blood sugar control by increasing the number and sensitivity of the insulin receptors on cell membranes. By facilitating glucose entry into cells, the glucose level in the bloodstream declines (76, 77).

Using weight control and a high-fiber diet in diabetics, Dr. James Anderson has lowered total cholesterol and LDL levels an average of 22% and 29% respectively, while boosting HDL 9% (78). He has also reduced or eliminated medications in most of his diabetic patients. Minimizing drugs is important because the use of early oral medications to control blood sugar resulted in an increase in coronary events in the University Group Diabetes Program (79) and insulin injections can suppress the body's own insulin secretion by the pancreas. Again, a total dietary and lifestyle approach is necessary to optimize health enhancement.

References

1. Warner, K.E. (1983). The economics of smoking: Dollars and sense. *New York State Journal of Medicine*, **83**, 1273-1274.
2. Warner, K.E. (1987). Health and economic implications of a tobacco-free society. *Journal of the American Medical Association*, **258**, 2080-2086.
3. Klein, L.W., Pichard, A.D., Holt, J., Smith, H., Gorlin, R., & Teicholz,

---

[2]That is, asymptomatic hyperglycemia is not an independent CHD risk factor once the confounding variables are accounted for in the statistical analysis.

L.E. (1983). Effects of chronic tobacco smoking on the coronary circulation. *Journal of the American College of Cardiology*, 1, 421-426.

4. Surgeon General of the United States. (1983). *The health consequences of smoking: Cardiovascular disease. A report of the Surgeon General* (Department of Health and Human Services Publication No. (PHS) 84-50204). Rockville, MD: Department of Health and Human Services.

5. Friedman, G.D., Dales, L.G., & Ury, H.K. (1979). Mortality in middle-aged smokers and nonsmokers. *New England Journal of Medicine*, 300, 213-217.

6. Shapiro, S., Rosenburg, L., Slone, D., Rosenberg, L., Kaufman, D.W., Stolley, P.D., & Miettinen, O.S. (1979). Oral-contraceptive use in relation to myocardial infarction. *Lancet*, 1, 743-746.

7. Pooling Project Research Group. (1978). Relationship of blood pressure, serum cholesterol, smoking habit, relative weight, and ECG abnormalities to incidence of major coronary events: Final report of the Pooling Project. *Journal of Chronic Diseases*, 31, 201-306.

8. Royal College of Physicians. (1977). *Smoking or health: The third report*. Tunbridge Wells: Pitman Medical.

9. Kannel, W.B., & Shurtleff, D. (1973). The Framingham study: Cigarettes and the development of intermittent claudication. *Geriatrics*, 28, 61-68.

10. Kannel, W.B. (1981). Update on the role of cigarette smoking in coronary artery disease. *American Heart Journal*, 101, 319-328.

11. Cryer, P.E., Haymond, M.W., Santiago, J.V., & Shah, S.D. (1976). Norepinephrine and epinephrine release and adrenergic mediation of smoking-associated hemodynamic and metabolic events. *New England Journal of Medicine*, 295, 573-577.

12. Aronow, W.S., Goldsmith, J.R., Kern, J.C., Cassidy, J., Nelson, W., Johson, L.L., & Adams, W. (1974). Effect of smoking cigarettes on cardiovascular hemodynamics. *Archives of Environmental Health*, 28, 330-332.

13. Tillmans, H., Sarma, I.S.M., Seeler, K., & Bing, R.I. (1974). Lipid metabolism in perfused human coronary arteries and saphenous veins. In Schettler, G., & Weizel, A. (Eds.), *Atherosclerosis*, III, (pp. 118-125). New York: Springer-Verlag.

14. Kaufman, D.W., Helmrich, S.P., Rosenberg, L., Miettinen, O.S., & Shapiro, S. (1983). Nicotine and carbon monoxide content of cigarette smoke and the risk of myocardial infarction in young men. *New England Journal of Medicine*, 308, 409-413.

15. DeBias, D.A., Banarjee, C.M., Birkhead, N.C., Greene, C.H., Scott, S.D., & Harrer, V.W. (1976). Effects of carbon monoxide inhalation on ventricular fibrillation. *Archives of Environmental Health*, 31, 38-42.

16. Nowak, J., Murray, J.J., Oates, J.A., & Fitz-Gerald, G.A. (1987). Biochemical evidence of a chronic abnormality in platelet and vascular

function in healthy individuals who smoke cigarettes. *Circulation*, **76**, 6-14.

17. Levine, P.H. (1973). An acute effect of cigarette smoking on platelet function: A possible link between smoking and arterial thrombosis. *Circulation*, **48**, 619-623.

18. Wald, N., Howard, S., Smith, P.G., & Kjeldsen, K. (1973). Association between atherosclerotic disease and carboxyhaemoglobin levels in tobacco smokers. *British Medical Journal*, **1**, 761.

19. Birnsting, M.A., Brinson, K., & Chakrabarti, B.K. (1971). The effect of short-term exposure to carbon monoxide on platelet stickiness. *British Journal of Surgery*, **58**, 837-839.

20. Surgeon General of the United States. (1982). *The health consequences of smoking. Cancer: A report of the Surgeon General.* Rockville, MD: Department of Health and Human Services.

21. Fielding, J.E. (1985). Smoking: Health effects and control. *New England Journal of Medicine*, **313**, 491-498.

22. Surgeon General of the United States. (1984). *The health consequences of smoking: Chronic obstructive lung disease. A report of the Surgeon General.* Rockville, MD: Department of Health and Human Services.

23. Kahn, H.A. (1966). The Dorn study of smoking and mortality among United States veterans: Report on 8 and one-half years of observation. In W. Haenszel (Ed.), *Epidemiologic approaches to the study of cancer and other chronic diseases* (National Cancer Institute Monograph No. 19) (pp. 1-125). Bethesda, MD: National Cancer Institute.

24. Allen, R.E. (1981). *Lifegain* (p. 61). Morristown, NJ: Human Resources Institute.

25. Surgeon General of the United States. (1988). U.S. Department of Health, Education, and Welfare. *Smoking and health: A report of the Surgeon General.* Washington, DC: U.S. Government Printing Office.

26. Surgeon General of the United States. (1988). *Health consequences of smoking: Nicotine addiction: A report of the Surgeon General.* DHHS Publication No. (CDC) 88-8406. Washington, DC: U.S. Government Printing Office.

27. American Heart Association. (1986). Public policy on smoking and health: Toward a smoke-free generation by the year 2000. *Circulation*, **73**, 381A-395A.

28. Kaufman, D.W., Palmer, J.R., Rosenberg, L., & Shapiro, S. (1987). Cigar and pipe smoking and myocardial infarction in young men. *British Medical Journal*, **294**, 1315-1316.

29. Surgeon General of the United States. (1986). *The health consequences of involuntary smoking: A report of the Surgeon General.* Bethesda, MD: Department of Health and Human Services.

30. Correa, P., Pickle, L.W., Fontham, E., Lin, Y., & Haenszel, W. (1983). Passive smoking and lung cancer. *Lancet*, **2**, 595-597.

31. Hirayama, T. (1981). Non-smoking wives of heavy smokers have a higher risk of lung cancer: A study from Japan. *British Medical Journal*, **282**, 183-185.

32. Bolhaven, C., & Niessen, H.J. (1961). Amounts of oxides of nitrogen and carbon monoxide in cigarette smoke, with and without inhalation. *Nature*, **192**, 458-459.

33. Lefcoe, N.M., Ashley, M.J., Pederson, L.L., & Keays, J.J. (1983). The health risks of passive smoking: The growing case for control measures in enclosed environments. *Chest*, **84**, 90-95.

34. Wolf, P.A., D'Agostino, R.B., Kannel, W.B., Bonita, R., & Balanger, A.J. (1988). Cigarette smoking as a risk factor for stroke: The Framingham Study. *Journal of the American Medical Association*, **258**, 1025-1029.

35. Kleinman, J.C., Feldman, J.J., & Monk, M.A. (1979). The effects of changes in smoking habits on coronary heart disease mortality. *American Journal of Public Health*, **69**, 795-802.

36. Doll, R., & Peto, R. (1976). Mortality in relation to smoking: Twenty years' observation of British doctors. *British Medical Journal*, **4**, 1525.

37. Hammond, E.C., & Garfinkel, L. (1969). Coronary heart disease, stroke, and aortic aneurysm. Factors in the etiology. *Archives of Environmental Health*, **19**, 167-182.

38. Aberg, A., Bergstrand, R., Johansson, S., Ulvenstam, G., Vedin, A., Wedel, H., Wilhelmsson, C., & Wilhelmsen, L. (1983). Cessation of smoking after myocardial infarction. Effects on mortality after 10 years. *British Heart Journal*, **44**, 416-422.

39. Gordon, T., Kannel, W.B., Dawber, W.R., & McGee, D. (1975). Changes associated with quitting cigarette smoking: The Framingham study. *American Heart Journal*, **90**, 322.

40. Rosenberg, L., Kaufman, D.W., Helmich, S.P., & Shapiro, S. (1985). The risk of myocardial infarction after quitting smoking in men under 55 years of age. *New England Journal of Medicine*, **313**, 1511-1514.

41. Rogot, E. (1974). Smoking and general mortality among U.S. veterans, 1954-1969. Department of Health, Education, and Welfare, Public Health Service. Publication No. NIH 74-544. Bethesda, MD.

42. Sholtz, R.J., Rosenman, R.H., & Brand, R.J. (1975). The relationship of reported parental history to the incidence of coronary heart disease in the Western Collaborative Group Study. *American Journal of Epidemiology*, **102**, 350.

43. Snowden, C.B., McNamary, P.M., Garrison, R.J., Feinleib, M., Kannel, W.B., & Epstein, F.H. (1982). Predicting coronary heart disease in siblings—a multivariate assessment: The Framingham Heart Study. *American Journal of Epidemiology*, **115**, 217.

44. Colditz, G.A., Stampfer, M.J., Willett, W.C., Rosner, B., Speizer, F.F., & Hennekens, C.H. (1986). A prospective study of parental history of myocardial infarction and coronary heart disease in women. *American Journal of Epidemiology*, **128**, 48-58.

45. Kannel, W.B. (1987). New perspectives on cardiovascular risk factors. *American Heart Journal*, **114**, 213-219.
46. Perkins, K.A. (1986). Family history of coronary heart disease: Is it an independent risk factor? *American Journal of Epidemiology*, **124**, 182.
47. Conroy, R.M., Mulcahy, R., Hickey, N., & Daly, L. (1985). Is family history of coronary heart disease an independent coronary risk factor? *British Medical Journal*, **53**, 378.
48. Robertson, T.L., Kato, H., Gordon, T., Kagan, A., Rhoads, G.G., Land, C.E., Worth, R.M., Belsky, J.L., Dock, D.S., Miyanski, M., & Kawamoto, S. (1977). Epidemiologic studies on coronary heart disease and stroke in Japanese men living in Japan, Hawaii, and California. *American Journal of Cardiology*, **39**, 244-249.
49. Keys, A. (1975). Coronary heart disease—the global picture. *Atherosclerosis*, **22**, 149-192.
50. Malmros, H. (1950). The relation of nutrition to health: A statistical study of the effect of the war-time on arteriosclerosis, cardiosclerosis, tuberculosis, and diabetes. *Acta Medica Scandinavica*, **138** (Suppl. 246), 137.
51. National Institutes of Health Consensus Development Conference. (1985). Lowering blood cholesterol to prevent heart disease. *Journal of the American Medical Association*, **253**, 2080-2090.
52. Goldstein, J.L., & Brown, M.S. (1982). The LDL receptor defect in familial hypercholesterolemia. Implication for pathogenesis and therapy. *Medical Clinics of North America*, **66**, 335.
53. Chait, A., Albers, J.J., & Brunzell, J.D. (1980). Very low density lipoprotein over-production in genetic forms of hypertriglyceridemia. *European Journal of Clinical Investigation*, **10**, 17-22.
54. Schaefer, E.J., & Levy, R.I. (1985). Pathogenesis and management of lipoprotein disorders. *New England Journal of Medicine*, **312**, 1300-1310.
55. Grundy, S.M. (1984). Hyperlipoproteinemia: Metabolic basis and rationale for therapy. *American Journal of Cardiology*, **54**, 20C-26C.
56. Bush, T.L., Fred, L.P., Barrett-Connor, E. (1988). Cholesterol, lipoproteins, and coronary heart disease in women. *Clinical Chemistry*, **34**, B60-B70.
57. Wahl, P., Walden, C., Knopp, R., Hoover, J., Wallace, R., Heiss, G., & Rifkind, B. (1983). Effect of estrogen/progestin potency on lipid-lipoprotein cholesterol. *New England Journal of Medicine*, **308**, 862-867.
58. National Cholesterol Education Program. (1987). So you have high blood cholesterol . . . (NIH Publication No. 87-2922). Bethesda, MD.
59. Castelli, W., & Anderson, K. (1986). Symposium on initial antihypertensive therapy. A population at risk: Prevalence of high cholesterol levels in hypertensive patients in the Framingham study. *American Journal of Medicine*, **80** (Suppl 2A), 23-32.
60. Hannekens, C.H., Evans, D., Peto, O. (1988). Oral contraceptive use,

cigarette smoking, and myocardial infarctions. *New England Journal of Medicine,* **319,** 1313-1317.

61. Sullivan, J.M., Vander-zwaag, R., Lemp, G.F., Hughes, J.P., Maddock, V., Kroetz, F.W., Ramanathan, K.B., & Mirvis, D.M. (1988). Postmenopausal estrogen use and coronary atherosclerosis. *Annals of Internal Medicine,* **108,** 358-363.

62. Lipson, A., Stoy, D.B., LaRosa, J.C., Muesing, R.A., Cleary, P.A., Miller, V.T., Gilbert, P.R., & Stadel, B. (1986). Progesterone and oral contraceptive-induced lipoprotein changes: A prospective study. *Contraception,* **34,** 121-134.

63. Marz, W., Gross, W., Gahn, G., Romberg, G., Taubert, H.D., & Kuhl, H. (1985). A randomized crossover comparison of two low-dose contraceptives: Effect on serum lipids and lipoproteins. *American Journal of Obstetrics and Gynecology,* **153,** 287-293.

64. Gruchow, H.W., Anderson, A.J., Barboriak, J.J., & Soboeinski, K.A. (1988). Postmenopausal use of estrogen and occlusion of coronary arteries. *American Heart Journal,* **115,** 954-963.

65. Bush, T.L., Barrett-Connor, E., Cowan, L.D., Criqui, M.H., Wallace, R.B., Suchindrin, C.M., Tyroler, H.A., & Rifkind, B.M. (1987). Cardiovascular mortality and non-contraceptive use of estrogen in women: Results from the Lipid Research Clinics Program Follow-up Study. *Circulation,* **75,** 1102-1109.

66. Henderson, B., Paganini-Hill, A., Ross, R.K., & Mack, T.M. (1987, September 14). Effects of estrogen on cardiovascular disease. *Postgraduate Medicine,* **82,** 31-37.

67. Stampfer, M.J., Willett, W.C., Colditz, G.A., Rosner, B., Speizer, F.E., & Hennekens, C.H. (1985). A prospective study of postmenopausal estrogen therapy and coronary heart disease. *New England Journal of Medicine,* **313,** 1044-1049.

68. Grundy, S.M. (1986). Cholesterol and coronary heart disease: A new era. *Journal of the American Medical Association,* **256,** 2849-2858.

69. Hopkins, P.N., & Williams, R.R. (1986). Identification and relative weight of cardiovascular risk factors. *Cardiology Clinics,* **4,** 3-32.

70. Eaton, S.B., & Konner, M. (1985). Paleolithic nutrition. *New England Journal of Medicine,* **312,** 283-289.

71. Kannel, W.B., & Gordon, T. (1974). *The Framingham Study. An epidemiologic investigation of cardiovascular disease. Section 30, some characteristics related to the incidence of cardiovascular disease and death: 18-year follow-up* (Publication No. 74-599). Washington, DC: U.S. Government Printing Office.

72. Stamler, R., & Stamler, J. (1979). Asymptomatic hyperglycemia and coronary heart disease. *Journal of Chronic Disorders,* **32,** 683-691.

73. Gordon, T., Castelli, W.P., Hjortland, M., Kannel, W.B., & Dawber, T.R. (1977). Predicting coronary heart disease in middle-aged and older persons. *Journal of the American Medical Association,* **238,** 497-499.

74. U.S. Department of Health, Education, and Welfare, Public Health Service. (1979). *Fact sheet. Arteriosclerosis* (DHEW Publication No. [NIH] 79-1421). Washington, DC: U.S. Government Printing Office.

75. Dawber, T.R. (1980). *The Framingham Study*. Cambridge, MA: Harvard University Press.

76. Richter, E.A., Ruderman, N.B., & Schneider, S.H. (1981). Diabetes and exercise. *American Journal of Medicine, 247*, 2674-2679.

77. Pederson, O., Beck-Nielsen, J., & Jeding, L. (1980). Increased insulin receptors after exercise in patients with insulin-dependent diabetes mellitus. *New England Journal of Medicine, 302*, 886.

78. Anderson, J.W., Story. L., & Sieling, B. (1984). Hypercholesterolemic effects of oat-bran or bean intake for hypercholesterolemic men. *American Journal of Clinical Nutrition, 40*, 1146-1155.

79. Miller, M., Knatterud, G.L., Hawkins, B.S., & Newberry, W.B. (1976). A study of the effects of hypoglycemic agents on vascular complications in patients with adult-onset diabetes VI. *Diabetes, 25*, 1129-1151.

Suggested Readings

Smoking Cessation

American Council on Science and Health. (1984). *Smoking or health: It's your choice*. New York: Author.

American Council on Science and Health. (1985). *Searching for a way out: Smoking cessation techniques*. New York: Author.

American Lung Association. (1990). *Freedom from smoking in 20 days: A self help quit smoking program*. New York: Author.

American Lung Association. (1990). *A lifetime of freedom from smoking: A maintenance program for exsmokers*. New York: Author.

Fagerstrom, K.O. (1978). Measuring degree of physical dependence to tobacco smoking with reference to individualization of treatment. *Addictive Behaviors, 3*, 235-241.

Ferguson, T. (1989). *The no-nag, no-guilt, do-it-your-own-way guide to quitting smoking*. New York: Ballantine.

Fortmann, S.P., Killen, J.D., Telch, M.J., & Newman, B. (1988). Minimal contact treatment for smoking cessation. *Journal of the American Medical Association, 260*, 1575-1580.

Kottke, T.E., Battista, R.N., DeFriese, G.H., & Brekke, M.L. (1988). Attributes of successful smoking cessation interventions in medical practice. A meta-analysis of 39 controlled trials. *Journal of the American Medical Association, 259*, 2882-2889.

National Heart, Lung, and Blood Institute. (1986, August). *Clinical opportunities for smoking intervention: A guide for the busy physician* (DHHS NIH Publication No. 86-2178). Hillside, NJ: Enslow.

Pomerleau, O., & Pomerleau, C. (1984). *Break the smoking habit: A behavioral program for giving up cigarettes*. Ann Arbor, MI: Behavioral Medicine Press.

U.S. Department of Health and Social Services. (1985). *Clearing the air: A guide to quitting smoking*. Washington, DC: U.S. Government Printing Office.

U.S. Department of Health and Social Services. (1986). *Clinical opportunities for smoking intervention: A guide for the busy physician*. Washington, DC: U.S. Government Printing Office.

U.S. Department of Health and Human Services. (1986). *Clinical opportunities for smoking intervention* (NIH Publication No. 86-2178). Washington, DC: U.S. Government Printing Office.

PART

III

THE NUTRITIONAL APPROACH TO CHOLESTEROL CONTROL

☐

Cholesterol awareness is growing at an unprecedented rate. As late as 1983, only a third of American adults reported that their cholesterol had ever been tested. Today it is difficult for anyone to ignore the cholesterol consciousness sweeping the country. Public cholesterol screenings now inform millions of Americans nationwide of their cholesterol numbers. Physicians are advised by the National Cholesterol Education Program (NCEP) to routinely obtain cholesterol levels from all patients over age 20. As a result, doctors, dietitians, and other health care providers are being called on to provide more nutritional education to their patients and clients.

Part III provides a simple yet precise guide for preventing cardiovascular diseases through nutrition. Foods are arranged into three major categories—fat, fiber, and fish—in chapters 7, 8, and 9, respectively. This categorization helps in understanding and implementing a cholesterol-lowering diet and differs slightly from the classification scheme used by the American Dietetic Association. The latter includes the following groupings: starchy foods (cereals, pasta, bread, beans, starchy vegetables), protein (meat, fish, cheese), milk, fruit, fats, and vegetables.

Chapter 7 focuses on how dietary fat and cholesterol contribute to atherosclerosis. Fatty foods include the worst arterial offenders, namely, saturated and tropical oils, red meats, full-cream dairy products, and nuts. These foods are high in cholesterol, fat, and calories and while they are not forbidden entirely, they should be limited in quantity and frequency of servings.

The second major nutritional category, discussed in chapter 8, is fiber-rich foods. This section encompasses legumes (beans and peas), grains, fruits, and vegetables. The more of these foods eaten, the better, because they are low in fat, contain no cholesterol, and supply fiber, vitamins, and minerals. Legumes are also high in protein and when combined with grains can be substituted for meat or dairy to satisfy the body's protein requirement.

Chapter 9 shows that incorporating more fish into the diet is an important heart-saving goal. Most finfish are very low in fat compared with red meats or poultry, and most of the fat present is unsaturated. Fish from cold Northern seas, such as mackerel, salmon, and halibut, are the best choices because of the omega-3 oils they contain.

Obviously, there is considerable overlap between the food groups in terms of their chemical makeup. They all contain protein, carbohydrate, and fat, though to widely varying percentages. The meat and dairy groups are good sources of protein, for example, but are generally high in fat and cholesterol. Legumes are high in protein and carbohydrate but low in fat and cholesterol-free.

Chapter 10 explores perhaps the most important and basic nutritional guideline, which is to consume a wide variety of natural foods. This assures that overall nutritional needs for protein, fat, carbohydrates, vitamins, minerals, and fiber are met. The section includes an explanation of menu planning to assist readers (and their clients) in selecting the proper amount of foods from each of these groups: meats, dairy products, fruits, vegetables, grains, and oils. The chapter closes with advice on recipe modification, along with some techniques and sample recipes that demonstrate how traditional favorites can be prepared in a heart-healthy manner.

Chapter

7

Dietary Fat and Cholesterol

A nutritious diet is the first and foremost vehicle to reduce blood cholesterol and its associated risk of CHD, stroke, and peripheral vascular disease. Heart-healthy foods are low in cholesterol and fat, particularly saturated fat. The polyunsaturated and monounsaturated fats help to lower blood cholesterol levels when they are substituted for saturated fats. Yet, their use should also be limited to keep total fat consumption at a normal level.

Dietary fat and cholesterol have a great impact on serum cholesterol levels, not only by increasing the LDL directly, but also by inhibiting the liver from performing its cleanup job. Foods high in cholesterol and saturated fat suppress the number of LDL receptors in the liver, reducing the clearance of cholesterol from the circulation.

Americans eat almost twice as much fat as the human body is designed to handle, making this our most dangerous dietary practice. Fats make up 37% to 40% of our total calories instead of the recommended 25% to 30% (1-3). We also eat far too much of the worst kind of fats, those that are saturated. These comprise 15% to 17% of our total calories but should be limited to under 10%.

There is no reason to eat so much fat. Actually, we can do quite well with only 1% to 2% of total calories from fat. We need this amount of linoleic acid for the synthesis of important messenger molecules called prostaglandins. It is the only essential fatty acid, so named because we cannot build it from smaller molecular units. Our bodies can synthesize every other type of fat that is needed.

Fat molecules consist of three fatty acids, which are chains of 12 to 26 carbon atoms attached to a glycerol molecule like an extended E. This is by far the most common form of fat and is called a triglyceride. Figure 7.1 is a chemical diagram of a triglyceride illustrating three fatty acids that are

```
     H
     |
  C-C-OH
     |
HO-C-C        Glycerol
     |
  C-C-OH
     |
     H
```

Stearic acid (saturated)

```
      H        H  H  H  H  H  H  H  H  H  H  H  H  H  H  H  H  H  H
      |        |  |  |  |  |  |  |  |  |  |  |  |  |  |  |  |  |  |
   H-C- OOC -C -C -C -C -C -C -C -C -C -C -C -C -C -C -C -C -C -C-H
      |        |  |  |  |  |  |  |  |  |  |  |  |  |  |  |  |  |  |
               H  H  H  H  H  H  H  H  H  H  H  H  H  H  H  H  H
```

Oleic acid (monounsaturated)

```
      H        H  H  H  H  H  H  H  H|H  H  H  H  H  H  H  H  H
      |        |  |  |  |  |  |  |  | |  |  |  |  |  |  |  |  |
   H-C- OOC -C -C -C -C -C -C -C -C ⁼C -C -C -C -C -C -C -C -C-H
      |        |  |  |  |  |  |  |  |    |  |  |  |  |  |  |  |
               H  H  H  H  H  H  H       H  H  H  H  H  H  H  H
```

Linoleic acid (polyunsaturated)

```
      H        H  H  H  H  H  H  H  H|H  H  H|H  H  H  H  H  H
      |        |  |  |  |  |  |  |  | |  |  | |  |  |  |  |  |
   H-C- OOC -C -C -C -C -C -C -C -C ⁼C -C -C ⁼C -C -C -C -C -C-H
      |        |  |  |  |  |  |  |  |    |        |  |  |  |  |
      H        H  H  H  H  H  H  H       H        H  H  H  H
```

Figure 7.1 Saturated fatty acids, such as stearic acid (top), have all available carbon (C) sites bound with hydrogen (H). Oleic acid (center) is a mono-unsaturated fatty acid and thus has one double bond (at arrow) that displaces two hydrogen atoms. Linoleic acid (bottom) and other polyunsaturated fatty acids have two or more double bonds (at arrows) along the carbon chain. Fatty acids are further classified biochemically according to the number and position of the double bonds along the carbon chain. O = oxygen.

important in human nutrition: stearic acid (saturated), oleic acid (mono-unsaturated), and linoleic acid (polyunsaturated).

The three strands are the fatty acids. Hydrogen atoms lie on either side of the carbon atoms in the chains. The terminal carbon has two oxygen (O) atoms and one hydrogen (H) atom attached, forming a carboxyl group that chemically bonds to one of the glycerol sites.

Because the glycerol molecule remains constant, the behavior of a triglyceride molecule is determined by the fatty acids present. Biochemists have grouped fatty acids into three main categories: saturated, mono-unsaturated, and polyunsaturated. Saturation refers to the amount of hydrogen present, a feature that significantly affects chemical and physiological properties. The three fatty acids of a given triglyceride molecule may be identical or, more commonly, may differ. The triglyceride may contain only saturated, only unsaturated, or any combination of fatty acids.

Saturated Fats

Saturated fats tend to be solid at room temperature because they are literally packed with hydrogen at all available sites along the carbon chain. Chemically, this requires that no double bonds exist between carbon atoms (Refer to the top fatty acid chain in Figure 7.1).

Saturated fats raise cholesterol levels more than anything else in the diet does (4). For every 1% of total calories that come from saturated fat, the blood cholesterol increases an average of 2.7 mg/dl (5). Saturated fat may even increase the incidence of CHD independent of its effect on blood cholesterol levels. Three of the proposed mechanisms include increasing blood glucose, blood pressure (6), and clotting tendencies (7).

Approximately 15% to 17% of our total calories are derived from saturated fat instead of the recommended 7% to 10% (8). Consuming the lesser amount, with no other dietary change, is calculated to reduce serum cholesterol levels by about 20 mg/dl. Intake of saturated fats can safely be minimized because they provide no essential nutrients.

Concentrated sources of saturated fat are red meats (beef, pork, mutton), egg yolks, and full-cream dairy products (that is, nonskimmed). Together these are responsible for three fourths of the saturated fat in the American diet (9). Hamburger is the single major contributor, and cheese holds the number-two position. Considerable amounts of cholesterol are found in all these foods as well.

Plant products are usually quite low in saturated fat. A notable exception is the tropical oil group—coconut, palm, and palm kernel oils. Of the three, coconut oil is the worst. It's even more saturated and therefore more of an artery clogger than lard. It is widely used for frying foods in restaurants and is found in most commercial bakery products, prepared foods, and even granola. Only a close look at the product label will alert the health-oriented shopper. Tropical oils comprise a small percentage of America's total fat intake but a significant percentage of some individuals' diets, especially those who rely on convenience food items. Figure 7.2 shows the relative saturation of common cooking oils (10).

Other sources of saturated fat that sneak into the diet are vegetable oils that have been hydrogenated. Hydrogenation is a chemical process that injects hydrogen into the structure of the fatty acid chains rendering them partially or fully saturated. These dangerous fats are almost ubiquitous in processed and baked food products. Hydrogenation increases a product's shelf life but has the opposite effect on human life.

One mechanism by which saturated fats may work to drive up blood cholesterol is by increasing the cholesterol absorption from the intestine.

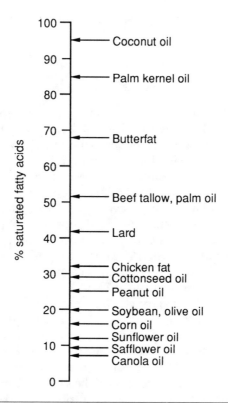

Figure 7.2   The proportion of saturated fat found in common cooking oils.

Without saturated fats, less of the cholesterol in foods is absorbed. Red meat, egg yolks, and full-cream dairy products contain both saturated fats and cholesterol and thus are doubly dangerous. Another factor is that the liver releases more cholesterol-containing VLDL in response to saturated fats in the diet.

The primary pathway by which saturated fats raise blood cholesterol, however, is indirect—by slowing cholesterol's clearance by the liver. When they enter the bloodstream after a meal, saturated fats reduce the number of LDL-cholesterol receptors along the surface of liver cells. As blood passes through the liver, fewer LDL particles are captured by cholesterol receptors. Thus, instead of being absorbed into the liver cells for reprocessing, cholesterol backs up into the bloodstream, forming plaque (11).

Not all saturated fatty acids have the same effect on lipids. One in particular, stearic acid, has been shown to be neutral in its effect on blood cholesterol (12). Stearic acid is rapidly converted in the body to oleic acid, a monounsaturated fatty acid. Chocolate is a rich source of stearic acid, but it also contains other saturated fats that do raise cholesterol. The chemical structure of stearic acid appears in Figure 7.1.

Unsaturated Fats

For many years, populations with relatively high intakes of unsaturated (as opposed to saturated) fats have been known to have lower blood pressures, lower glucose and cholesterol values, and lower rates of heart attack and stroke (13, 34). In controlled experiments, substituting unsaturated oils for saturated fats significantly lowered LDL cholesterol levels (14, 15). They also lower blood pressure by 6% to 10% (16, 17).

An excessive amount of unsaturated fat, however, is not necessarily better. The amount of calories derived from fats should be limited to 25% to 30% of the total daily intake (18). Margarine, for instance, is much less saturated than butter but is still 99% fat and thus should be limited.

The broad category of unsaturated fats is divided into monounsaturated fatty acids and polyunsaturated fatty acids. They are referred to as oils because they are liquid at room temperature. These are generally derived from plant sources. They are also present in smaller concentrations in meats and dairy products.

Polyunsaturated Fats

Polyunsaturated fats are categorized into either the omega-6 vegetable oils, which include sunflower, corn, safflower, soybean, and canola, or the omega-3 fish oils, eicosapentaenoic acid (EPA) and docosahexaenoic acid (DHA). Figure 7.3 illustrates this classification scheme.

Polyunsaturated fatty acids have two or more double bonds along the carbon backbone and even more hydrogen atoms absent.

Recent enthusiasm has highlighted the health benefits of the omega-3 polyunsaturates found in many cold-water fish. The fish oils EPA and DHA

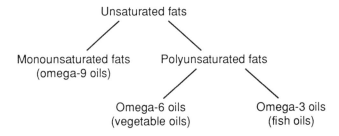

Figure 7.3 The basic classification scheme for dietary fats. Fats are grouped according to the degree of hydrogenation: either fully saturated, or mono- or polyunsaturated. They are further classified by the placement of the last double bond in the carbon chain. The double bond is three carbon atoms from the end in the omega-3 fatty acids (fish oils and certain land plants), six from the end in omega-6 polyunsaturates (some animal and most vegetable oils), and nine from the terminal carbon in monounsaturates (omega-9 oils).

seem to exert a protective effect on arteries, reduce clotting tendencies, and improve cholesterol and triglyceride levels. The health benefits of fish and other omega-3 oils are discussed in chapter 9.

Some animal experiments have raised concern that large amounts of polyunsaturated fats may possibly promote cancer. No evidence to date indicates that this occurs in humans; there are no populations known to consume large amounts of polyunsaturated fats. Nevertheless, polyunsaturated fats should contribute no more than 10% of total (daily) calories. Reducing total fat consumption will lower the overall risk of cancer, particularly cancer of the breast, colon, and prostate.

Monounsaturated Fats

Formerly thought to be neutral in respect to blood cholesterol, monounsaturated fatty acids have been credited with cholesterol-lowering properties when they replace saturated fatty acids (19). Mensink and Katan substituted monounsaturated fat for some of the saturated fat in the diet of 31 women and 27 men (20). The experimental diet had 15% of total calories from monounsaturated fats, 13% from saturated fats, and 8% from polyunsaturated fats. At the end of the 36-day trial, LDL levels had fallen an average of 18%.

Other benefits ascribed to these fats are that they lower blood pressure (21), blood glucose (34), decrease blood clotting tendencies, and protect the arterial walls from cholesterol influx (22). Furthermore, they lower LDL without appreciably lowering the beneficial HDL, as may diets high in polyunsaturates (23, 24) and carbohydrates (25).

In their chemical structure, monounsaturated fatty acids have a single double bond between carbon atoms, which displaces two hydrogen atoms (see Figure 7.1, center). When heat is applied during cooking, monounsaturates have less tendency to become saturated than polyunsaturates do (26).

Oleic acid is by far the most common monounsaturated fatty acid in nature. Olive oil is a particularly rich source of oleic acid, which helps explain why Mediterranean populations, which consume olive oil as their primary source of fat, have such low rates of hypertension, diabetes, and atherosclerosis. People living on the island of Crete, for example, obtain 40% of their calories from fat yet have very low cholesterol levels and rates of CHD (13). (Processed olives are also high in monounsaturated fatty acids but are extremely high in sodium.)

Other good sources of monounsaturates are canola oil (rapeseed), peanut oil, and avocados. Health-conscious shoppers have already noticed the presence of high-oleic safflower oil in an increasing number of health foods. At present, most Americans obtain the bulk of their monounsaturates from red meat, a source that frequently includes too much saturated fat and cholesterol. Cutting back on these sources will allow more liberal use of the other foods rich in monounsaturates.

Selecting Low-Fat Foods

The most important element in a heart-healthy diet is reducing the amount of dietary fat, especially saturated fat. The richest sources of saturated fats in common foods are red meats such as beef, pork, and lamb, and nonskim dairy products. Other high-fat foods are oils, spreads, and nuts, though these are frequently higher in polyunsaturated and mono-unsaturated fatty acids and thus less atherogenic.

Tables 7.1 to 7.4 categorize foods by poor, better, and best choices, relative to their fat content, for meats, dairy products, oils, and nuts/seeds, respectively.

Persons following the Step One and Step Two eating plans, which are discussed in chapter 10, can use these tables to help them stay within the guidelines of these plans. Step One limits fat consumption to 30% of total daily calories. Food choices in this plan include items from the "better" and "best" groups. Step Two, which limits fat consumption to about 25% of total daily calories, includes primarily "best choice" items. The "poor choice" column lists foods high in saturated fat, cholesterol, or both. These can be included on special occasions (once or twice a month) without adverse effect on serum cholesterol. Note that the food tables for fiber and fish in chapters 8 and 9 follow a similar pattern.

Cholesterol is found to varying degrees in all meats, dairy foods, and other animal products. Making "better" and "best" choices in these groups will automatically reduce dietary cholesterol. Some additional tips to trim dietary cholesterol include the following:

- Use only one to three egg yolks each week, including those in bakery products such as pies, cakes, custard, soufflés, crepes, blintzes, pancakes, and waffles (average: 1/4 to 1/2 yolk per serving).
- Avoid organ meats such as liver, kidney, sweetbreads, and brain.
- Minimize regular salad dressings and creams, including sour cream, ice cream, and cream cheese.
- Limit shrimp, lobster, and other shellfish to one serving a week or less (see Table 9.3, Fish chapter).

Meat Group

Meats are an excellent source of protein, B vitamins, iron, zinc, and other minerals. Vitamin B_{12} (cobalamin) is found only in animal products such as beef, chicken, fish, and dairy foods. The leanest sources of these foods are recommended (unless B_{12} supplementation is used).

Unfortunately, most cuts of beef, pork, and lamb are concentrated sources of saturated fat and cholesterol. The health impact is clear: People who regularly consume red meat have higher average blood pressure and LDL levels than vegetarians. Subsequently, they develop heart attack, stroke, and cancer twice as frequently as do vegetarians (27).

This does not mean that we must become vegetarians to be healthy. Cholesterol-lowering diets using lean meat have been developed (28). For hundreds of thousands of years, our Paleolithic ancestors hunted animals whose flesh made up a major part of their diet (29). But game meat contains only 6% to 7% fat (by weight), whereas domesticated beef is 20% to 30% fat or more (30).

If the beef industry succeeds in its plan to breed and raise cattle that have lower fat levels, we can be more liberal in our beef intake (9). At present, however, most beef and pork must be purchased as lean as possible and eaten in portions of only 3 to 4 ounces. Mutton still has a high fat content in nearly all cuts, except leg.

Successful cholesterol-lowering diets using lean red meat have been developed. Participants in an English study, for example, lowered their cholesterol levels by nearly 20%. Six ounces (170 gm) of well-trimmed, low-fat meat was included daily, but the total fat content was held to 27% of total calories. Also included was enough fiber to adhere to the Step One guidelines that are described in chapter 10 (28).

Shoppers should note that *prime* beef is the most expensive and the fattiest. Much of its fat is within the meat as marbling and thus cannot be trimmed (although some can be cooked out). *Choice* beef has less marbling, but more than *select* cuts, which are the leanest (*select* was formerly called *good*). Acceptable hamburger meat can be procured by purchasing ground lean round, sirloin, or any other lean cut. Most processed meats should be avoided, but acceptable brands may be available that have only 1 gm of fat per 30 calories. Table 7.1 lists the poor, better, and best choices for red meats and poultry relative to their fat content.

Adults should have no more than 6 ounces (170 gm) or two servings of meat a day. A serving of meat is not the typical 12-ounce sirloin found on restaurant menus—that is at least three servings! An adult serving of meat is 3 to 3-1/2 ounces (85 to 100 gm) or, when cooked, roughly the size of a deck of playing cards. (Meat loses approximately one fourth of its weight during cooking.) A small food scale is a useful tool to help people make accurate portion sizes (weights).

Examples of appropriate adult servings of meat include the following:

- 2 slices (4 × 2 × 1/4 inch or 10 × 5 × 0.6 cm) of any roasted or baked meat
- 1 medium loin chop cut 3/4 inch (2 cm) thick

Table 7.1 Meat Group: Poor, Better, and Best Choices[a]

Poor choices More than 50% of total calories from fat	Better choices Approximately 35%-50% of total calories from fat	Best choices Less than 35% of total calories from fat
Beef "Regular" ground beef, ground sirloin, spare ribs, short ribs, corned beef, brisket, meatballs, ribeye roast or steak cuts, all frozen creamed beef entrees, all USDA "Prime" cuts of beef with fat marbled throughout	**Beef** Flank steak, veal cutlets, rump roast, chuch roast (round bone), "lean" hamburger, cube steak, club steak, rib steak, T-bone steak, porterhouse steak, filet mignon, stew meat, short loin, tenderloin, USDA "Choice" cuts of beef with little fat marbling	**Beef[b]** Eye of round and full cut and top round, sirloin, sirloin tip, chipped beef, flank steak, lean veal, shank crosscuts, USDA "Select" cuts of beef with no fat marbling
Pork Spareribs, ground pork, pork sausage, bacon, Boston butt, shoulder butt, rump chuck	**Pork** Loin chops, roast cutlets, blade, shoulder (arm or picnic), Canadian bacon	**Pork** USDA "Select" center-cut ham (fresh and cured), tenderloin
Poultry Domestic goose and duck, self-basting chicken or turkey, processed poultry products like bologna and hot dogs	**Poultry** Chicken or turkey loaf, ground turkey (the skin is usually included), cornish hen without skin	**Poultry** Range fed chicken and turkey, especially white meat (without skin), canned poultry packed in water
Lamb Ground lamb patties, shoulder	**Lamb** Chops, roast	**Lamb** Leg
Very poor choices		
Processed meats Hot dogs, frankfurters, bologna, canned sandwich spreads, canned luncheon meats, knockwurst, bratwurst, organ meat such as brain and liver	**Processed meats** Turkey ham, sliced chicken or turkey	**Processed meats** Meats with no more than 1 gm of fat per ounce, 95% fat-free meats (by weight) such as lean boiled ham, chicken, or turkey

(Cont.)

Table 7.1   (Continued)

Poor choices More than 50% of total calories from fat	Better choices Approximately 35%-50% of total calories from fat	Best choices Less than 35% of total calories from fat
		Large Wild Game All
	Protein alternative Old-fashioned peanut butter	Protein alternatives Tofu, tempeh, or other soy products; egg whites or egg substitutes; all dried beans and legumes

ªBased on two 3-ounce servings per day.

ᵇEven these cuts may vary widely in fat content. To assure a healthy selection, choose only well-trimmed USDA "Select" cuts with little or no fat marbling.

Note. Meats need not be absolutely forbidden, only limited in their amount and frequency and cooked without frying.

- 1 lean ground beef patty 3 inches across and 1/2 inch (9 × 1 cm) thick when cooked (4 patties per pound, or 9 per kg, of raw meat)
- One piece (4 × 2 inches or 10 × 5 cm) of steak
- 3/4 cup (200 ml) diced meat or chicken (loosely packed)
- 3/4 cup (200 ml) cooked, flaked, or chopped meat or poultry
- Half a medium-sized chicken breast, skinned and cooked
- One chicken thigh plus one drumstick, skinned and cooked
- Two thin slices of lean roast beef (3 inches × 3 inches × 1/4 inch or 8 × 8 × 0.5 cm)

Dairy Group

Dairy foods are leading sources of calcium, protein, vitamins A and D, and some of the B-complex vitamins (riboflavin and B_{12}). Unfortunately, most are high in fat, especially saturated fat. Regular full-cream cheese gets 70% to 80% of its calories from fat, a percentage that is higher than in nearly all meats. Except for low-fat varieties, cheese intake should be minimized.

Cheese ranks as the second-major source of saturated fat in the American diet today. Though beef intake declined, per-capita consumption of cheese doubled between 1966 and 1986. The United Dairy Industry Association predicts that cheese intake may triple the 1966 level to more than 28 pounds per person per year by 1992 (31).

Many Americans are under the false impression that all dairy products are healthy. Table 7.2 shows that most dairy products fall outside the Step One and Step Two eating plans. Even the "better" choices have 3 to 5 gm of fat (mostly saturated) in a 1-ounce serving. The "best choice" cheeses have less than 3 gm of fat per serving. These are limited to a precious few—low-fat cottage cheese (including pot cheese or farmer's cheese), part-skim ricotta, and select brands of diet cheese.

Low-fat or nonfat dairy products have similar nutrients as whole-milk products. In fact, skim milk has even more calcium than whole milk.[1] The fat-soluble vitamins A and D are removed with the fat in the processing, then added back. These products are frequently labeled "fortified

---

[1]Other heart-healthy sources of calcium include low-fat yogurt; blackstrap molasses; almonds; broccoli; kale, spinach, and other greens; tofu; oysters; and canned sardines and salmon with bones.

Table 7.2 Dairy Group: Poor, Better, and Best Choices[a]

Poor choices	Better choices	Best choices
Whole milk, chocolate milk, goat milk, evaporated whole milk	Low-fat milk (2%), low-fat chocolate milk, soybean milk, low-fat buttermilk	Skim milk (1/2%-1%), evaporated skim or nonfat milk, artificially sweetened cocoa or milkshakes
Whole-milk yogurt	Low-fat yogurt, fruited or plain	Nonfat yogurt, fruited or plain
Ice cream, especially gourmet varieties	Low-fat ice cream and ice milk	Ice milk, frozen low-fat or nonfat yogurt, sherbet, sorbet
Cheeses (60%-70% fat calories or more than 5 gm of fat per serving)	(50%-60% fat calories or 3-5 gm of fat per serving)	(Less than 50% fat calories or 3 or fewer gm of fat per serving)
Creamed and regular cottage cheese, Jarlsberg, Parmesan, Feta, Camembert, Romano, Swiss, and most processed cheeses		

(Cont.)

Table 7.2   (Continued)

Poor choices	Better choices	Best choices
Very poor choices[b]		
Greater than 70% fat— Brie, brick, blue, Gorgonzola, Roquefort, cheddar, Colby, Edam, Gouda, Monterey Jack, Muenster, Havarti, New Holland cheeses, mozzarella and ricotta (whole milk), provolone, and cream cheese	Reduced fat cottage cheese[c], Kraft Light block cheese (cheddar, Colby, Swiss, and Monterey Jack); part-skim mozzarella, Parmesan, feta, Romano, and low-fat processed cheese	Low-fat (.5% or 1%) cottage cheese, part-skim cheese such as ricotta, all soy imitation "cheeses,"[d] and cheeses using fat substitutes

[a]Based on two to three servings a day.

[b]These food choices are very high in saturated fats and should be eaten very infrequently and in small portions. On days when one of these is eaten, cut back on one meat serving.

[c]Hoop cheese, pot cheese, and baker's cheese are virtually identical to cottage cheese and are available in .5% to 4% fat contents (by weight).

[d]Technically, the word "cheese" can apply only to milk-derived products. Though soy "cheese" may have up to 4 gm of fat per serving, it appears here because it is low in saturated fat and has no cholesterol.

Note. A serving of milk is one 8-ounce cup. A single cheese serving is 1 ounce, which is the size of a matchbox or one slice of processed cheese. As with meat, a 1-ounce serving of cheese is much smaller than the serving size to which we are accustomed.

with vitamins A and D." Imitation or filled milk contains many additives but only a fraction of the nutrients that milk has.

Most adults and children need two servings of dairy products daily. Teenagers, active adults, and pregnant or breastfeeding women need three servings. An adult serving is generally regarded as 1 ounce (28 gm) of cheese, 8 ounces (225 gm) of yogurt, or 1 cup (237 ml) of milk.

Although they are not dairy products per se, soybean "cheeses" such as Soya Kaas, Soy Nu, and others are excellent low-fat and cholesterol-free substitutes for cheese. They are produced in various flavors such as mozzarella, Monterey Jack, jalapeno, and cheddar.

Oils, Spreads, Nuts, and Seeds

Salad dressings, margarines, and nuts are usually very high in fat and calories and should be used sparingly. Fortunately, many products are now available that use unsaturated oils such as the soft or liquid margarines. Dressings labeled "diet" or "low-fat" contain less than 5 grams of fat per tablespoon (15 cc). Nuts are high in monounsaturated fat, which contributes to their high fat and calorie content.

Tables 7.3 and 7.4 show that the poorest choices in this section are products that contain large amounts of tropical oils. Although these are plant products and are free of cholesterol, many—such as coconut oil, palm oil, or palm kernel oil—contain alarming amounts of saturated fat.

Consumption of oils, spreads, and nut products, even those comprised largely of unsaturated fat, should stay within the total fat limits of the

Table 7.3 Oils and Spreads: Poor, Better, and Best Choices

Poor choices	Better choices	Best choices
Butter	Stick margarine	Squeeze or soft tub margarine
Lard or beef tallow, solid or hydrogenated vegetable shortening, palm oil, palm kernel oil, coconut oil	Most vegetable oils, including corn, safflower, sesame, cottonseed, walnut, soy, and sunflower oils	Canola and olive oils
Salad dressings with sour cream, egg yolks, and/or cheese	Reduced-calorie salad dressings (10-20 calories per tablespoon) using any of the better-choice oils	Low-calorie dressings (less than 10 calories per tablespoon), vinegar
Cream and sour cream		Nonfat yogurt, blenderized low-fat cottage cheese
Regular meat gravies, butter sauces, or white cream sauces	Low-fat sour cream substitutes such as Hood Light, Lean Cream	Gravies made without fat
Regular mayonnaise, tartar sauce	Gravies made with low-fat ingredients	Canola or soy mayonnaise
Hydrogenated nut butters	"Light" mayonnaise	Tahini, almond or other nut butters, apple butter, honey, jams, jellies, preserves
Liver pate, nondairy creamers, chocolate or cocoa butter	Freshly ground peanut butter or peanut butter in which the oil separates to the top	Avocado
	Black olives, green olives	

Note. Choosing from the "better" and "best" columns will help lower serum cholesterol. The "poor" choices are high in saturated fat, cholesterol, or both and have the greatest propensity to raise blood cholesterol. A serving in the oils group is 1 teaspoon (15 ml) unless otherwise stated, and provides 45 calories, though smaller quantities are recommended (32).

Table 7.4   Nuts and Seeds: Poor, Better, and Best Choices

Poor choices	Better choices	Best choices
Coconut and macadamia	Brazil nuts, pecans, pinenuts, and cashews	Almonds, filberts (hazelnuts), peanuts, and pistachios
Sugared or salted roasted nuts	Dry roasted seeds, including sunflower, sesame, and pumpkin	Walnuts (high in monounsaturates)

Note. Nuts and seeds are high in fiber and other nutrients but still very high in fat. The better and best choices here are heart healthy but must be used in moderation because of their high fat content.

Step One or Step Two plans. Instead of high-fat foods, choose items from the other groups, especially the fruits, grains, and vegetables. Substituting saturated fat with protein or carbohydrate has been shown by angiography to have a greater effect in preventing atherosclerotic plaque than if the saturated fat is substituted with polyunsaturated or monounsaturated fat (33). Other fat-reducing tips include

- adding equal amounts of water to dressing; mix in blender,
- experimenting with flavored vinegars, such as Balsamic, herb, or raspberry, and
- pouring off the oil layer in nut butters and replacing it with applesauce or juice.

A nutritious diet is the first and most basic vehicle to reducing blood cholesterol and its associated risk of CHD, stroke, and peripheral vascular disease. As with other lifestyle improvements, changing one's eating pattern is best done gradually.

The average American needs to cut back on cholesterol and total fat intake by at least one third of the present consumption and reduce saturated fat by one third to one half. This will reduce blood cholesterol levels an average of 30% to 40%—enough to dramatically curtail atherosclerosis. Though medications may be necessary in addition to these guidelines, eating a healthy diet can only benefit an individual.

References

1. American Heart Association. (1988). Position statement. Dietary guidelines for healthy American adults. *Circulation, 69*, 721A-724A.
2. Expert Panel of the National Cholesterol Education Program. (1988). Report of the National Cholesterol Education Program Expert Panel

on detection, evaluation, and treatment of high blood cholesterol in adults. *Archives of Internal Medicine*, **148**, 36-39.

3. American Heart Association. (1984). Special report. Recommendations for treatment of hyperlipidemia in adults. *Circulation*, **69**, 1065A-1090A.

4. Grundy, S.M. (1987a). Dietary therapy for different forms of hyper-lipoproteinemia. *Circulation*, **76**, 523-528.

5. Keys, A., Anderson, J.T., & Grande, F. (1965). Serum cholesterol response to changes in the diet. *Metabolism*, **14**, 747-787.

6. Puska, P., Nissinen, A., Vartiainen, E., Dougherty, R., Mutanen, M., Iacano, J.M., Korhonen, H.J., Pietinen, P., Leino, U., Moisio, S., & Huttunen, J. (1983). Controlled, randomized trial of the effect of dietary fat on blood pressure. *Lancet*, **1**, 4-5.

7. Jakubowski, J.A., & Ardlie, N.G. (1978). Modification of human platelet function by a diet enriched in saturated or polyunsaturated fat. *Atherosclerosis*, **31**, 335-344.

8. Grundy, S.M., Bilheimer, D., Blackburn, H., Brown, W.U., Kwitervich, P.O., Jr., Mattson, F., Schonfeld, G., & Weidman, W.H. (1982). Rationale for the diet-heart statement of the American Heart Association. *Circulation*, **65**, 839A-854A.

9. Committee on Technological Options to Improve the Nutritional Attributes of Animal Products. (1988). *Board of Agriculture*, National Research Council. Designing foods. Animal product options in the marketplace. Washington, DC: National Academy Press.

10. U.S. Department of Agriculture, Human Nutrition Information Service. (1981). *Nutritive Value of Foods*. Home and Garden Bulletin Number 72. Washington, DC: U.S. Government Printing Office, p. 16.

11. Grundy, S.M. (1986a). Cholesterol and coronary heart disease: A new era. *Journal of the American Medical Association*, **256**, 2849-2858.

12. Bonanome, A., & Grundy, S. (1988). Effect of dietary stearic acid on plasma cholesterol and lipoprotein levels. *New England Journal of Medicine*, **318**, 1244-1248.

13. Keys, A. (1970). Coronary heart disease in seven countries. *Circulation*, **41**(Suppl. 1), 1-211.

14. Nichaman, M.Z., & Hamm, P. (1987). Low-fat, high-carbohydrate diets and plasma cholesterol. *American Journal of Clinical Nutrition*, **45**, 1155-1160.

15. Ehnholm, C., Huttunen, J.K., Pietinen, P., Leino, U., Mutanen, M., Kostiainen, E., Iacono, J.M., Dougherty, R., & Puska, P. (1984). Effect of a diet low in saturated fatty acids on plasma lipids, lipoproteins, and HDL subfractions. *Arteriosclerosis*, **4**, 265-269.

16. Rouse, I., Armstrong, B., Beilin, L.J., & Vandingen, R. (1983). Blood-pressure-lowering effect of a vegetarian diet: Controlled trial in norma-tive subjects. *Lancet*, **1**, 5-6.

17. Smith-Barbaro, P.A., & Pucak, G.J. (1983). Dietary fat and blood pressure. *Annals of Internal Medicine, 98,* 828-831.

18. Brussaard, J.H., Katan, M.B., Groot, P.H.E., Havekes, L.M., & Houtvast, J.G.A.J. (1982). Serum lipoproteins of healthy persons fed a low-fat diet or a polyunsaturated fat diet for three months. A comparison of two cholesterol-lowering diets. *Atherosclerosis, 42,* 205-219.

19. Grundy, S.M. (1986b). Comparison of monounsaturated fatty acids and carbohydrates for lowering plasma cholesterol. *New England Journal of Medicine, 314,* 745-748.

20. Mensink, R.P., & Katan, M.B. (1989). Effect of a diet enriched with monounsaturated or polyunsaturated fatty acids on levels of low-density and high-density lipoprotein cholesterol in healthy women and men. *The New England Journal of Medicine, 321,* 436-441.

21. Williams, P.T., Fortmann, S.P., Terry, R.B., Garay, S.C., Vranizan, K.M., Ellsworth, N., & Wood, P.D. (1987). Associations of dietary fat, regional adiposity, and blood pressure in men. *Journal of the American Medical Association, 257,* 3251.

22. Stender, S., Leth-Espensen, P., & Kjeldsen, K. (1987). Olive oil inhibits atherogenesis in cholesterol fed rabbits by a mechanism not mediated through changes in plasma cholesterol concentrations. *Circulation, 76,* IV-34.

23. Grundy, S.M. (1987b). Monounsaturated fatty acids, plasma cholesterol, and coronary heart disease. *American Journal of Clinical Nutrition, 45,* 1168-1175.

24. Mattson, F.H., & Grundy, S.M. (1985). Comparison of effects of dietary saturated, monounsaturated, and polyunsaturated fatty acids on plasma lipids and lipoproteins in man. *Journal of Lipid Research, 26,* 194-202.

25. Mensink, R.P., & Katan, M.B. (1987). Effect of monounsaturated fatty acids versus complex carbohydrates on high-density lipoproteins in healthy men and women. *Lancet, 1,* 122.

26. O'Keefe, J.H., Jr., Lavie, C.J., & O'Keefe, J.O. (1989). Dietary prevention of coronary artery disease. *Postgraduate Medicine, 85,* 243-261.

27. Sacks, F.M., Donner, A., Castelli, W.P., Gronemeyer, J., Pletka, P., Margolius, H.S., Landsberg, L., & Kass, E.H. (1981). Effect of ingestion of meat on plasma cholesterol of vegetarians. *Journal of the American Medical Association, 246,* 640-644.

28. Watts, G.F., Ahmed, W., Quiney, J., Houlston, R., Jackson, P., Iles, C., & Lewis, B. (1988). Effective lipid lowering diets including lean meat. *British Medical Journal, 296,* 235-237.

29. Eaton, S.B., & Konner, M. (1985). Paleolithic nutrition. *New England Journal of Medicine, 312,* 283-289.

30. Illingworth, D.R., & Connor, S.L. (1987). Cholesterol content of game

meat. (Questions and answers). *Journal of the American Medical Association*, **258**, 1532.

31. United Dairy Industry Association. (1988). Cheese varieties and types 1968-1987 per capita civilian consumption trends and extensions to 1992. Rosemont, IL: United Dairy Industry Association.

32. American Diabetes Association & American Dietetic Association. (1989). *Exchange Lists for Meal Planning*. Alexandria, VA.

33. Blankenhorn, D.H., Johnson, R.L., Mack, W.J., El Zein, H.A., & Vailas, L.I. (1990). The influence of diet on the appearance of new lesions in human coronary arteries. *Journal of the American Medical Association*, **263**, 1646-1652.

34. Trevisan, M., Krogh, V., Freudenheim, J., Blake, A., Muti, P., Panico, S., Farinaro, E., Mancini, M., Menotti, A., Ricci, G., & the Research Group ATS-RF2 of the Italian National Research Council. (1990). Consumption of olive oil, butter, and vegetable oils and coronary disease risk factors. *Journal of the American Medical Association*, **263**, 688-692.

Chapter

8

Fiber

Dietary fiber is now a prominent topic in human nutrition. Because fiber is indigestible and thus not a nutrient, it has been mistakenly dismissed in the past as having no health benefits. Today, most health professionals and even laypersons realize that high-fiber foods help alleviate and prevent intestinal problems. Not as well known, however, is that soluble fiber can lower serum cholesterol by as much as 25%, cutting the risk of heart attack in half.

The pioneering work of Burkitt and Trowell in the 1960s introduced this neglected dietary component to the medical community. Working in Africa, they were impressed by the rarity of the chronic diseases that are so common in advanced societies. Heredity didn't explain the difference, because tribe members who moved into cities and adopted modern lifestyles soon began to develop these diseases as well (1, 2).

By making extensive comparisons of differences in diets, they hypothesized that fiber-depleted diets were at least partially responsible. During the 1960s and 1970s, they and other investigators found an association between low-fiber diets and coronary heart disease, hypertension, cancer, obesity, and a variety of gastrointestinal diseases.

Fiber, as well as dietary fat, was an early suspect to explain some of the widely varying CHD rates between countries (3, 4). Advanced societies that consume refined foods have higher cholesterol levels and more atherosclerosis. In a review of 20 countries, Japan had the highest fiber intake and the lowest CHD rate (5). The United States had the lowest fiber intake and the highest CHD rate. Autopsy studies revealed that groups consuming more fiber had less extensive coronary atherosclerosis (6).

Surveys within populations also indicate that dietary fiber has a cardio-protective effect. In the Netherlands, researchers determined that people who consumed the least amount of cereals had four times more heart attacks than those in the high-fiber group (these two groups made up the lower and upper thirds of the sample) (7). This finding was duplicated in the United States by a study following men of Irish descent (8). Vegetarians seem to be spared heart disease as a result of their high fiber intakes as well as their low consumption of saturated fats and cholesterol (9-12).

Even more convincing were clinical trials in which fiber supplementation helped reduce atherosclerosis (13, 14). Fiber has greatly facilitated the control of other chronic diseases including diabetes (15), hypertension (16, 17), and obesity (18).

Definition of Fiber

Fiber is that part of food not broken down by the body in digestion. It has also been called "roughage" or "bulk." Burkitt and Trowell found that the daily stool output of rural Africans weighed over one pound (470 gm) compared to 3.8 ounces (108 gm) in the British. Fiber and moisture accounted for the difference in weight.

How fiber came to be measured is an intriguing story in itself. When food was analyzed by chemical methods, fiber was originally defined as the residue present after the food had been boiled in strong acid and alkali. It was then called crude fiber, aptly named considering this rough method of analysis. We now know that this chemical digestion destroyed the type of fiber responsible for lowering blood cholesterol—the soluble kind. Thus the analysis underestimated the total fiber present, particularly the heart-healthy variety found in fruits, beans, and oats.

In the early 1970s chemists developed techniques to analyze food for all its fiber, opening a new door into fiber research. We now know that there are two basic categories of dietary fiber, soluble and insoluble, based on the physical ability to dissolve in water. Each has physiological qualities that complement the other's. Insoluble fiber, found in plant cell walls, primarily helps intestinal problems. Soluble fiber, found in oats, beans, and fruits, helps control diabetes and blood cholesterol.

In 1984 the new system of measuring all the fiber in food, now termed total dietary fiber, was officially accepted by the U.S. Food and Drug Administration. This was a boon not only to researchers but also to consumers interested in healthy food choices. Food labels began to list information about total dietary fiber. The older, outdated listing of crude fiber is still on many packages, but this accounts for insoluble fiber only.

Food sources do not contain just one class of fiber but rather a mixture of the two, usually with a preponderance of one kind or the other. Because soluble and insoluble fiber differ slightly in their health effects, a healthy diet includes both types.

The insoluble fibers are so named because they are insoluble in water. They include the celluloses, hemicelluloses, and lignin. In the body, they cause the food to move more rapidly through the intestine, encouraging regularity. These fibers are found within the plant cell wall. This is why wheat bran (which includes the outer coating of the kernel) and the skins of fruits and vegetables are such good fiber sources.

Highly refined foods are digested so completely that only a small residue remains in the intestine. For purely mechanical reasons, a smaller caliber stool requires greater effort to move through the bowels. This in turn promotes constipation, diverticulosis, hemorrhoids, and cancer.

Burkitt found that food eaten by the Africans took 36 hours to traverse the length of the digestive tract, whereas in Britain it took 77 hours. By remaining undigested, insoluble fiber adds bulk to the stool, expediting its passage along 23 feet of intestines. This gives the colon (large intestine) less time to reabsorb water from the stool.

Because it makes bowel movements larger, softer, and therefore able to pass with more ease and regularity, insoluble fiber prevents constipation, hemorrhoids, and diverticulosis. Diverticulosis is an outpouching at weak areas along the walls of the colon caused by chronically higher pressures within it. When pieces of food material become trapped in the pouches, or diverticuli, they become inflamed and result in diverticulitis. This is a common cause of abdominal pain in older Americans, over half of whom have colon diverticuli.

Insoluble fiber, and perhaps soluble fiber as well, also protects against gallstones, peptic ulcers, overweight, colitis, irritable bowel syndrome, hypertension, and breast cancer (19). Excellent sources of insoluble fiber are wheat bran, whole wheat, pears, and peas.

Because insoluble fiber was the first kind of fiber to have its health benefits described in the medical literature, we have come to associate ''fiber'' primarily with wheat bran, which is rich in insoluble fiber only. Water-soluble fiber, however, has the greatest potential for controlling blood cholesterol and diabetes and preventing atherosclerosis. Health professionals and the general public need to become familiar with the properties and sources of soluble fiber as well.

Subcategories of soluble fiber are the pectins, gums, and mucilages. Pectins are abundant in bananas, oranges, carrots, and apples. Because of their gelling property, they have been used for centuries in the preparation of jams. Gums are found in dried beans and grains such as oats, rye, and barley. Guar gum, derived from the seed of the Indian cluster bean *Cyamopsis tetragonoloba*, is used as a thickener in sauces and a stabilizer in many commercially prepared foods.

The third subclass of soluble fiber is the mucilages, found in psyllium seed products (such as Metamucil) that are commonly used to treat constipation. They can lower LDL 10% to 20% or more when several grams are used (20, 21). As a supplement to dietary sources of soluble fiber, psyllium may have a role in cholesterol therapy alongside the bile acid sequestrants. Both have a similar mechanism of action in reducing cholesterol levels.

How Soluble Fiber Affects Cholesterol

Soluble fiber is thought to exert its effect at least partially by reducing the intestinal absorption of bile acids and dietary cholesterol. The fibers absorb water in the stomach, which imparts a gel-like consistency to the food. The gelling insulates the food somewhat from digestive enzymes, and slightly less cholesterol is absorbed (22, 23).

Soluble fiber also binds the cholesterol-rich bile in the lower small intestine. Normally 97% of the total bile output, including about 1,000 mg of cholesterol a day, is reabsorbed by the lower small intestine. By binding with bile acids, the soluble fiber interrupts this enterohepatic retrieval system (24). The liver then starts pulling cholesterol out of the bloodstream, reducing its concentration.

Another proposed mechanism is that soluble fiber decreases the rate at which the liver produces its own cholesterol. It is thought that certain by-products of soluble fiber (probably short-chain fatty acids) directly inhibit cholesterol synthesis in the liver (25, 26).

In 1975, Jenkins and co-workers in London reported a dramatic lowering of subjects' cholesterol levels by supplementing their diets with 36 gm of guar or 30 gm of pectin per day. After only 2 weeks, cholesterol levels were lowered 30 mg/dl by pectin and 36 mg/dl by guar gum in spite of the high quantities of meat, eggs, and dairy products in the subjects' typical British diet. The subjects' cholesterol levels changed from an average 230 mg/dl before the fiber was added to under 200 mg/dl afterward (6 to 5.1 mmol/L). Their risk of heart attack dropped from borderline high to desirable (NIH definition) with this single dietary change. The fiber-cholesterol connection was strengthened further when the subjects' cholesterol levels rose again after the soluble fiber was withdrawn from their diet (27).

Even more striking results were obtained when Anderson combined high-fiber foods with foods that were also reduced in fat and cholesterol (28). After 21 days of a low-fat diet supplemented with 17 gm daily of soluble fiber, subjects achieved a 20% drop in total cholesterol and a 24% decrease in LDL cholesterol. When subjects were followed for longer than 3 weeks, the cholesterol levels continued to fall to 30%. HDL eventually rose 10%.

Thirty grams of soluble fiber a day has been successful in reducing total cholesterol by up to 25% and LDL by up to 30% (28, 30, 31). Statistically, such a decrease reduces the risk of heart attack by 50%.

Another bonus of making fiber a staple in the diet is that beneficial HDL cholesterol may eventually increase. Some of Anderson's subjects were followed for almost 2 years, and at the end of this period their HDL cholesterol levels were a third higher (10 mg/dl or 0.3 mmol/L). This long-term benefit to HDL had not been generally recognized before, because most fiber studies had been completed within 2 months (33).

Fiber and Diabetes Control

Fiber should be an integral part of every diabetic's diet for improving blood glucose control. Soluble fiber helps to stabilize blood sugar by slowing the absorption of carbohydrate (starches and sugars), thereby acting as a time-release mechanism (29, 32, 34). Because unprocessed food breaks down more slowly, the rise in blood glucose after a meal is more gradual and less of a shock to the body's regulatory system. Beans and lentils seem to blunt the blood sugar and insulin surge more effectively than do oats (33). Insoluble fiber may assist diabetic control by speeding the movement of the food, spreading its absorption over a greater length of intestine (35).

At the University of Kentucky, Anderson has used high-fiber diets successfully for many years to treat diabetics. Patients with Type I (juvenile onset) diabetes have been able to decrease their insulin dosage by 30% to 40%. Of the Type II (adult onset) patients who had required insulin, 80% were able to discontinue their injections (15). Almost 90% of the diabetics who had been taking pills for glucose control were withdrawn from all medication.

In Philadelphia, adult-onset diabetics followed by Ray and associates gained control over their diabetes and cholesterol by adding 20 gm of guar gum and 10 gm of wheat bran to their daily diets (36). Their fasting blood glucose levels fell from an average of 301 to 184 mg/dl (16.7 to 10.2 mmol/L), while blood cholesterol levels fell from 277 to 193 mg/dl (7.2 to 5.0 mmol/L) during the two months of the study.

By eating foods rich in soluble fiber, the diabetic almost immediately becomes more sensitive to insulin and requires less medication. Thus, when a diabetic person increases soluble fiber intake, the physician should closely follow him or her to adjust dosages as necessary.

Diabetics with high blood triglycerides (hypertriglyceridemia) also may benefit from a fiber-enriched diet. The decrease in triglycerides varies with each individual but ranges between 10% and 25%. The rise in triglyceride levels after a meal is affected even more than the fasting level.

Weight Control and Other Benefits

In experiments using fiber to control blood glucose or cholesterol, some subjects lost weight without consciously trying. Inadvertently, the investigators discovered that fiber aids in weight control by increasing satiety. When the soluble fiber soaks up water in the stomach, it takes longer to move out into the intestine. This gives a more rapid, more noticeable, and longer lasting feeling of fullness (18, 25, 37).

Weight reduction, in turn, augments fiber's tendency to control serum cholesterol, blood pressure, and diabetes. In the National Diet Heart Study, persons who lost as little as 10 pounds were able to boost fiber's cholesterol-lowering ability (38). Weight loss is also promoted by fiber-rich foods because they are generally low in calories and take longer to chew.

Another benefit is that fiber has a modest tendency to lower both systolic and diastolic blood pressure (17, 39, 40). It also helps protect against some of the most common cancers in America, including colon, breast, uterus, lung, oral cavity, larynx, esophagus, stomach, bladder, and prostate (7, 41, 42).

Recommendations for Fiber Intake

Most of us should double our fiber intake from the current average of 10 to 20 gm to at least 40 gm a day. Specific recommendations for dietary fiber vary, and as yet it has no Recommended Dietary Allowance (RDA). But many health organizations, including the American Cancer Society, the National Cancer Institute, the American Heart Association, and the Senate Select Committee on Nutrition and Human Needs, are calling for an increase in dietary fiber.

The National Cancer Insitute currently recommends 20 to 30 gm of fiber a day for the general public. Some clinicians recommend a total of 40 to 60 gm a day for people with high blood cholesterol, diabetes, or constipation. For smaller persons or those on low-calorie diets, the recommended amount is 20 to 30 gm of fiber for every 1,000 calories eaten (26).

The optimum ratio of soluble to insoluble fiber depends on individual health status. For most Americans, especially those with cholesterol levels above 180 mg/dl (4.7 mmol/L), preventing atherosclerosis is best achieved by consuming more soluble fiber. Individuals with hypercholesterolemia or diabetes should consume fiber in a ratio of at least one soluble to three insoluble. For those plagued by constipation, hemorrhoids, or diverticulosis or who have a family history of colon cancer, insoluble fiber is more important. Table 8.1 lists the amounts of total and soluble fiber in a number of fiber-rich foods.

Many people find it difficult to obtain these higher quantities of fiber with our current food sources. I recommend that anyone with borderline or high blood cholesterol attempt as a realistic goal to reach 40 gm of total fiber per day, 10 gm of which should be soluble. This has been included in the Step One eating plan described in chapter 10.

The goal of 40 gm of fiber a day can easily be achieved by eating more whole grains, beans, and fruits; for example, two slices of whole-wheat bread, one ounce (30 gm) of high fiber cereal, one unpeeled apple or pear, five figs or prunes, and a serving each of broccoli and beans.

Table 8.1 Foods Highest in Soluble and Total Fiber Per Gram and Per Serving

Food	Fiber g/100g Total	Soluble	Serving size	Grams/serving	Soluble fiber/serving
Cereals					
All Bran	30.8	5.1	1/3 c	28	1.4
Heartwise	20.3	10.5	1 c	28	2.9
Oat bran, uncooked	14.4	7.2	1/3 c	28	2.0
Oat Bran Crunch	16.4	9.3	1/2 c	28	2.6
Oat bran hot cereal with apples and cinnamon, uncooked	8.8	4.8	1/4 c	28	1.3
Oatmeal, uncooked	9.5	4.9	1/3 c	28	1.4
Grains					
Barley, pearl, uncooked	11.8	3.4	2 T	25	0.9
Flour, oat	9.5	5.5	2-1/2 T	19	1.0
Flour, rye	12.9	3.9	2-1/2 T	20	0.8
Macaroni, whole wheat, uncooked	9.0	2.1	1/4 c	26	0.5
Wheat bran	41.0	3.4	1/2 c	30	1.0
Wheat germ	17.5	3.2	3 T	22	0.7

(Cont.)

189

Table 8.1 (Continued)

Food	Fiber g/100g		Serving size	Grams/ serving	Soluble fiber/ serving
	Total	Soluble			
Breads & Crackers					
Bread, cellulose	9.9	1.1	2 slices	46	0.5
Bread, pumpernickel	8.4	3.9	1 slice	32	1.2
Bread, rye	6.6	3.0	1 slice	28	0.8
Bread, whole wheat	5.5	1.2	1 slice	28	0.3
Crackers, whole wheat	10.9	1.8	4	18	0.3
Melba toast, wheat	8.9	1.8	5 slices	20	0.4
Fruits					
Apricots, dried	7.9	4.4	7 halves	25	1.1
Blackberries, fresh	3.4	1.0	3/4 c	108	1.1
Dates, dried	4.4	1.2	2-1/2 medium	21	0.3
Figs, dried	8.2	4.0	1-1/2	28	1.1
Mango, fresh	2.8	1.6	1/2 small	104	1.7
Prunes, dried	6.6	3.8	3 medium	25	1.0

Vegetables

Broccoli, cooked	3.1	1.5	1/2 c	78	1.2
Brussels sprouts, cooked	4.9	2.5	1/2 c	78	2.0
Cabbage, winter, fresh	3.8	2.8	1 c	70	1.4
Parsnip, cooked	4.2	2.3	1/2 c	78	1.8
Peas, frozen, cooked	5.4	1.6	1/2 c	80	1.3
Turnip, cooked	6.1	2.2	1/2 c	78	1.7

Legumes

Black beans, cooked	7.1	2.8	1/2 c	86	2.4
Butter beans, cooked	7.3	2.9	1/2 c	94	2.7
Chick peas, cooked	5.3	1.6	1/2 c	82	1.3
Kidney beans, dark red, cooked	7.8	3.2	1/2 c	88	2.8
Navy beans, cooked	7.1	2.4	1/2 c	91	2.2
Pinto beans, cooked	6.9	2.2	1/2 c	85	1.9

Concentrated fibers

Citrucel	33.3	33.3	1 T	6	2.0
Citrus pectin	55.4	55.2	1 T	10	5.5
Effer-syllium	35.0	26.7	1 t	7	1.9
Flax fiber	33.8	13.0	2 T	17	2.2
Metamucil, sugar-free	74.5	65.2	1 t	4	2.6

Note. From Anderson, James W., M.D. *Plant Fiber in Foods.* (1990). HCF Nutrition Research Foundation, Inc., P.O. Box 22124, Lexington, Kentucky, 40522, 1986.

Oats and beans, rich in soluble fiber, are approximately equal to each other in their cholesterol-lowering effect. A dramatic improvement of blood cholesterol can be achieved simply by including a half cup (120 cc) of oat bran or a half cup of beans (red, kidney, pinto, and others) into the daily diet (43-45). Smaller quantities of oats and beans are needed if an individual also eats fresh or dried fruits, which are good sources of pectin. (Capsules of processed fiber supplements are not recommended except under special circumstances as advised by the treating physician.)

Selecting High-Fiber Foods

Fiber plays an important role in human nutrition despite the fact that it is not a true nutrient. People who need to increase daily fiber intake to 40 gm can achieve this by eating four to six servings of fiber-rich foods each day. One way to help clients with this dietary change is to suggest that they eat more of the high-fiber foods they like, and then introduce other high-fiber foods with which they may be unfamiliar. Chapter 10, page 221, offers more tips.

Table 8.2　Fruit Group: Poor, Better, and Best Choices for Soluble Fiber

Poor choices	Better choices	Best choices
Grapes, melon, fruit juices*, fruit drinks, ades, punch	Fresh apples, bananas, blackberries, boysen-berries, raspberries, cranberries, rhubarb, cherries, pineapple, apricots, mangos	Fresh fruit in season, especially those high in soluble fiber: citrus fruits, dates, figs, granadilla (passion fruit), pears, plums, prunes, peaches, and currants
Candied fruits, fruit canned in heavy syrup, frozen fruit with added sugar	Fruit canned in light syrup, sweetened applesauce, sweetened dried or sulfured fruits (check label), pure and unsweetened juices	Canned fruit in water or juice, unsweetened applesauce, plain (unsulfured) dried fruit, unsweetened frozen fruit

*These are not unhealthy but are listed here because they are relatively low in soluble fiber.

Note. Most in the better column and many in the poor column are high in vitamins and carbohydrates, if not fiber.

The transition to fiber-fich foods should be gradual to avoid problems such as bloating, gas, cramps, or diarrhea. If at least some fiber is incorporated into all meals, the digestive system will become accustomed to it, and these side effects will be minimized. Consuming the entire day's supply of fiber in one sitting or, worse, the entire week's supply in one day is much more likely to cause bloating and flatulence.

Excellent sources of fiber include fresh and dried fruits, grains, legumes (peas, beans), and vegetables. These foods are also low in fat and high in vitamins, potassium, and other minerals. The legume group is a good source of protein as well. The best sources for soluble fiber include rolled oats, oat bran, beans, barley, psyllium seeds, and citrus fruits.

Tables 8.2, 8.3, and 8.4 list fiber-rich foods in the fruit, grain/legume, and vegetable food groups. As with the fatty food groups, the healthiest selections are in the "better choice" and "best choice" categories. People

Table 8.3 Grain, Starchy Vegetable, and Legume Group: Poor, Better, and Best Choices for Soluble Fiber

Poor choices	Better choices	Best choices
	Breads and Grains	
Artificially colored wheat bread, low-calorie diet bread, commercial quick breads, doughnuts, butter rolls, egg bagels, cheese breads	Whole-wheat, sprouted, cracked-wheat, multi-grain breads, rolls, buns, or muffins[a]	Cereals, granola, breads, rolls, or muffins made with oats, oat bran, rolled oats, whole cornmeal, dark rye, barley
Flour tortillas made with saturated fats, pre-fried corn tortillas	Flour tortillas, corn or blue corn tortillas made with nonhydrogenated oil	Vegetable soups, including gazpacho, onion, and tomato (1 cup per serving)
	Cereals	
Highly sugared commercial cereals, processed hot cereals, commercial granola-type cereals made with saturated oils (usually these have 4 or more grams of fat per serving)	Most dry cereals made with "white" or "wheat" flour, usually with 1 to 2 gm of fat per serving; instant hot cereals[a]	Some high-fiber commercial cereals, such as All-Bran or Heartwise oat bran (Kellogg's), corn bran, Bran Chex or Bran Buds, 100% bran, Grape Nuts (General Foods), puffed wheat, wheat germ

(Cont.)

Table 8.3 (Continued)

Poor choices	Better choices	Best choices
Crackers		
Most snack crackers like cheese crackers or butter crackers, which are made with saturated oils; potato chips, Cheetos; most microwave popcorn	Crackers that use acceptable non-hydrogenated oils	Whole-grain and low-fat crackers like graham and matzo, bread sticks, Rye Krisp, zwiebacks, oyster, flat-breads, crisp breads, pretzels, rice cakes
Legumes		
Refried beans made with lard or hydrogenated fats, beans with pork or franks		All dried beans, especially navy, kidney, pinto, and black beans; soybeans, black-eyed peas, chick-peas, split peas, and lentils; vegetarian refried beans with no hydrogenated fat used; quinoa, amaranth[b]
Mixes		
Commercial pancakes, biscuits, waffles, baking mixes, French toast	Homemade pancakes and waffles made with acceptable oils	Low-fat pancakes, French toast, or waffles made with egg whites, whole-wheat or oat bread
Pasta and rice		
Artificially colored pasta mixes; pasta prepared with cream, butter, or cheese sauces; egg noodles, chow mein noodles	White rice, instant rice	Brown or wild rice, basmati rice, millet, barley (steamed or boiled), unbuttered popcorn
Prepackaged seasoned rice mixes, fried rice	White enriched pasta (macaroni, spaghetti, manicotti, etc.)	Vegetable or whole-grain pasta

Poor choices	Better choices	Best choices
	Vegetables	
Starchy vegetables with cheese or butter sauces, canned vegetables	Frozen starchy vegetables, "instant" potatoes, packaged potato mixes	All fresh starchy vegetables such as corn, hominy, mixed vegetables, peas, potatoes, pumpkin, winter squash
Commercially fried potatoes, onion rings	Potatoes fried in acceptable oils	Baked potatoes, baked French "fries"

[a]These are not listed as "best choice" because they are not high in soluble fiber.
[b]These beans are a complete protein source and can be used alone as substitutes for meat.

Table 8.4 Vegetable Group: Poor, Better, and Best Choices for Fiber

Poor choices	Better choices	Best choices
Frozen vegetables with butter, cream, or other sauces; breaded and fried vegetables	Fresh or frozen vegetables (plain) such as artichoke, asparagus, beets, green or yellow beans, beets, garden cress, leeks, mushrooms, mustard greens, okra, onion, parsley, potato (with skin), rutabaga, squash, tomatoes, spinach, cucumbers[a]	Fresh vegetables in season, especially those high in soluble fiber and vitamins: broccoli, brussels sprouts, carrots, cabbage (especially Chinese), cauliflower, corn, kale, parsnips, peas, turnips, and yams
Low-fiber vegetables: celery, chicory, collards, cucumbers, eggplant, iceberg lettuce, green or red pepper, sweet potato (canned), pumpkin, radishes		
Canned creamed vegetables, high-salt vegetables: pickles, sauerkraut, cole slaw, pickled vegetables, most commercial vegetable juices	Canned plain vegetables, drained of canning water; vegetable juices, unsalted	

[a]These vegetables may be rich in vitamins but are low in soluble fiber.
Note. Avocados and olives have been placed in the Oils and Spreads Group because of their high fat content.

following the Step One eating plan can select fairly evenly between the "better" and "best" columns. Those on the Step Two eating plan should choose primarily from the "best choice" category. The "poor choice" foods contain little or no fiber and are often high in sugar, salt, and preservatives.

References

1. Burkitt, D.P., & Trowell, H.C. (1975). *Refined carbohydrate foods and disease*. New York: Academic Press.
2. Trowell, H.C. (1978). The development of the concept of dietary fiber in human nutrition. *American Journal of Clinical Nutrition, 31*, S3-S11.
3. Morris, J.N., Marr, J.W., & Clayton, D.G. (1977). Diet and heart: A postscript. *British Medical Journal, 2*, 1307-1314.
4. Keys, A., Grande, F., & Anderson, J.T. (1961). Fiber and pectin in the diet and serum cholesterol in man. *Proceedings of the Society of Experimental Biology of New York, 106*, 555-8.
5. Liu, K., Stamler, J., Trevisan, M., & Moss, D. (1982). Dietary lipids, sugar, fiber, and mortality from coronary heart disease. *Arteriosclerosis, 2*, 221-227.
6. Moore, M.C., Guzman, M.A., Schilling, P.E., & Strong, J.P. (1976). Dietary-atherosclerosis study on deceased persons. Relation of selected dietary components to raised atherosclerotic lesions. *Journal of the American Dietetic Association, 68*, 216-223.
7. Kromhout, D., Bosschieter, E.B., & de Lezenne Coulander, C. (1982). Dietary fibre and 10-year mortality from coronary heart disease, cancer, and all causes. *Lancet, 2*, 518-522.
8. Kushi, L.H., Lew, R.A., Stare, F.J., Ellison, C.R., el Lozy, M., Bourke, G., & Daly, L. (1985). Diet and 20-year mortality from coronary heart disease. The Ireland-Boston Diet-Heart Study. *New England Journal of Medicine, 312*, 811-818.
9. Thorogood, M., Carter, R., Benfield, L., McPherson, K., & Mann, J. (1987). Plasma lipids and lipoprotein cholesterol concentrations in people with different diets in Britain. *British Medical Journal, 295*, 351-353.
10. Burr, M.L., & Sweetnam, P.M. (1982). Vegetarianism, dietary fiber, and mortality. *American Journal of Clinical Nutrition, 36*, 873.
11. Fraser, G.E., & Swannell, R.J. (1981). Diet and serum cholesterol in Seventh-Day Adventists: A cross sectional study showing significant relationships. *Journal of Chronic Disorders, 34*, 487.
12. Sacks, F.M., Castelli, W.P., & Donner, A. (1975). Plasma lipids and lipoproteins in vegetarians and controls. *New England Journal of Medicine, 292*, 1148-1151.

13. Arntzenius, A.C., Kromhout, D., & Barth, J.D. (1985). Diet, lipo-proteins, and the progression of coronary atherosclerosis. The Leiden Intervention Trial. *New England Journal of Medicine, 313*, 805-811.
14. Miettinen, M., Turpeinen, O., Karvonen, M.J., Elosuo, R., & Paavilainen, E. (1972). Effect of cholesterol-lowering diet on mortality from coronary heart-disease and other causes: A twelve-year clinical trial in men and women. *Lancet, 2*, 835-838.
15. Anderson, J.W., & Bryant, C.A. (1986). Dietary fiber: Diabetes and obesity. *American Journal of Gastroenterology, 81*, 898-906.
16. Lindahl, O., Lindwall, L., & Spangberg, A. (1984). A vegan regimen with reduced medication in the treatment of hypertension. *British Journal of Nutrition, 52*, 11-20.
17. Wright, A., Burstyn, P.G., & Gibney, M.J. (1979). Dietary fibre and blood pressure. *British Medical Journal, 2*, 1541-1543.
18. DiLorenzo, C., Williams, C.M., Hajnal, F., & Valenzuela, J.E. (1988). Pectin delays gastric emptying and increases satiety in obese subjects. *Gastroenterology, 95*, 1211-1215.
19. Burkitt, D. (1984). Fiber as protective against gastrointestinal diseases.
      52.
      T.K., & Hunninghake,
      psyllium hydrophilic
      iation, 261, 3419-3423.
      T., Tietyen-Clark, J.,
      rol-lowering effects of
      erolemic men. *Archives*

      citrus pectin on blood
      erican Journal of Clinical

      f pectin on serum cho-
      nolipidemic and hyper-
      9, 471-477.
      ds. *American Journal of*

      abolic effects of dietary

      es, E.D., Chen, W.J.,
      take selectively lowers
      ncentrations of hyper-
      l Nutrition, 34, 824-829.
      Cummins, J.H. (1975).
      on serum-cholesterol.

      n overview. *American Journal of Gastroenterology, 81*, 982-987.

29. Jenkins, D.J., Wolever, T.M., & Leeds, A.R. (1983). The glycaemic index of foods tested in diabetic patients: A new basis for carbohydrate exchange favouring use of legumes. *Diabetologia*, **24**, 257-264.
30. Hilman, C., Peters, S.G., Fisher, C.A., & Pomare, E.W. (1985). The effects of the fiber components pectin, cellulose and lignin on serum cholesterol levels. *American Journal of Clinical Nutrition*, **42**, 207-213.
31. Jenkins, D.J., Reynolds, D., Slavin, B., Leeds, A.R., Jenkins, A.L., & Jepson, E.M. (1980). Dietary fiber and blood lipids: Treatment of hypercholesterolemia with guar crispbread. *American Journal of Clinical Nutrition*, **33**, 575-581.
32. Thorne, M.J., Thompson, L.U., & Jenkins, D.J.A. (1983). Factors affecting starch digestibility and the glycemic response with special reference to legumes. *American Journal of Clinical Nutrition*, **38**, 481-488.
33. Anderson, J.W., Story, L., Sieling, B., Chen, W.J., Petro, M.S., & Story, J. (1984). Hypocholesterolemic effects of oat-bran or bean intake for hypercholesterolemic men. *American Journal of Clinical Nutrition*, **40**, 1146-1155.
34. Simpson, H.C.R., Simpson, R.W., Lousley, S., Carter, R.D., Geekie, M., Hockaday, T.D., & Mann, J.I. (1981). A high carbohydrate leguminous fibre diet improves all aspects of diabetic control. *Lancet*, **1**, 1-4.
35. Wahlqvist, M.L. (1987). Dietary fiber and carbohydrate metabolism. *American Journal of Clinical Nutrition*, **45**, 1232-1236.
36. Ray, T.K., Mansell, K.M., Knight, L.C., Malmud, L.S., Owen, O.E., & Boden, G.B. (1983). Long-term effects of dietary fiber on glucose tolerance and gastric emptying in noninsulin dependent diabetic patients. *American Journal of Clinical Nutrition*, **37**, 376-381.
37. Haber, G.B., Heaton, K.W., Murphy, D., & Burroughs, L.F. (1977). Depletion and disruption of dietary fiber. Effects on satiety, plasma glucose and serum insulin. *Lancet*, **2**, 679.
38. National Diet Heart Study Research Group. The national diet heart study final report. *Circulation*, **37** (Suppl I):1-421.
39. Anderson, J.W., & Tietyen-Clark, J. (1986). Dietary fiber: Hyperlipidemia, hypertension, and coronary heart disease. *American Journal of Gastroenterology*, **81**, 907-919.
40. Fehily, A.M., Milband, J.E., Tarnell, J.W., Hayes, T.M., Kubiki, A.J., & Eastham, R.D. (1982). Dietary determinants of lipoproteins, total cholesterol, viscosity, fibrinogen, and blood pressure. *American Journal of Clinical Nutrition*, **36**, 890-896.
41. National Academy of Sciences. (1982). *Diet, nutrition, and cancer*. Washington, DC: National Academy Press.
42. Bingham, S., Williams, D.R.R., Cole, T.J., & James, W.P. (1979). Dietary fibre and regional large-bowel cancer mortality in Britain. *British Journal of Cancer*, **40**, 456-463.

43. Turnbull, W.H., & Leeds, A.R. (1987). Reduction of total and LDL-cholesterol in plasma by rolled oats. *European Journal of Clinical Nutrition, 41.*

44. Van Horn, L.V., Liu, K., Parker, D., Emidy, L., Liao, Y.L., Pan, W.H., Giuinetti, D., Hewitt, J., & Stamler, J. (1986). Serum lipid response to oat product intake with a fat-modified diet. *Journal of the American Dietetic Association, 86,* 759-764.

45. Anderson, J.W., Story, L., Sieling, B., & Chen, W. (1981). Hypocholesterolemic effects of plant fiber: Short-term and long-term effects of oat bran or beans. *Clinical Research, 29,* 754A.

Suggested Readings

Burkitt, D.P., & Trowell, H.C. (1975). *Refined carbohydrate foods and disease.* New York: Academic Press, 1975.

Connor, W.E., & Bristow, J.D. (1985). (Eds.). *Coronary heart disease: Prevention, complications and treatment.* Philadelphia: J.B. Lippincott.

Kaplan, N., & Stamler, J. (1983). *Prevention of coronary heart disease.* Philadelphia: W.B. Saunders.

Levine, R. (1981). Fiber as a binding agent. In M. Winick (Ed.), *Nutrition and the killer diseases.* (pp. 173-187). New York: John Wiley.

Levy, R., Rifkind, B., Dennis, B., & Ernst, N. (Eds.) (1979). *Nutrition, lipids and coronary heart disease: A global view.* New York: Raven Press.

Spiller, G.A. (1986). *Handbook of dietary fiber in human nutrition.* Boca Raton, FL: CRC Press.

Spiller, G.A. (1986). *Handbook of dietary fiber in human nutrition.* Boca Raton, FL: CRC Press.

Trowell, H., Burkett, D., & Heaton, K. (Eds.) (1985). *Dietary fibre, fibre-depleted foods and disease.* London: Academic Press.

Vahouny, G.V., & Kritchevsky, D. (Eds.) (1986). *Basic and clinical aspects of dietary fiber.* New York: Plenum Press.

Chapter

9

Fish

Curiosity about the nutritional value of fish was kindled when epidemiologists noted very low rates of heart attack in fishing societies. Greenland Eskimos, for example, enjoy near-complete freedom from atherosclerosis. Even though they eat large amounts of seal blubber, Eskimos have blood cholesterol levels 10% to 40% lower than their Danish neighbors (1-3). CHD claims the lives of only 3% of Eskimos compared to 40% of the Danes (4).

Eskimos do not simply inherit a tendency for low blood cholesterol; those who migrate to Denmark quickly develop the same or even higher cholesterol and triglyceride levels as the typical Dane. Eskimos consume much less saturated fat and much more polyunsaturated fat than members of coronary-prone countries. In addition Eskimos consume large quantities of a distinctive type of polyunsaturated fat, the omega-3 oils. These surveys gave the first epidemiologic evidence that these fatty acids can exert a protective effect on the heart.

The health benefits of eating fish received another strong endorsement from a study from the Netherlands. Kromhout and co-workers carefully analyzed the diets of 852 middle-aged men, then followed their health status for the next 20 years (5). The men who consumed one or two fish meals a week (averaging one ounce, or 28 gm, of fish each day) had fewer than half as many deaths from heart attack as those who avoided fish. Even smaller amounts of fish had some benefit, though not as much. The two groups had similar blood cholesterol levels indicating that at least some of the health benefits from eating fish occur independently of serum cholesterol level. Fish consumption has also been found to offer protection against atherosclerosis in studies from Britain (6), Sweden (7), United States (8) and Japan (9).

The Effects of Omega-3 Oils

Research over the past two decades has verified that certain marine fats have unique metabolic properties that thwart plaque formation and its complications. In several animal studies, omega-3 oils helped suppress atherosclerosis (10). They seem to protect the endothelial lining from high cholesterol levels (11) and resist arterial narrowing (vasoconstriction) as a response to stress (12).

Omega-3 fatty acids tend to suppress blood pressure, cholesterol, triglycerides, and blood clotting (13-16). Supplementing the diets of persons with CHD already present with omega-3 fatty acids may decrease the symptoms of angina chest pain and increase exercise tolerance (17, 18). They are now being used with some success to prevent clot formation after balloon angioplasty (19). Nevertheless, the use of commercially prepared fish oil capsules should be limited to special medical conditions under the guidance of a physician.

Fish Sources of Omega-3 Fatty Acids

The two most common omega-3 fatty acids are eicosapentaenoic acid (EPA) and docosahexaenoic acid (DHA). The whale and seal eaten by the Eskimos are rich in these fatty acids.

Commercial fish containing the highest concentrations of EPA and DHA include mackerel, halibut, salmon (especially chinook), albacore tuna, and whitefish. The fish don't actually make the omega-3 oils; they incorporate the oils into their flesh from their food supply (plankton). Table 9.1 lists the omega-3 content in 21 types of fish (20).

All varieties of fish are excellent sources of protein, vitamins, and minerals. Fish is slightly lower than red meat in its cholesterol content and generally much lower in fat content. And, unlike meat, the fat in fish is mostly unsaturated. As a comparison, only 25% of the total calories in cod are from fat, with 7% of those calories from saturated fat. Salmon, a relatively fatty fish, has 32% of its calories from fat, 8% of which are saturated. Ribeye steak, on the other hand, derives 80% of its calories from fat, 40% from saturated fats.

Nonfish Sources of Omega-3 Fatty Acids

Omega-3 polyunsaturated fats can also be found in other food groups. The fat of wild game such as deer and antelope contains approximately 4% EPA, compared with trace amounts in domesticated animals (21).

Land plants contain small amounts of another omega-3 fat, linolenic acid, in their photosynthesizing chloroplasts. Some of the linolenic acid is slowly converted in the body to EPA via a chain of chemical reactions. Figure 9.1 shows the chemical structures of linolenic acid and EPA.

Table 9.1   Polyunsaturated (Omega-3) Content of Fish

Species	gm/100 gm (3.5 oz)
Salmon, chinook, canned	3.04
Mackerel, Atlantic	2.18
Salmon, chinook, fresh	2.10
Salmon, pink	1.87
Tuna, albacore, canned (light)	1.69
Salmon, coho, canned	1.50
Salmon, sockeye, canned	1.50
Whitefish, lake	1.50
Sablefish	1.39
Herring, Atlantic	1.09
Trout, rainbow	1.08
Squid	.85
Oyster, Pacific	.84
Bass, striped	.64
Catfish, channel	.61
Crab, Alaskan King	.57
Perch, ocean	.51
Halibut	.46
Shrimp, on average	.39
Flounder, yellowtail	.30
Haddock	.16

Note. From Hepburn, F.N. et al., "Provisional Tables on the Content of Omega-3 Fatty Acids and Other Fat Components of Selected Foods." Adapted from *Journal of the American Dietetic Association*, vol. 86: 788, 1986.

Plants that are relatively high in linolenic acid are listed in Table 9.2 (20). In particular, notice the high omega-3 fat content (linolenic acid) of soy products, oat germ, walnuts, chia seeds, and canola oils. The omega-3 content of these foods is much lower than that of most fish, and any health benefits from consuming terrestrial omega-3 sources remains unproven.

How Fish Affects Cholesterol

Since the 1950s it has been known that both omega-3 and omega-6 polyunsaturated fats tend to lower blood cholesterol levels (22, 23). Not until

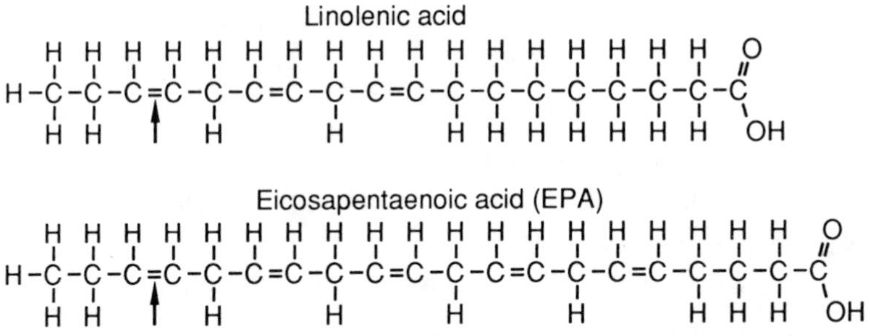
Linolenic acid
Eicosapentaenoic acid (EPA)

Figure 9.1 Linolenic acid (top) is an omega-3 fatty acid found in certain land plants. A small percentage of it can be transformed in the body to EPA (bottom). Both are omega-3 fatty acids because their first double bond from the terminal end (at arrow) occurs at the third carbon atom.

Table 9.2 Omega-3 Content of Selected Foods

Low-fat plant sources	gm/100 gm
Oat germ	1.4
Wheat germ	0.7
Chia seeds, dried	3.9
Soybeans, sprouted, cooked	2.1
Soybean kernels, roasted	1.5
Butternuts, dried	8.7
Walnuts, black	3.3
Walnuts, English/Persian	6.8
High-fat plant sources	**gm/1 Tbsp or 15 ml**
Rapeseed (canola) oil	1.6
Walnut oil	1.5
Wheat germ oil	1.0
Soybean oil	0.95
Soybean lecithin	0.71
Salad dressing, soybean	0.64
Salad dressing, regular blue cheese	0.52
Salad dressing, regular Italian	0.46
Soybean oil (partially hydrogenated)	0.36

Note. From Hepburn, F.N. et al., "Provisional Tables on the Content of Omega-3 Fatty Acids and Other Fat Components of Selected Foods." Adapted from *Journal of the American Dietetic Association*, vol. 86: 788, 1986.

the 1980s, however, were the omega-3s investigated for special properties. Research now indicates that they may have an even greater effect on cholesterol and triglycerides than the other polyunsaturates (24).

EPA can lower total cholesterol by 25% even in people with average levels (24). The decrease is primarily in LDL and triglycerides and is dose-related—it increases as greater amounts of fish are eaten (26-28).

The effects of increasing the amount of fish in the diet vary considerably from one person to another. Some individuals have a significant drop in serum cholesterol within 2 weeks if 2 to 4 fish meals each week are substituted for high-fat meat meals. Those with the highest cholesterol or triglyceride levels stand to gain the most from adding fish to their diet. In persons with hypertriglyceridemia, triglycerides may be lowered by up to 85%. In contrast, the omega-6 oils (most vegetable polyunsaturates) may raise triglycerides.

Some individuals obtain an increase in protective HDL levels from fish (27, 29, 30). Vegetable oils, however, frequently depress HDL levels (31, 32). Either response is highly individualized and is usually not seen for several months.

Phillipson and associates announced encouraging results from adding fish oil to the diets of subjects affected by both high cholesterol and high triglycerides (25). All subjects experienced a benefit—total cholesterol levels fell an average of 36%, and triglycerides fell an average of 72%. This occurred in spite of the fact that the diet also contained 350 mg of cholesterol a day.

Even if an individual's blood cholesterol and/or triglycerides are acceptable or borderline high, fish may be helpful in reaching an even safer level (15, 24, 27). However, this may require larger amounts of omega-3s taken for a longer time. In a study from Oregon, healthy persons lowered their total cholesterol by 23% and triglycerides by 43% when 4 ounces of purified salmon oil was added to their diet (33). However, because the salmon oil represented about 30% of their total fat intake, such a diet must be considered experimental.

Other Benefits From Eating Fish

Research has shown that in addition to improving cholesterol and triglyceride levels, fish consumption lowers blood pressure and reduces the clotting tendencies of blood (30, 34). Such improvements occur when fish is substituted for typical red-meat meals. Again, omega-3 fatty acids are thought to dilate small arteries, which causes the drop in blood pressure (17, 29, 35-37). Another likely reason for blood pressure reduction is that fish, particularly finfish, is lower in sodium than most red meat.

In one study, researchers lowered the blood pressure of 32 subjects by 7 mmHg (systolic) and 4 mmHg (diastolic) with high doses (50 ml) of EPA supplements (38). The pressures continued to decline when the study ended after four weeks, indicating an even greater long-term benefit.

The membranes of blood platelets undergo changes as well when 3 to 5 gm a day of EPA is consumed (30, 36, 39). The properties of these omega-3 fatty acids reduce the stickiness of the platelets, and this in turn decreases their tendency to aggregate and form clots along damaged arteries (40). Another anticlotting agent is prostacylin (from the endothelial cells), which keeps arterial linings smooth.

Blood viscosity is also reduced by omega-3 fatty acids (41). Reductions have been confirmed with as little as 1.4 gm of EPA a day (34). When such changes in viscosity are combined with those of the blood platelets, clots tend to form less often, thus reducing plaque buildup.

Risks for other diseases and health problems appear to decrease when omega-3 fatty acid intake is increased. Omega-3 oils may be beneficial in rheumatoid arthritis for example (42). Taken in doses of at least 3 gm a day, EPA inhibits the production of leukotriene B4, a substance that causes joint-damaging inflammation. Fish oils may also ameliorate psoriasis (43), atopic (allergic) dermatitis, asthma, and autoimmune disorders (34, 44). Evidence from more than a dozen studies, mostly in animals, suggests that omega-3 oils may suppress cancer.

Table 9.3 separates fish species into poor, better, and best choice categories in terms of their omega-3 content. All the fish in the "better choice" column are heart-healthy, although they may not be as rich in omega-3s as the "best choice" fish. The "poor" choices include fish high in cholesterol and/or environmental pollutants. Avoid the mustard of crab, or the tamali of lobster because these tissues are very high in fat and may have high concentrations of any pollutants to which the animal was exposed (45). Shellfish is high in cholesterol but can be eaten in moderation when baked, boiled, or steamed because it is low in saturated fat.

In summary, Eskimos and other fishing societies have an enviably low rate of heart attack, less than one fifth the rate found in the United States. They have low levels of cholesterol and triglycerides and a very low prevalence of diabetes. The HDL levels of Eskimos are nearly 50% higher than those of Europeans. Their blood flows easily (low viscosity) under low pressures and they have relatively slow clotting times. All these factors largely result from diet and are no doubt responsible for the rarity of CHD in Eskimo populations.

Studies have shown that fish consumption can protect the heart and blood vessels independent of its effect on blood cholesterol. Eating as little as a half ounce (14 gm) fish a day, or one to two fish meals a week, appears to cut the risk of heart attack by 50%.

The mechanisms behind fish's cardioprotection involve several avenues of plaque inhibition. These include a significant drop in cholesterol and triglycerides and sometimes a boost to HDL. The omega-3 fatty acids are two to five times more potent in lowering cholesterol and triglycerides

Table 9.3   Fish Group: Poor, Better, and Best Choices for Omega-3 Fatty Acids

Poor choices	Better choices	Best choices
Any fried fish or shellfish; especially when breaded; oil-packed sardines, shrimp, lobster, crab, crayfish, or squid (limit to 3 oz per week)[a]	Most fresh or frozen finfish (3-4 oz or 1/2 cup per serving), bass (freshwater), cod, flounder, monkfish, butterfish, red snapper, mahi mahi, sardines (fresh or frozen, 9 medium), most mollusks such as oysters and mussels (12 medium)	Salmon, mackerel, herring, water-packed tuna, halibut, sablefish, whitefish, perch, trout[b]
Fish that may be contaminated with pollutants, such as catfish, swordfish, shark, and sometimes striped bass and bluefish		Tuna or salmon, canned in water (1/2 cup)[c]

[a]Especially avoid the "mustard" in blue crabs or the "tamali" in lobsters.

[b]These varieties are especially healthful if shipped from Canada or Alaska, because they will contain more omega-3 fatty acids.

[c]The water used in packing should be drained, even if it does not contain salt.

Note. The omega-3 content of the same species of fish will vary according to supply of plankton upon which the fish feed.

than are the omega-6 vegetable oils. In addition, omega-3s may improve blood pressure and viscosity and inhibit clotting tendencies, cancer, and immunological diseases.

References

1. Bang, H.O., Dyerberg, J., & Sinclair, H.M. (1980). The composition of the Eskimo food in northwestern Greenland. *American Journal of Clinical Nutrition, 33,* 2657-2661.
2. Kromann, N., & Green, A. (1980). Epidemiological studies in the Upernavik district, Greenland. *Acta Medica Scandinavica,* **208,** 401-406.

3. Bang, H.O., & Dyerberg, J. (1972). Plasma lipids and lipoproteins in Greenlandic west-coast Eskimos. *Acta Medica Scandinavica*, **192**, 85-94.
4. Bang, H.O., & Dyerberg, J. (1980). Lipid metabolism and ischemic heart disease in Greenland Eskimos. *Advances in Lipid Research*, **3**, 1-22.
5. Kromhout, D., Bosschieter, D.B., & de Lezenne Coulander, C.L. (1985). The inverse relation between fish consumption and 20-year mortality from coronary heart disease. *New England Journal of Medicine*, **312**, 1205-1209.
6. Thorogood, M., Carter, R., Benfield, L., McPherson, K., & Mann, J. (1987). Plasma lipids and lipoprotein cholesterol concentrations in people with different diets in Britain. *British Medical Journal*, **295**, 351-353.
7. Norell, S.E., Ahlbom, A., Feychting, M., & Pedersen, N.L. (1986). Fish consumption and mortality from coronary heart disease. *British Medical Journal*, **293**, 426.
8. Shekelle, R.B., Paul, O., Shryock, A., & Stamler, J. (1985). Fish consumption and mortality from coronary heart disease. *New England Journal of Medicine*, **313**, 820.
9. Hirai, A., Terano, T., Saito, H., Tamura, Y., Yoshida, S., Sajiki, J., & Kumagai, A. (1984). Eicosapentaenoic acid and platelet function in Japanese. In W. Lovenberg & Y. Yamori (Eds.), *Nutritional prevention of cardiovascular disease* (pp. 231-239). New York: Academic Press.
10. Harris, W.S. (1989). Can fish oil retard atherosclerosis? *Practical Cardiology*, **15**, 25-32.
11. Weiner, B.H., Ockene, I.S., Levine, P.H., Cuenoud, H.F., Fisher, M., Johnson, B.F., Daoud, A.S., Jarmolych, J., Hosmer, D., & Johnson, M.H. (1986). Inhibition of atherosclerosis by cod-liver oil in a hyperlipidemic swine model. *New England Journal of Medicine*, **315**, 841-846.
12. Shimokawa, H., & Vanhoutte, P.M. (1988). Dietary cod-liver oil improves endothelium-dependent responses in hypercholesterolemic and atherosclerotic porcine coronary arteries. *Circulation*, **78**, 1421-1430.
13. Lavie, C.J., Squires, W., & Gau, G.T. (1987). What is the role of fish and fish oils in the primary and secondary prevention of cardiovascular disease? *Journal of Cardiopulmonary Rehabilitation*, **7**, 526-533.
14. Nestel, P.J. (1987). Polyunsaturated fatty acids (n-3, n-6). *American Journal of Clinical Nutrition*, **45**(Suppl. 5), 1161-1166.
15. Sanders, T.A.B. (1986). Nutritional and physiological implications of fish oils. *Journal of Nutrition*, **116**, 1857-1859.
16. Sanders, T.A., Sullivan, D.R., Reeve, J., & Thompson, G.R. (1985). Triglyceride-lowering effect of marine polyunsaturates in patients with hypertriglyceridemia. *Arteriosclerosis*, **5**, 459-465.
17. Mehta, J.L., Lopez, L.M., Lawson, D., Wargovich, T.J., & Williams, L.L. (1988). Dietary supplementation with omega-3 polyunsaturated

fatty acids in patients with stable coronary disease: Effects on indices of platelet and neutrophil function and exercise performance. *American Journal of Medicine*, **84**, 45-52.

18. Saynor, R., Verel, D., & Gillott, T. (1984). The long-term effect of dietary supplementation with fish lipid concentrate on serum lipids, bleeding time, platelets and angina. *Atherosclerosis*, **50**, 3-10.

19. Slack, J.D., Pinkerton, C.A., & VanTassel, J. (1987). Can oral fish oil supplement minimize restenosis after percutaneous transluminal coronary angioplasty? [Abstract] *Journal of the American College of Cardiology*, **9**, 64A.

20. Hepburn, F.N., Exler, J., & Weihrauch, J.L. (1986). Provisional tables on the content of omega-3 fatty acids and other fat components of selected foods. *Journal of the American Dietetic Association*, **86**, 788-793.

21. Eaton, S.B., & Konner, M. (1985). Paleolithic nutrition. *New England Journal of Medicine*, **312**, 283-289.

22. Malmros, H., & Wigand, G. (1957). The effect on serum cholesterol of diets containing different fats. *Lancet*, **2**, 1-8.

23. Bronte-Stewart, B., Antonis, A., Eales, L., & Brock, J.F. (1956). Effects of feeding different fats on serum cholesterol levels. *Lancet*, **1**, 521-526.

24. Harris, W.S., Connor, W.E., & McMurry, M.P. (1983). The comparative reductions of the plasma lipids and lipoproteins by dietary polyunsaturated fats: Salmon oil versus vegetable oils. *Metabolism*, **32**, 179-184.

25. Phillipson, B.E., Rothrock, D.W., Connor, W.E., Harris, W.S., & Illingworth, D.R. (1985). Reduction of plasma lipids, lipoproteins and apoproteins by dietary fish oils in patients with hypertriglyceridemia. *New England Journal of Medicine*, **312**, 1210-1216.

26. Ballard-Barbash, R., & Callaway, C.W. (1987). Marine fish oils: Role in prevention of coronary heart disease. *Mayo Clinic Proceedings*, **62**, 113-118.

27. Lossonczy, T.O. von, Ruiter, A., Bronsgeest-Schoute, H.C., Gent, C.M. van, & Hermus, R.J.J. (1978). The effect of a fish diet on serum lipids in healthy human subjects. *American Journal of Clinical Nutrition*, **31**, 1340-1346.

28. Chait, A., Onitiri, A., Nicoll, A., Rabaya, E., Davies, J., & Lewis, B. (1974). Reduction of serum triglyceride levels by polyunsaturated fat. *Atherosclerosis*, **20**, 347-364.

29. Singer, P., Wirth, M., Berger, I., Voigt, S., Gerike, U., Gödicke, W., Köberle, U., & Heine, H. (1985). Influence on serum lipids, lipoproteins and blood pressure of mackerel and herring diet in patients with Type IV and V hyperlipoproteinemia. *Atherosclerosis*, **56**, 111-118.

30. Sanders, T.A.B., & Roshani, F. (1983). The influence of different types of omega-3 polyunsaturated fatty acids on blood lipids and platelet function in healthy volunteers. *Clinical Science*, **64**, 91-99.

31. Turner, J.D., Le, N.A., & Brown, W.B. (1981). Effect of changing

dietary fat saturation on low density lipoprotein metabolism in man. *American Journal of Physiology*, **241**, E57-E63.

32. Shepherd, J., Packard, D.J., Grundy, S.M., Yeshurun, D., Gotto, A.M., & Taunton, O.D. (1980). Effects of saturated and poly-unsaturated fat diets on the chemical composition and metabolism of low density lipoproteins in man. *Journal of Lipid Research*, **21**, 91-99.

33. Illingworth, D.R., Harris, W.S., & Connor, W.E. (1984). Inhibition of low density lipoproteins synthesis by dietary omega-3 fatty acids in humans. *Arteriosclerosis*, **4**, 270-275.

34. Yetiv, J.Z. (1988). Clinical applications of fish oils. *Journal of the American Medical Association*, **260**, 665-670.

35. Lorenz, R., Spengler, U., Fischer, S., Duhm, J., & Webber, P.C. (1983). Platelet function, thromboxane formation and blood pressure control during supplementation of the Western diet with cod liver oil. *Circulation*, **67**, 504-511.

36. Mortensen, J.Z., Schmidt, E.B., Nielsen, A.H., & Dyerberg, J. (1983). The effect of N-6 and N-3 polyunsaturated acids on hemostasis, blood lipids and blood pressure. *Thrombosis Haemostasis*, **50**, 543-546.

37. Lockette, W.E., Webb, R.C., Cuuop, B.R., & Pitt, B. (1982). Vascular reactivity and high dietary eicosapentaenoic acid. *Prostaglandins*, **24**, 631-639.

38. Knapp, H.R., & Fitzgerald, G.A. (1989). The antihypertensive effects of fish oil. *New England Journal of Medicine*, **320**, 1037-1043.

39. Goodnight, S.H., Harris, W.S., Connor, W.E., & Illingworth, D.R. (1982). Polyunsaturated fatty acids, hyperlipidemia, and thrombosis. *Arteriosclerosis*, **2**, 87-113.

40. Dyerberg, J., Bang, H.O., Stoffersen, E., Moncada, S., & Vane, J.R. (1978). Eicosapentaenoic acid and prevention of thrombosis and atherosclerosis? *Lancet*, **2**, 117-119.

41. Cartwright, L.J., Pockley, A.G., Galloway, J.H., Greaves, M., & Preston, F.E. (1985). The effects of dietary omega-3 polyunsaturated fatty acids on erythrocyte membrane phospholipids, erythrocyte deformability and blood viscosity in healthy volunteers. *Atherosclerosis*, **55**, 267-281.

42. Kremer, J.M., Jubiz, W., Michalek, A., Rynes, R.I., Bartholomew, L.E., Bigaoutte, J., Timchalk, M., Beeler, D., & Lininger, L. (1987). Fish-oil fatty acid supplementation in active rheumatoid arthritis. *Annals of Internal Medicine*, **106**, 497-503.

43. Bittiner, S.B., Tucker, W.F.G., Cartwright, I., & Bleeheu, S.S. (1988). A double-blind trial of fish oil in psoriasis. *Lancet*, **1**, 378-380.

44. Lee, T.H., Hoover, R.L., Williams, J.D., Sperling, R.I., Ravalese, J., Spur, B.W., Robinson, D.R., Coroy, E.J., Lewis, R.A., & Austen, K.F. (1985). Effect of dietary enrichment with eicosapentaenoic and docosa-hexaenoic acids on in vitro neutrophil and monocyte leukotriene

generation and neutrophil function. *New England Journal of Medicine,* **312**, 1217-1224.

45. Lefferts, L.Y. (1988). Good fish . . . bad fish. *Nutrition Action Health Letter* (Available from the Center for Science in the Public Interest), **15**, 5-7.

Suggested Readings

Glomset, J.A. (1985). Fish, fatty acids, and human health. *New England Journal of Medicine,* **312**, 1253-1254.

Lands, W.E. (1986). *Fish and human health.* San Diego: Academic Press.

McCarthy, M.A., & Matthews, R.H. (1984). *Composition of foods: Nuts and seed products.* U.S. Department of Agriculture Handbook 8-12.

Reeves, J.B., & Weihrauch, J.L. (1979). *Composition of foods: fats and oils,* U.S. Department of Agriculture Handbook 8-4.

Simopoulos, A.P., Kifer, R.R., & Martin, R.E. (Eds.) (1986). *Health effects of polyunsaturated fatty acids in seafoods.* Orlando, FL: Academic Press.

Chapter

10

Putting It
All Together

By present estimates, at least 100 million Americans need to change their eating habits to lower their blood cholesterol (1,2). During the 1990s, vast numbers of people will approach the medical system for guidance. To this end, the American Heart Association and the National Cholesterol Education Program (NCEP) suggest a two-tiered approach, the Step One and Step Two eating plans. The food tables in chapters 7, 8, and 9 list foods that are within the limits of Step One and Step Two as "better choice" and "best choice" selections.

What Are the Step One and Step Two Eating Plans?

The Step One plan is truly a first step toward the prevention of cardio-vascular diseases (as well as cancer, obesity, diabetes, and gastrointestinal diseases). It is not a special diet but a recommended eating guide for every-one over two years of age. If this plan were universally accepted, our society's epidemic of chronic, incurable, diet-related diseases would decrease dramatically.

The data in Table 10.1 compare Steps One and Two to the traditional American diet. Saturated fat should only comprise a small piece of the dietary pie. Carbohydrates are the largest slice. The histogram data compare the recommended intake of cholesterol, fiber, and sodium with the traditional intake (3-5).

Here is a summary of the Step One eating plan:

1. Decrease total fat to less than 30% of total calories.
2. Decrease saturated fat intake to no more than 10% of total calories.

Table 10.1   Summary of the Step One and Step Two Eating Plans,[a] Compared to the Typical American Diet

Diet	Step One	Step Two	Typical American diet
Fat	<30%	<25%	35%-40%
Saturated fat	<10%	<7%	15%-17%
Polyunsaturated fat	Up to 10%	Up to 10%	20%-25%
Monounsaturated fat[b]	10%-15%	10%-15%	10%-15%
Protein	15%	15%	20%-40%
Carbohydrate	50%	60%	25%-35%
Cholesterol intake (mg/day)	<300	<200	450-500
Total dietary fiber (gm)	40	60	10-20
Soluble fiber (gm)	10	20	4-6
Sodium (gm)	<2	<1.5	6-18

[a]The Step One and Step Two plans shown here differ slightly from those used by the NCEP. Fiber and sodium recommendations are included here, and the total fat content in Step Two is reduced to 25% of total calories.

[b]Most of the monounsaturated fats in today's American diet are taken in with red meats. Thus, if these food sources are reduced, other sources of monounsaturates such as olive oil can be added.

Note. Carbohydrates should make up the bulk of the total diet, whereas saturated fat should comprise only a small portion. Adapted from references (3), (4), and (5).

For example, a person needing 1,500 calories a day would consume 17 gm of saturated fat; for 2,000 calories, 22 gm; for 2,500 calories, 28 gm.

3. Decrease cholesterol intake to less than 300 mg a day (a bit more than is contained in one egg yolk).
4. Increase fiber intake, especially soluble fiber. The goal for total dietary fiber, soluble plus insoluble, is 40 gm. This should include at least 10 gm of soluble fiber.
5. Limit sodium intake to 2 gm.

Step Two is more stringent but not severely so. It approximates the average diet in countries that have a very low incidence of CHD. This plan is recommended if an individual's cholesterol level remains unacceptable after 3 to 6 months on Step One. The NCEP defines unacceptable cholesterol as LDL levels remaining over 160 mg/dl (4.1 mmol/L) in the absence of CHD or two or more other cardiovascular risk factors. In my opinion, if atherosclerosis is already evident, or if two other risk factors are present (such as high blood pressure, smoking, diabetes, severe obesity, male gender, or HDL less than 35 mg/dl or 0.9 mmol/L), an LDL level over 100 mg/dl (2.6 mmol/L) is unacceptable. An LDL level over 130 mg/dl (3.36 mmol/L) is unacceptable even if other risk factors are not present. Support from family members is critical in maintaining this eating plan. A registered dietitian may also provide support and assistance. In addition, people who wish to guard themselves against atherosclerosis can use Step Two as a guide to optimum health. Here is a summary of the Step Two eating plan:

1. Keep total fat intake under 25% of total calories with an upper limit of 10% of total calories from polyunsaturates and up to 10% to 15% from monounsaturates.
2. Decrease saturated fat to less than 7% of total calories. For someone consuming 1,500 calories a day, saturated fat should total no more than 12 gm/day. For 2,000 calories, this would be 16 gm; and for 2,500 calories, 19 gm.
3. Decrease cholesterol to less than 200 mg a day.
4. Increase total dietary fiber to 50 to 60 gm a day, or 20 to 30 gm per 1,000 calories consumed. This should include 15 to 20 gm of soluble fiber.
5. If hypertension persists, limit sodium intake to under 1.5 gm.

Protein intake is the same for Step One and Step Two: 10% to 15% of total calories. Recommended carbohydrate intake (starches and sugars) is 50% to 70%, depending on fat intake and the individual's energy requirements. People in vigorous exercise programs who do not need to lose weight should include more carbohydrates in their diets. Starchy vegetables and fruits should replace most of the foods high in saturated fat. Total caloric intake should be adjusted if necessary to achieve and maintain ideal weight. These guidelines need not be met every day, but rather as an average.

The average result of the Step One plan is a reduction in cholesterol levels by 30 to 40 mg/dl (0.8 to 1 mmol/L), cutting the average American's risk of heart attack by one third. The average result of Step Two is an additional 15 mg/dl (0.4 mmol/L) reduction in cholesterol level. This represents half the CHD risk if an individual started with a cholesterol level of 200 mg/dl (5.2 mmol/L) or higher. The average cholesterol level in U.S. adults today is 215 mg/dl (5.5 mmol/L).

How quickly can cholesterol levels be expected to fall? In general, an individual adhering to either plan can expect to see beneficial decrements in serum cholesterol within a few weeks (see Figure 10.1). However, considerable individual variation exists, delaying the drop in cholesterol in some persons for several months to one year. These persons need reassurance that the benefits to serum cholesterol will eventually be seen.

In a small minority of persons, even Step Two will be insufficient to adequately control cholesterol. Again, the minimum goals are to maintain

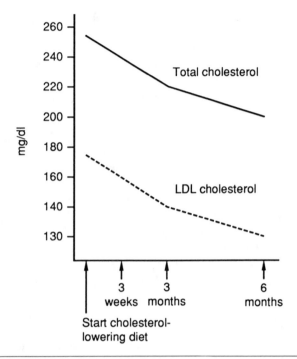

Figure 10.1   Expected changes in blood cholesterol level after beginning a cholesterol-lowering diet.

Note. From *So You Have High Blood Cholesterol* (p.15), 1987. *So You Have High Blood Cholesterol* was originally published by the National Heart, Lung, and Blood Institute. Copyright 1987 by the National Heart, Lung, and Blood Institute. Reprinted by permission.

LDL under 130 to 160 mg/dl (3.36 to 4.1 mmol/L) in the absence of athero-sclerosis or two other risk factors, or under 100 to 130 mg/dl (2.6 to 3.36 mmol/L) if clinical disease or two risk factors are present. Total fat, satu-rated fat, and cholesterol in the diet may need to be restricted even further, and soluble fiber, fish, and exercise increased even more. In this instance, the help of a registered dietitian should be enlisted.

If LDL is still over 190 mg/dl (4.9 mmol/L) after 6 months on the Step Two plan or is above 160 mg/dl (4.1 mmol/L) with atherosclerosis already present or with two or more other risk factors, drug therapy should be considered (3). See Appendix B for more complete decision guidelines in cholesterol management.

Menu Planning

The overall eating plan must be based on individual caloric needs and enough servings from all the food groups. Begin by determining the

Table 10.2 Recommended Energy Intake Guidelines

	Age	Multiplier	Weight (kg)	Examples Energy needs (calories)
Males	19-24	40	70	2,800
	25-50	37		
	51+	30		
Females	19-24	38	50	1,900
	25-50	36		
	51+	30		

Note. Resting energy requirements decrease with age due to lower metabolic rates. From *Recommended Dietary Allowances,* © 1989, by the National Academy of Sciences, National Academy Press, Washington, DC. Adapted by permission.

number of calories needed for an average day by using a multiplier based on the individual's age and multiplying it by the ideal weight in kilograms (1 kg = 2.2 lbs) (see Table 10.2). Add an additional 25% for those who are moderately active and 50% for those who are very active (7). A moderately active person exercises three times a week for 30 to 40 minutes in activities such as running, vigorous cycling, swimming, racquetball, or singles tennis. A very active person exercises vigorously five or more times a week for 40 to 60 minutes. Bear in mind that these are rough guidelines as caloric needs vary from person to person.

The next step is to determine the recommended number of servings from each food group to include in the daily menu. Active people need proportionally more carbohydrates, which are found in fiber-rich foods: grains, legumes, fruits, and vegetables. The recommended servings from the various food groups at different caloric intakes are given in Table 10.3.

This table is intended only as a guide for desirable food intakes averaged over several days. Specific food-group servings need not be precise each day or even each week. Modifications to this regimen can easily be arranged according to individual food preferences. The number of dairy servings, for example, can be increased liberally if nonfat or skim products are used. Low-fat dairy products or legumes are excellent substitutes for meats. Starchy vegetables can replace grains as carbohydrate sources, and fruits can substitute for vegetables if vitamin intake remains adequate.

In order to keep within calorie limits and fit the Step One or Step Two eating plan, it is assumed that the food choices will be taken from the "better choice" and "best choice" columns in the food tables found in chapters 7, 8, and 9.

Serving sizes vary from one food group to another. Examples include 3 to 3.5 ounces (85 to 100 gm) for meat, one cup (240 ml) milk or yogurt,

Table 10.3   Daily Portions of Food Groups in Ounces

Food group	Daily total caloric need (in calories)						
	2,500	2,000	1,800	1,600	1,400	1,200	1,000
Protein[a] (oz)	6	6	6	5	5	5	4
Dairy[b]	3	2	2	2	2	1	1
Grains	11	9	7	6	5	4	4
Fruits	7	4	4	4	3	3	3
Vegetables	5	4	4	4	4	3	2
Fats	8	7	6	5	4	3	2

[a]Dietary protein—red meat, poultry, fish, or legumes.
[b]You may substitute one serving of grains or one fruit plus one vegetable serving for each dairy serving.

one-half cup (120 ml) for most grains, one slice of bread, one-third to one-half cup (70 to 120 ml) for fruit juice, and one-half cup (120 ml) for cooked or one cup (240 ml) for raw vegetables. A single serving for fruits varies considerably: for example, two figs or plums; one apple, orange, peach, or pear; one half grapefruit, mango, or banana; and one cup (240 ml) of raspberries, papaya, or cubed melon. One serving for oils and spreads delivers 5 gm of fat, although smaller amounts are to be encouraged to keep total fat intake low. Examples include one teaspoon (5 ml) of regular margarine, mayonnaise, or cooking oil; one tablespoon (15 ml) of diet margarine and mayonnaise or regular salad dressings; one eighth of a medium avocado (8).

Flexibility in meal planning is important to allow for occasional splurges without feelings of guilt or failure. At the end of every week determine if the appropriate number of servings from each food group were included. If not, adjust the following week's menus to increase or decrease particular foods. Table 10.4 provides an example of a Step One menu plan for an individual requiring 2,000 calories a day (this corresponds to the second column from the left in Table 10.3).

Recipe Modification[1]

The key to recipe modification is knowing how to spot ingredients that are less desirable for health's sake and how to reduce, eliminate, or substitute for these ingredients—-without sacrificing flavor and palatability.

---

[1]The author extends his sincere appreciation to Mary Taylor for developing the modified recipes in this section.

Table 10.4   Example of a 2,000 Calorie Step One Menu Plan

Breakfast

1/2 cup unsweetened canned fruit or juice; or 1 small piece fresh fruit (1 fruit portion)

1/2 cup hot cereal, or 3/4 cup unsweetened dry cereal plus 2 oatbran muffins (3 grain)

2 teaspoons margarine (2 fat)

1 tablespoon peanut butter (1 protein)

1 cup skim milk or plain, nonfat yogurt (1 dairy)

Coffee or tea (no sugar or cream)

Noon meal

2 ounces fish, poultry, or lean beef; or 1/2 cup water-packed tuna (2 protein)

2 slices bread; or 1 cup potatoes; or pasta; or 2/3 cup rice (2 grain)

1 teaspoon margarine or mayonnaise plus 1 tablespoon salad dressing (2 fat)

1/2 cup unbuttered, cooked vegetables; or lettuce salad; or vegetable sticks (1 vegetable)

1/2 cup unsweetened, canned fruit or juice; or 1 small piece fresh fruit (1 fruit)

1 cup skim milk; or plain, nonfat yogurt; or 2 ounces low-fat cheese; or 1/2 cup low-fat cottage cheese (1 dairy)

Coffee or tea (no sugar or cream); or sugar-free beverage

Snack

1/2 cup unsweetened, canned fruit or juice; or 1 small piece fresh fruit (1 fruit)

Evening meal

3 ounces fish, poultry, or lean beef; or 3/4 cup water-packed tuna (3 protein)

1 slice bread plus 1 cup potatoes or pasta; or 2/3 cup rice (3 grain)

2 teaspoons margarine or mayonnaise plus 1 tablespoon salad dressing (3 fat)

1 cup unbuttered, cooked vegetables; or lettuce salad; or vegetable sticks (1 vegetable)

1/2 cup unsweetened, canned fruit or juice; or 1 small piece fresh fruit (1 fruit)

Coffee or tea (no sugar or cream); or sugar-free beverage

Snack

3 cups unbuttered air-popped popcorn; or 3 graham cracker squares; or 1 oatbran muffin (1 grain)

Coffee or tea (no sugar or cream); or sugar-free beverage

To modify a typical recipe, preview the list of ingredients for the items that you want to avoid; most often these are high in fat. Be sure to treat items such as meat and cheese as condiments rather than major ingredients.

Next, choose the ingredients that add a desirable quality to the dish, such as protein, vitamins, fiber, taste, texture, or color. Refer to the food tables in chapters 7, 8, and 9 for additional "better" and "best choice" selections.

At the end of this chapter are two versions of three recipes that illustrate how simply a standard recipe can be modified to become a healthier selection.

Some Tips for Reducing Fat and Cholesterol

There are a number of ways to reduce or eliminate fat and cholesterol from standard recipes. Some of the more common ways include

- trimming visible fat from meat,
- removing the skin from poultry,
- sautéing items in a liquid other than oil, and
- changing the cooking technique from frying to baking, broiling, grilling, steaming, or poaching.

Lean cuts of meat are generally less oily than high-fat cuts and benefit from slower (longer) cooking times. To retain the juices and enhance the flavor, cover or baste lean meats with wine, defatted broth, or tomato or lemon juice. After preparing a stew or gravy, let it cool in the refrigerator and skim off the solidified fat layer. About half of this fat can be replaced with another liquid.

One of the major sources of dietary cholesterol is the yolk of an egg. In most recipes, two egg whites or a quarter cup of egg substitute[2] can replace one whole egg. If a yellow color is desired, add a pinch of turmeric or saffron to the recipe.

In dishes with dairy products, substitute the low-fat or nonfat counterparts for the whole-milk varieties. Evaporated nonfat milk is an excellent choice for cream soups, sauces, and baked goods. For casseroles containing high-fat cheese, try replacing about half of the cheese with pureed low-fat cottage cheese, nonfat yogurt, or tofu. These alternatives also work well for dips and spreads that use sour cream, mayonnaise, or cream cheese. Herbs add a distinct flavor to these types of recipes.

Whipped cream is another dairy product that is often high in fat. To make a nonfat version, combine one-third cup of water, one tablespoon of lemon juice, three fourths of a teaspoon of vanilla, and one-third cup of nonfat milk powder. Beat for 10 minutes until stiff, then add two tablespoons of sugar. A less sweet but acceptable topping calls for pureed cottage cheese that is spooned into a strainer lined with a coffee filter or a cheesecloth. Cover and refrigerate for a day or two before using.

---

[2]Commercial egg substitutes are basically egg whites; they are high in protein and vitamins yet free of fat and cholesterol. They can be made in the home by simply blending egg whites. They should be frozen or used within 2 to 4 days.

In most baked goods, one third to one half of the total fat can be reduced without affecting the flavor of the product. To maintain the moisture content in these recipes, substitute about an equal amount of water, juice, milk, chopped fruit, or pureed vegetables. Use nonstick baking pans (or sheets) or lightly coat them with vegetable cooking spray, or cornmeal. Another alternative is baking parchment.

Finally, rather than cooking vegetables in oil, try steaming them and serve with herbs or lemon juice instead of butter. Or, when stir-frying is desired, select one of the "best choice" oils from the food table in chapter 7.

Some Tips for Adding Fiber to Recipes

Another way to make a recipe more nutritious is to increase its fiber content, especially with soluble fiber. Perhaps the most effective way is to substitute legumes for meat in casseroles or as main dishes. Pinto beans or other dried beans work well for beef in tacos, burritos, and other similar dishes. To facilitate the cooking and digestibility of beans and legumes, soak them for a day, or boil them, remove from heat, and then let them sit until the liquid is absorbed.

Although regular cooking doesn't appear to appreciably reduce fiber content, overcooking does destroy a percentage. Excessive pureeing is an even greater threat to fiber composition. For this reason, raw, steamed, or sauteed vegetables are recommended for eating. Whole and fresh fruits are also preferable to fruit juices because of their beneficial effects on blood sugar and cholesterol control. Blood sugar and insulin surges are twice as high after drinking juice than after eating fresh fruit (9).

Dried fruits are another source of fiber. Raisins, figs, dates, and apricots are good replacements for some of the sugar in recipes so long as some additional liquid is included. Of course, dried fruits alone are excellent high-fiber snacks.

Vegetarian meals often provide high-fiber options. However, to ensure that a given meal supplies all of the essential amino acids (for adequate protein), ingredients must be included in the appropriate combinations. Grains are deficient in lysine and legumes are deficient in methionine. Thus, these two food sources complement one another in providing a complete source of protein. Many cultures have relied on these nutritionally sound staples for centuries.

To increase the soluble fiber in baked goods, a gradual approach is the best advice. For example, begin by replacing 30% to 50% of the refined flour with a high-fiber flour. Add oat bran, ground psyllium seeds, or both whenever possible.[3] Cornmeal and millet flour add a delightful

---

[3]The fiber in wheat bran is 8% soluble and 92% insoluble, whereas in oat bran it is 50% soluble and 50% insoluble. Eighty-five percent of the fiber in psyllium is soluble, while 15% is insoluble. Fiber constitutes 80% of the total weight of psyllium seed husks.

texture, but egg whites are needed to sustain the structure of these products. Recipes require more liquid because of the water-absorbing property of fiber.

Psyllium is the richest known source of soluble fiber and may be purchased at better health food stores as seeds or in powder form. Add to ground meat dishes, casseroles, breads, muffins, and other baked goods that use flour. Begin by adding a small amount, about 1 or 2 teaspoons (5 to 10 ml) per serving, and then experiment with higher amounts. Include up to an equal amount of additional liquid per serving in the recipe. Psyllium also goes well on cereals, salads, and in fruit drinks, such as shakes.

Barley, oats, millet, and potatoes are excellent high-fiber ingredients for many dishes. Rolled oats are a popular choice for crunchy toppings on desserts, casseroles, or as a coating on baked fish and poultry. Oat bran and pureed potatoes (such as yams) will thicken soups and stews and go well in casseroles.

Fortunately, soluble fiber is not destroyed by milling, as is the insoluble fiber in wheat. Even finely ground oat flour retains its soluble fiber and its ability to slow the absorption of sugar, fat, and cholesterol within the intestine.

Some Tips for Adding Fish to Meals

Many persons, especially in inland areas, need assistance in increasing the amount of fish in their diets. Some claim that they do not care for the taste of fish, perhaps because they recall eating fish that was overcooked and dry, or stale and thus "fishy" tasting. Others may have grown tired of eating the same type of fish prepared time after time with the same seasonings or cooking techniques. But scores of different fish varieties are available, each of which may be prepared in many ways.

Fish is an excellent source of protein and vitamins and is low in saturated fat and cholesterol. It can replace fatty meats in a wide range of dishes including soups, casseroles, and salads. The fish is added later because of its short cooking time. With creativity and practice, fish can be substituted in many favorite traditional recipes.

The many varieties of fish and methods of preparation create endless possibilities for delicious meal combinations. With a few culinary techniques and favorite recipes, anyone can cook fish well. Also, fish satisfies without causing drowsiness, so it's perfect for lunch or a light dinner.

Cooking fish is actually quite simple and very quick. The "10-minute rule" applies to most methods of preparation. Cook the fish 10 minutes for each inch (2.5 cm) of thickness at its thickest point. This rule applies to baking at 350 °F (170 °C), broiling 4 inches from the heat, poaching in a shallow pan, or steaming on a rack. Cooking times in microwave ovens vary, but average 4 to 8 minutes for a one pound (450 gm) fillet. Arrange the fish in a single layer and cover with plastic wrap to retain moisture. Use the food tables in chapter 9 as a guide for selecting fish.

Examples of Recipe Modification

The recipes on the following six pages illustrate the concepts of reducing the fat content of a cake, substituting a low-fat, high-fiber alternative to meat in chili, and changing the cooking technique from deep frying to oven frying.

References

1. Wilson, P.W.F., Christiansen, J.C., Anderson, K.M., & Kannel. W.B. (1989). Impact of national guidelines for cholesterol risk factor screening: The Framingham Offspring Study. *Journal of the American Medical Association*, **262**, 41-44.
2. Consensus Conference. (1985). Lowering blood cholesterol to prevent heart disease. *Journal of the American Medical Association*, **253**, 2080-2086.
3. Expert Panel. National Cholesterol Education Program. (1988). Report of the National Cholesterol Education Program Expert Panel on detection, evaluation, and treatment of high blood cholesterol in adults. *Archives of Internal Medicine*, **148**, 36-69.
4. American Heart Association. Special Report. (1984). Recommendations for treatment of hyperlipidemia in adults. *Circulation*, **69**, 1065A-1090A.
5. Anderson, J.W., & Tietyen-Clark, J. (1986). Dietary fiber: Hyperlipidemia, hypertension, and coronary heart disease. *American Journal of Gastroenterology*, **81**, 907-919.
6. U.S. Department of Health and Human Services. (1987). *So you have high blood cholesterol*. NIH Publication No. 87-2922, p. 15.
7. National Research Council. (1989). *Recommended dietary allowances*. 10th Edition. Academic Press, p. 33.
8. American Diabetes Association, & American Dietetic Association. (1989). *Exchange lists for meal planning*. Alexandria, VA.
9. Haber, G.B., Heaton, W.K., Murphy, D., & Burroughs, L.F. (1977). Depletion and disruption of dietary fibre. Effects on satiety, plasmaglucose, and serum-insulin. *Lancet*, **2**, 679-682.

Carrot Cake

serves 15

standard version

2 cups sugar
1-1/2 cups oil
4 eggs
1/2 teaspoon salt
2-1/2 teaspoons baking powder
2-1/2 teaspoons baking soda
2 teaspoons cinnamon
3 cups flour
2 cups grated carrot
1/2 cup chopped walnuts

Cream Cheese Frosting
1 8-ounce package cream cheese
1 teaspoon milk
1 16-ounce box powdered sugar

□

NUTRIENT COMPARISON

Carrot Cake		Carrot Applesauce Cake	
Cholesterol	83 mg	Cholesterol	25 mg
Total fat	32 g	Total fat	12 g
Saturated	9 g	Saturated	1 g
Monounsaturated	8 g	Monounsaturated	2g
Polyunsaturated	15 g	Polyunsaturated	9 g
Calories	555	Calories	338
Fiber	1.5 g	Fiber	3.7 g
Sodium	198 mg	Sodium	161 mg
Potassium	131 mg	Potassium	309 mg

serves 10

Carrot Applesauce Cake

modified version

1 cup unbleached white flour
1 cup whole-wheat flour
2 teaspoons ground cinnamon
1/2 teaspoon ground nutmeg
1/2 teaspoon salt
1-1/2 teaspoon baking soda
1/2 cup teff or flour
1/2 cup canola oil
1 cup applesauce
1 cup maple syrup
1 whole egg
1/3 cup raisins
3 cups grated carrots
4 egg whites
1/4 teaspoon cream of tartar

☐

Preheat oven to 350 °F (175 °C). Spray or lightly oil a 9-inch tube pan or line with parchment. Combine flours, cinnamon, nutmeg, salt, soda, and teff in a mixing bowl. Set aside.

Beat together the oil, applesauce, maple syrup, and whole egg until light. Combine raisins and carrots with dry ingredients. Add to applesauce mixture.

Beat egg whites until fluffy. Add cream of tartar and continue beating until stiff peaks form. Carefully fold whites into carrot mixture and transfer to prepared cake pan. Bake 25 to 30 minutes or until a tester comes out clean. Cool in pan for 15 minutes, then invert onto cake rack and cool completely.

Serve with fruit and nonfat yogurt as a topping.

Preparation time: 20 minutes
Cooking time: 25-30 minutes

Chili

serves 8

standard version

3 tablespoons butter or bacon
  drippings
2 pounds ground beef
1/2 cup chopped onion
1-1/4 cup canned tomatoes
1 tablespoon sugar
12 ounces shredded cheddar cheese
3-4 cup canned kidney beans
1 tablespoon salt
1/2 bay leaf

NUTRIENT COMPARISON

Standard Chili		Vegetarian Chili	
Cholesterol	106 mg	Cholesterol	0 mg
Total fat	34.1 g	Total fat	1.3 g
Saturated	20 g	Saturated	0.3 g
Monounsaturated	14 g	Monounsaturated	0.2 g
Polyunsaturated	0.1 g	Polyunsaturated	0.8 g
Calories	505	Calories	153
Fiber	7 g	Fiber	11 g
Sodium	1059 mg	Sodium	253 mg
Potassium	627 mg	Potassium	597 mg

serves 8

Vegetarian Chili

modified version

1-1/2 cups chopped red onion
3 cups cooked kidney beans
1 cup cooked pinto beans
1/4 teaspoon black pepper
2 cups canned tomatoes, drained
1 bay leaf
3 cloves garlic
1/4 teaspoon cumin
1/2 teaspoon salt
2 tablespoons chili powder
1/4 cup minced cilantro

☐

Combine all ingredients except cilantro in a large saucepan. Bring to a boil. Cover and simmer, stirring frequently for 1 hour. Stir in cilantro, taste, and adjust seasonings.

Preparation time: 15 minutes.
Cooking time: 1-1/2 hours.

Pan-Fried Fish

serves 4

standard version

2 cups corn flour or all-purpose
  flour
2 teaspoons onion powder
2 teaspoons salt
1 teaspoon dried tarragon, crushed
1 teaspoon ground black pepper
1 egg, beaten
1/2 cup milk
1 pound fresh or thawed frozen fish
  fillets
2 tablespoons cooking oil or
  shortening

NUTRIENT COMPARISON

Pan-Fried Fish		Salmon Almondine	
Cholesterol	127 mg	Cholesterol	54 mg
Total fat	30 g	Total fat	9 g
Saturated	12 g	Saturated	3 g
Monounsaturated	7 g	Monounsaturated	3 g
Polyunsaturated	11 g	Polyunsaturated	3 g
Calories	630	Calories	231
Fiber	3 g	Fiber	1 g
Sodium	1328 mg	Sodium	154 mg
Potassium	728 mg	Potassium	547 mg

serves 4

Salmon Almondine

modified version

4 pounds fresh salmon, preferably
  fillets (can substitute other fish)
1/8 cup nonfat milk
1 egg white
1/8 cup dry whole-wheat bread
  crumbs
1 tablespoon rolled oats
Pinch of salt and pepper
1 lemon, halved
1-1/2 tablespoons toasted slivered
  almonds
1/2 tablespoon minced parsley

☐

Preheat oven to 425 °F (218 °C). Soak fish in milk for 10 minutes. Beat egg white until frothy. Combine bread crumbs, oats, salt, and pepper on a piece of waxed paper.

Drain fish and discard milk. (Or use the milk in a fish-flavored soup or sauce.) Brush on egg white. Dust fillets with bread crumb mixture and place on a nonstick baking sheet. Squeeze half of lemon over fish. Bake until breading has browned and meat flakes but is still very moist. Allow 10 minutes of cooking for each inch of thickness. Remove to serving plate, sprinkle with almonds and parsley, and serve with remaining half of lemon cut into wedges.

Preparation time: 5 minutes.
Cooking time: 10-12 minutes.

PART

IV

PUBLIC HEALTH PROMOTION

☐

These are exciting times for the prevention of atherosclerosis, our nation's major health problem. We now know for certain that intervening to reduce cardiovascular risk factors, especially blood cholesterol, can and will reduce rates of CHD. Research continues to identify the types of foods that are either harmful or healthy. New food products are being developed that make a healthy diet both convenient and tasty. Technological advances have made fast and accurate testing devices available to monitor cholesterol. Powerful new drugs have been released that together with a healthy diet can restrain even the most recalcitrant cholesterol level. We now have the knowledge and tools to resist cholesterol-related death and disability.

Part IV of this book addresses the public health or population-based approach to cholesterol control. The magnitude of the cholesterol problem requires this strategy to complement the cases identified one-by-one in physicians' offices. In the United States alone, 100 million citizens are in need of intervention for blood cholesterol.

As larger segments of our society become aware of the cholesterol peril, more organizations will surely support measures to control it. Medical providers, wellness directors, fitness instructors, and health educators will be called upon to provide comprehensive and effective heart and cholesterol programs for their clients. Part IV of this book builds on the information presented in Parts I through III to help the health professionals design and manage cholesterol programs in hospitals, corporations, schools, and communities.

Chapter 11 describes how to plan and implement a cholesterol screening —the important first step in cholesterol control. Properly trained personnel, accurate measurement techniques, and adequate promotion of the event are crucial to ensure success. Lists of necessary equipment and supplies are included for each station at the screening site.

Chapter 12 outlines the four steps in establishing a comprehensive cholesterol-control program—design, marketing, implementation, and evaluation. The implementation phase focuses on a lesson plan for teaching a 5-week cholesterol course, including tips on presentation, group activities, supplies, and handout materials.

The final chapter summarizes the rationale and action plan for a societal approach to prevent cardiovascular death and disability. A mass of evidence exists confirming that lifestyle changes have already begun to arrest the CHD epidemic. But even more changes must be made, by health professionals, corporations, communities, and the food industry as well as private individuals.

Chapter

11

Cholesterol Screening

According to the guidelines set by the National Cholesterol Education Program (NCEP), 36% of American adults, or 60 million, are at high risk for developing premature heart disease because of elevated cholesterol levels and other risk factors (1-3). Another 25%, or 40 million, need dietary and lifestyle advice because they are at borderline high-risk for CHD.

The NCEP's Expert Panel recommends that all Americans over the age of 20 have their blood cholesterol measured (4). As of late 1988, however, only 59% of adults recalled ever having had a cholesterol test, and only 17% could state their results (5). Nearly one quarter of U.S. adults are unaware that their cholesterol levels place them at high risk for CHD. Men in their 20s to 40s are particularly vulnerable because of infrequent visits to physicians.

Many public and private organizations are taking steps to improve this situation by holding low-cost public cholesterol screenings in convenient locations. These screenings will identify persons at high risk; further diagnosis for hypercholesterolemia must be completed by a physician after repeat testings.

Accurate and immediate results can be obtained on-site using finger-stick blood samples and portable spectrophotometric equipment. Fasting is not required for these tests, which need only measure total cholesterol and not the separate lipoprotein fractions (6).[1]

Thousands of individuals can be tested when such programs are carefully planned (7). In fact, in three one-day screenings held during April of

---

[1] Fasting is required only for the measurement of triglycerides, which increase dramatically after a meal due to circulating chylomicrons. LDL and HDL are not appreciably affected by a single meal (6).

1988 and 1989 the Voluntary Hospitals of America screened 850,000 persons during its "Countdown USA" campaign following a well-organized national plan.

Planning the Screening

Anyone involved in the planning process should keep in mind the following five objectives of cholesterol screenings:

1. To detect individuals with elevated blood cholesterol and inform them of their increased risk and the need for permanent control
2. To increase general awareness of cholesterol and its central role in causing CHD, peripheral vascular disease, and stroke among such target groups as the public, employees, health club members, physicians, and other health care providers
3. To raise public consciousness about the impact of diet on CHD risk factors, particularly blood cholesterol, blood pressure, diabetes, and obesity
4. To facilitate appropriate referral to dietitians, educational classes, and medical supervision
5. To provide a mechanism to reach people who might otherwise not have their blood cholesterol measured

A small group of people should meet several months in advance to plan the screening. Though prior experience is not necessary, a willingness to work together and commit time and energy is crucial. Early in the planning process, choose an overall coordinator with good organizational skills. Select a site coordinator for each testing area and someone to be in charge of volunteers, training, budget, and the technical equipment. Outline and clarify job responsibilities to the satisfaction of each member of the planning committee.

The screening site should be convenient, clean, attractive, and large enough to accommodate the expected number of participants. It should have parking available, secure overnight storage, and adequate electrical outlets. Possible locations include shopping malls, supermarkets, hospitals, nursing homes, exercise clubs, schools, hotels, municipal buildings, businesses, and churches. Sites usually need to be booked months in advance.

Arrange the screening site to ensure privacy and confidentiality of results to participants. Find out if the site is already adequately insured for this type of function. If not, start early to acquire coverage, which can be expensive and difficult to obtain.

The date you select should correspond to a special anniversary or event. February is a good choice because it is National Heart Month, March is

National Nutrition Month, and September is designated as National Cholesterol Education Month. Local Red Cross or American Heart Association chapters are particularly responsive to outreach activities at these times. Determine the number of days that the screening will take place. Screenings that take place over several days involve much more planning, especially in keeping an adequate number of trained personnel on-site.

Cholesterol Testing Equipment

Rapid and accurate finger-stick blood sampling is now possible thanks to technological improvements in cholesterol-analyzing machines. Finger-stick measurements tend to run somewhat lower than venous samples (8).

The portable testing devices, reflectance spectrophotometers, use enzymatic methods to measure the cholesterol present in blood. At least a dozen are currently available that use separate cards or cassettes for each test. This simplifies the procedure, reduces the possibility of human error, and eliminates reagent mixing and the potential for spills. Each device has individual advantages and disadvantages, depending on the needs of the particular institution sponsoring the screening.

The most advanced of these portable machines that meet the government's present accuracy goal are shown in Figure 11.1. All use finger-stick blood samples, give immediate results, and—when used properly—are accurate to within 5% of the true values (7).

Kodak's DT-60 is an accurate, relatively inexpensive, and portable device that can perform a variety of tests on serum or plasma (9). It is the only one of these devices that requires spinning of the blood to obtain plasma. This introduces complexity into the procedure as well as the possibility for operator error, especially if the machine is used infrequently by non-technical personnel. The DT-60 can analyze up to 50 tests per hour, printing the results on a paper strip. Calibration is done by the operator and is quite simple.

Abbott Laboratory's Vision is the only one of these three analyzers that uses wet instead of dry chemistry. It spins a small plastic cassette containing a reagent solution before reading the result. The Vision is the most versatile of the machines because it can perform dozens of different blood tests simultaneously using whole blood or plasma. It is very useful for a medium to large medical department or physician's office. It is the fastest of the three, analyzing up to 70 tests per hour, but is also the most expensive, costing about twice as much as the other two. The Vision and the Kodak DT-60 are the only machines of their class that have already met the NCEP's 1992 goal of accuracy, reporting cholesterol levels that are within 3% of the true value (10).

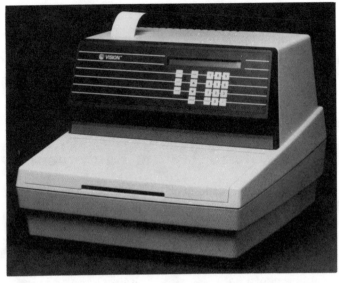

a

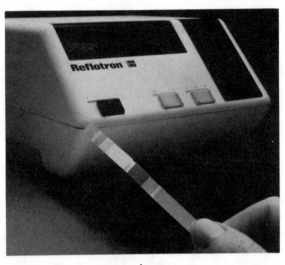

b

(Cont.)

Figure 11.1   Three accurate portable cholesterol testing machines: Abbott Laboratories' Vision®, Boehringer Mannheim's Reflotron®, and Kodak's Ecktachem DT-60®.

Note. Reprinted by courtesy of Abbott Laboratories, Boehringer Mannheim (Reflotron® is a registered trademark of Boehringer Mannheim GmbH), and Eastman Kodak Company.

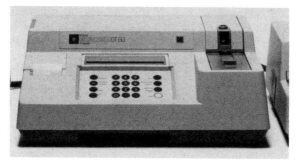

c

Figure 11.1   (Continued)

Boehringer Mannheim's Reflotron is perhaps the simplest machine to use and is thus well-suited for screenings when nontechnical personnel take the measurements. It can measure cholesterol content in whole blood, plasma, or serum (plasma minus clotting factors). It is limited in the number of parameters other than cholesterol that it can measure. Depending on operator training and quality control measures, the accuracy of the Reflotron has been shown to range from high (11) to borderline acceptable (10). Calibration is done by the manufacturer with each lot of test strips. Because the Reflotron is somewhat slower than the other two devices (15 to 20 tests per hour), multiple machines must be leased for a large screening. An optional printer is now available, allowing participants to receive a hard copy of their cholesterol number.

When the machines are properly calibrated with the manufacturers' disposable cards, and if control samples are done that can be traced to the Centers for Disease Control's methods, the testing machines are reliable and accurate devices. The growing percentage of offices and screenings that use this equipment are thus becoming standardized, and their results should be accurate to within 5% of the true values (12).

Contact the manufacturer representative for a demonstration and decide to lease or buy depending on your particular needs. For example, will you be doing mass screenings on occasion and need rapid results? Will many other tests besides cholesterol measurement be done frequently? How portable should the device be?

Cholesterol testing machines are best kept on-site so that participants can receive immediate results. This reduces the cost and simplifies the logistics of shipping and handling specimens and mailing the test results. The person in charge of technical/medical details should be familiar with the previous section on cholesterol measuring devices and the section on quality control (see below). If the measuring device uses plasma samples, the results should be adjusted to serum levels to be consistent with the recommendations of the National Cholesterol Education Program (see conversion calculations, p. 26). The manufacturer of the equipment you have chosen will provide assistance with other materials required for the machine.

If an outside lab is used for the screening, the physician or technician in charge should confirm that the lab is both standardizing its testing device and using reagents (chemicals) that have been standardized for the lab's particular machine. Consider, too, the convenience of the lab to your site. Accuracy of HDL values declines with prolonged transit time unless the samples remain frozen. In addition, consistently using the same laboratory will further minimize the variability of results.

Ensure Accuracy for Your Testing

A 1985 report of the College of American Pathologists found large variations in cholesterol results between laboratories (13). This is unacceptable because the recommendations for cholesterol management are now uniform throughout the country. A cholesterol measurement of 240 mg/dl in New York must equal a 240 mg/dl cholesterol result in California.

To address this issue, the Laboratory Standardization Panel was formed within the National Cholesterol Education Program (14). The panel's recommendations are that both precision (measured as the coefficient of variation) and accuracy (bias) variability within labs should now be within ±5%. By 1992, the panel hopes that all labs will maintain the accuracy of their cholesterol values within a 3% range of the gold standard, which is the definitive reference method. Most manufacturers, including the three already mentioned, have acted quickly to conform to these recommendations for uniform standardization.

Five areas of concern in establishing accurate cholesterol results include the calibration of instruments, standardization of the equipment, proper training of personnel, internal quality control, and external quality control checks using reference labs.

Calibration.   The manufacturer supplies materials to calibrate the instrument each day before it is used and periodically during the day of the screening. This is like setting a bathroom scale to zero before stepping on it. These materials should come only from the machine's manufacturer and should be traceable to the CDC reference method. The Reflotron calibrates itself automatically and must be shipped to the manufacturer if readings are inaccurate (as judged by using control specimens).

Standardization.   In the past, the major problem with accuracy has been not in the technical precision of the machines (the consistency of repeated measurements of the same sample), but in their standardization to the true value. This caused much of the variation from one lab to another. Manufacturers used slightly different reference values, akin to setting a bathroom scale to an inaccurate standard weight. The true cholesterol level, or reference value, is determined by the National Reference System for Cholesterol (NRS/CHOL).[2]

Training. Staff must be adequately trained and committed to running the testing machines and identifying and correcting problems when they occur. Operating a portable cholesterol measurement device requires some training but no specialized laboratory experience (11). Supervisors should note that most inaccurate test results occur when equipment operators are improperly trained (15). A potential problem also arises when a person operates the testing equipment on an irregular basis and may forget important details from one screening to the next. The manufacturer's recommended maintenance program for the instrument must be strictly adhered to and documented in the quality control log.

Internal Quality Control. Samples from the manufacturer are available to verify that proper lab technique is being used and to ensure that the machine is working properly. The results should have been determined by or should be traceable to the NRS/CHOL method. These are run in the usual manner by the staff or lab supervisor. A control sample should be done and recorded at the beginning of each day the instrument is used and after every 20 to 50 participants during the day. The results obtained, as well as the "true" value, are recorded in a logbook. The accuracy (bias) should remain less than 5%; otherwise the machine should be withdrawn until corrected.

External Quality Control. To further assure accuracy, compare your lab's results with an NRS/CHOL reference laboratory using split blood samples. This backup is essential to good quality control if you use reagents and components from different suppliers. The addresses of the nine designated reference labs across the country are listed in the Resource section at the end of this book.

To summarize, the medical director or head technician in charge of your screening should confirm that the lab is calibrating its equipment according to the CDC's reference materials; is using reagents that have been manufactured for its particular machine; has effective internal quality control measures; uses uniform specimen collection, handling, and storage; and employs competent, motivated staff to perform the testing. The cost of

---

[2]The NRS/CHOL is a joint project of the Centers for Disease Control and the National Institute of Standards and Technology (the latter formerly the National Bureau of Standards) using the modified Abell-Kendall method.

these quality control procedures will add an additional 10% to the total program cost and should be considered in the pricing.

Personnel for the Screening

The planning committee and its advisors will coordinate the management of and direction for the screening. They usually recruit clerical, technical, and possibly computer staff. Volunteer nursing organizations may be contacted and can supplement the core staff for screenings. Cosponsoring hospitals can also supply staff to assist. Determine each participant's time restrictions, and set up a reasonable duration for a shift.

Personnel should be trained for the screening no more than a few days in advance so that details remain fresh in everyone's memory. The medical supplier often provides training for the technical staff. Backup consultation and supervision of staff must be arranged with health professionals in clinical laboratories.

The staff will need breaks during most screenings. If the advertising has been successful, the screening will be quite busy. Two or three breaks in an 8-hour period is essential to keep staff morale high and attitudes friendly. When relying on volunteers, overstaff by 20% to allow for no-shows due to sickness, previous commitments, or forgetfulness. Be prepared to orient and retrain volunteers during the screening. Have people arrive 15 minutes before the scheduled start of their shifts.

Those operating the testing devices should be thoroughly trained in the machine they will be using and should demonstrate competence before the screening.

Advertising and Publicity

For screenings of a mixed population, obtain an analysis of the intended audience through surveys, census data, or local chamber of commerce reports. The most effective channels for reaching people depend on their demographic characteristics such as age, occupation, education, family size, social structure, and lifestyle. Different methods exist for reaching different segments of the population (16).

If the screening is targeted to a particular segment of the population, use a medium that will reach this group. Special recruitment efforts will be needed for minorities and low-income or low-educational groups, because these people have consistently been found to have more CHD risk factors and less access to health care.

Try to elicit cosponsorship of screenings with local newspapers, radio or television stations, and hospitals to increase exposure and keep costs down. Public service announcements (PSAs), especially if they feature prominent local politicians, entertainers, athletes, and so forth, will attract interest. Radio and television stations frequently broadcast PSAs free of charge for public or nonprofit organizations. In addition, radio and television talk programs can provide exposure not only to the screenings, but also to the effectiveness of treatment for elevated cholesterol levels.

Posters advertising the screening are most effective if placed in "life path points" such as grocery stores, drugstores, shopping malls, banks, churches, work sites, schools, and social clubs. Figure 11.2 is a sample screening poster. The announcements should include the location, dates, times, cost, and sponsoring organization. Emphasize that no fasting is

Cholesterol
SCREENING

♥ **DATES:** September 12 – 17

♥ **TIME:** 10:30 a.m. – 6:30 p.m.

♥ **LOCATION:** 5910 S. University (at Orchard) in Littleton, and 1651 Broadway (at Arapahoe) in Boulder

♥ **COST:** $5.00 . . . Quick and easy — no fasting required

♥ **Heart-Healthy Tasting Buffet** will be available for all cholesterol screening participants ♥ Recipes & other heart-healthy information ♥ Custom Gift Basket give-away; enter a free raffle

Figure 11.2 An example cholesterol screening poster, including complete information on the screening.

required, because many people think fasting is necessary and will therefore not attend, or a large number of people will overload the screening in the early morning.

Some ideas that have proven helpful for promoting cholesterol screenings in communities include the following:

- Have low-cost flyers placed in shopping bags at local supermarket checkouts during the week prior to the screening. Contact the store manager in advance for approval.
- Make use of public service announcements. If your group is a not-for-profit organization, a local radio or television station may provide a short slot in their programming free of charge. Stations are required to broadcast a certain number of PSAs each day. Use newspaper PSA space as well.
- Many radio and television stations have health shows. Arrange to have a representative appear in person to explain the rationale and significance of cholesterol testing as well as announce the time and place of the screening.
- Set up interviews with the local newspapers. A newspaper article showing a photo of the town mayor, the company CEO, or another well-known official being tested will pique reader interest.
- Seek political support of the mayor, county commissioners, and local health department.
- Send short press releases to newspapers and radio and television stations. Again, a photo will have much more impact.
- Put up posters in stores, the library, the senior center, and other prominent locations around town. Try to reach a variety of audiences.
- Check with your county's public information director, if there is one, and enlist her or his support and advice.
- If funds permit, take out a newspaper advertisement in a Sunday edition.
- Alert the medical community through letters or phone calls to physicians, hospitals, drug representatives, pharmacists, and dentists. This may also be an opportunity to seek out volunteers from their staff members.
- For multiday screenings, have a local radio or television station do a live remote from the site.

After the screening, a letter to the editor or other public statement thanking the volunteers and community is important. In the workplace, a similar note of appreciation should appear in the next newsletter. Personal phone calls to officials who were particularly important or helpful will help ensure an enthusiastic response for future screenings.

For screenings at corporations and other large organizations, effective promotional methods include the following:

- Payroll stuffers
- Posters in the cafeteria, on the notice board, and in other prominent locations
- Newsletters, especially with a message of support from the director, president, or CEO
- Word of mouth from the medical, benefits, or personnel department
- Presentations on cholesterol and nutrition given by a member of the medical department or an outside consultant
- Nutrition displays, perhaps with taste samples
- Heart-healthy recipe cards and/or coupons for nutritious food items

Logistics of the Screening Day

Numerous details must be worked out in advance to ensure a smooth process on the day of the screening. Depending on the size and duration of the screening, the number of analyzer machines, and staffing, you may wish to use an appointment system to better predict and control the flow rate of participants.

If the appointment system is not used, movement into and through the area will vary, so backup personnel should be scheduled to appear at peak hours. A plan that has worked well in my experience is to have on hand one or more staff persons trained and experienced in all aspects of the screening procedure who know how to expedite the stream of participants.

The flow of human traffic from registration to blood drawing, to the results table, to the counseling and referral area, and to the exit will be critical. One-way movement of participants is optimal. Prepare a diagram for the organizational staff and send a copy to the facility's maintenance staff, mall manager, and other applicable personnel for their approval and suggestions. These people usually have a good understanding of the normal flow of human traffic through the building. Figure 11.3 illustrates three possible screening set-ups.

Stations must be staffed appropriately, and personnel rotated between them if possible to alleviate boredom. For every 50 participants each hour, you will need approximately two registrars, four phlebotomists, two to four analyzer operators (depending on the type of machine), three or four counselors, two people giving out results, one site supervisor, and one extra "float" nurse who can work at any station.

Allow two to three hours to set up the stations for the first day. Tables must be brought in, set up, and covered with paper and plastic before the machines are installed and calibrated. Other essential items are chairs for the waiting area, name tags for volunteers, a phone, staplers, pens, clipboards for registration, cholesterol handouts, and referral lists for doctors and dietitians. The responsibility for the acquisition, transport,

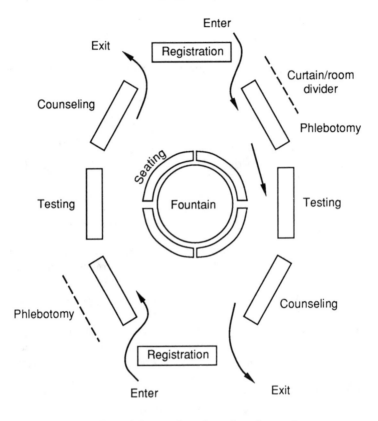

Round site, such as in a shopping mall

a   (Cont.)

Figure 11.3 Suggested floor plans for cholesterol screening areas.

and return of these materials must be delegated in advance. For multi-day screenings, a plan for secure overnight storage must be made.

A comprehensive checklist appears at the end of this chapter to help organizers with the supplies needed for the registration, phlebotomy, analyzing, and counseling stations.

Registration Station

A release-of-responsibility waiver should be required before an individual participates in any cholesterol screening. General liability coverage for the sponsoring organization is also advised unless approval has been obtained from the insurance carrier. Adequate coverage can be difficult

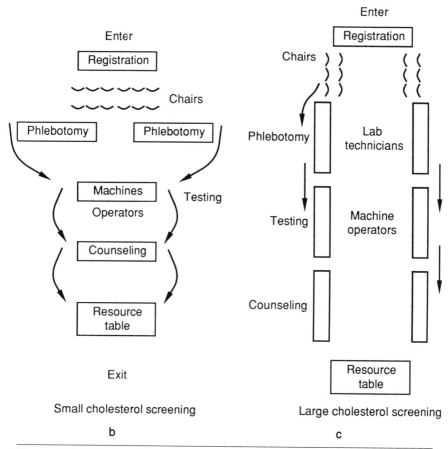

Figure 11.3 (Continued)

to obtain, so this should be investigated early. As more screenings are done and their safety verified, it is hoped the insurance problem will lessen.

The waiver can also serve as a questionnaire to obtain participants' demographics such as age, sex, marital status, and address. The questionnaire should be as detailed as necessary but not unduly so, as filling it out could impede the flow of traffic. Participants should sit and complete the questionnaire/waiver in an area adjacent to the phlebotomy station.

Statistics of height, weight, blood pressure, smoking, and other lifestyle habits will be important at the counseling and referral station and can help plan future health promotion activities. Information on how the individual learned of the screening is useful so that advertising strategies can be evaluated. See the sample waiver form.

Sample Waiver

I hereby request that a finger-stick cholesterol test be performed for me by the _____ screening program. I release _____ from any and all liability to me arising out of the performance of such test. I further understand the following:

1. The result of the test is to be considered preliminary only and in no way conclusive in assessing my risk for heart disease.
2. I am responsible for initiating follow-up should my screening cholesterol be elevated.
3. Data may be used by _____ for statistical and follow-up purposes only. My identity will remain confidential and no commercial use will be made of any of the data obtained.

I certify that I am of legal age and that I have read and understood the preceding paragraphs.

I do _____ do not _____ give my approval for the release of these results to my family physician, Dr. _____.

(Signature)   (Date)

(Address)

(City)   (State)   (Zip Code)   (Phone)

(Signature of parent/legal guardian for minors under 18 years)

Phlebotomy Station

Once they are registered, participants move to the blood drawing area. Ideally they should sit for 5 minutes before blood is taken (17). During this time the phlebotomist checks the waiver form for completeness and may answer any questions that participants have about the procedure. The risk of contracting AIDS is one of the most common questions. The phlebotomist should explain that new, sterile needles are used for each participant, thus eliminating any risk of contracting the virus. If the Autoclix is used, participants may be assured that its design precludes ever using the same lancet for more than one participant.

The Autoclix device is a spring-loaded cylinder into which a lancet is placed. The lancet end is then positioned against the participant's finger. The plunge of the lancet is rapid, rendering it essentially painless; perhaps 10% of the time the lancet will plunge near a nerve ending and cause a slight pinching sensation. Larger lancets are available for participants with heavily calloused fingers; however, technicians with experience may prefer to use the lancet manually.

To ensure safety, the phlebotomist and others who may have contact with blood should wear latex gloves during the entire testing procedure. These gloves should be changed with each participant or at least wiped clean with isopropyl alcohol.

The following five-step procedure for a finger-stick blood sample should take about 2 to 4 minutes.

1. Warm and cleanse any fingertip of the nondominant hand with an alcohol wipe. Remove excess alcohol with a cotton ball.
2. Obtain the blood sample by pricking either side of the fingertip (about 1/2 inch from the tip) with a small, sterile, razor-tipped lancet. Make sure the puncture is on the side facing the smaller fingers, because this area has fewer nerve endings. Wipe away any drops of blood that appear on the work station with isopropyl alcohol, either on cotton balls or in prepackaged wipes.
3. Wipe off the first bit of blood with a cotton ball, allowing a large drop to form. If necessary, gentle milking of the finger—not squeezing—is acceptable. Very little blood is needed for the new analyzers, only about .2 ml. (When blood is donated for a transfusion, the quantity is 2,000 times greater.)
4. Hold a glass capillary tube (if one is required) horizontally or slightly upward and move it to the edge of the blood. The blood will move up the tube spontaneously by capillary action. If the tube is held downward or moved out of the drop of blood, an air bubble will appear and the tube must be discarded. The analyzer representative will suggest a mechanism for closing the end of the tube. To fill a tiny vial, hold it beneath the finger, centered on the drop of blood, and move it sideways to pull in the blood.
5. Hand the participant a cotton ball to hold over the puncture site for a few minutes, and then cover it with a bandage. Instruct the participant to take the sample and/or registration paper to the results table. Allow those participants experiencing light-headedness to remain seated in a head-down position for a few minutes. Be sure to clean the plastic tip of the Autoclix with alcohol after each use.

Blood should not remain in certain capillary tubes for more than 10 minutes or it will clot. EDTA is the best anticoagulant for capillary tubes because it imparts a 3% to 4.7% difference between plasma and serum.

Other anticoagulants cause an increased spread, including oxalate (9%), citrate (14%), and fluoride (18%) (18).

To lessen the chances of blood clotting in tubes, the site coordinator should closely monitor the analyzing station for delays and slow the phlebotomy station if necessary. In addition, the coordinator must work closely with the chief phlebotomist to maintain adequate supplies because this station often becomes extremely busy. All personnel must be aware that blood-contaminated materials cannot be thrown into regular trash disposal systems. Contact a local hospital or health department for assistance in handling and disposing of biological waste.

The incidence of fainting is extremely low during this procedure, especially when the Autoclix is used. To be on the safe side, however, be sure to have a supply of cots and ammonia inhalants. Also, keep emergency phone numbers on hand, make arrangements to have an ambulance available on-site, and inform personnel of emergency protocol. Such precautions will ensure a safe screening.

Analyzing Station and Results Table

After blood is drawn, participants move to the analyzing station. They may hand the specimen to the analyzer technician themselves or be given a number and told to wait.

A process must be in effect to assure participants that the results of the cholesterol test are indeed their own. Some screenings encourage participants to carry their capillary tubes of blood directly to the machine operator and wait a minute or two for the results. This works well with the Reflotron or DT-60 because they process one test at a time.

If this is not practical in a large screening, a system for labeling the specimen must be devised. One option is a triple-label system. At registration, one of three identically numbered labels is placed on the capillary tube, and another on the registration form that is used in follow-up. A third label is given to the participant on a wallet card, which also lists the ranges for normal, borderline, and high blood cholesterol. Packets of labels are available from the manufacturers or can be printed in advance on sheets of 1/4-inch by 1/2-inch labels.

The analyzer operator records the cholesterol test results on the registration form, which is kept, and then records the participant's label number on the machine's cholesterol results ticket. A staff member uses this number to call a participant, who will match it to the wallet card number. This system assures all participants that the results are indeed their own.

Many people will have questions when they get their results. A staff member may be able to answer brief questions, but most should be handled at the counseling and referral table.

Counseling and Referral Station

Depending on the flow, participants can either obtain their cholesterol values directly from the analyzer station (in a small screening) or, more commonly, wait for the results in a designated area. Volunteers can then dispense the results as they are processed.

A graphic way to convey the result is to write the cholesterol number on a wallet card that lists the National Institutes of Health's categories for desirable, borderline, and high levels of cholesterol (4). You may want to add my categories of ideal, acceptable, and extremely high:

Cholesterol Categories

Ideal	Acceptable	Borderline	High	Extremely high
<160	160-200	200-240	240-280	>280 mg/dl
<4.1	4.1-5.2	5.2-6.2	6.2-7.2	>7.2 mmol/L

You must consider yourself in the next higher category if you have already had a heart attack or stroke or if you possess two or more of the following risk factors:

1. Male gender
2. Smoking
3. High blood pressure
4. Diabetes
5. Severe obesity (more than 30% above ideal weight)
6. HDL cholesterol less than 35 mg/dl (0.9 mmol/L)
7. History of heart attack before age 55 in a parent or sibling

---

After receiving their cholesterol results, participants are directed to the counseling and referral station. They will be curious at this point as to what the numbers mean. Counselors should advise that a diagnosis of borderline or high blood cholesterol can be made only by the participant's physician, using a fasting lipid profile and perhaps a thyroid test or other investigations.

Participants with ideal cholesterol levels (lower than 160 mg/dl or 4.1 mmol/L) and no other risk factors should be congratulated. Their lifestyle, heredity, or both are providing them with near-certain protection from atherosclerosis. Advise them to have their blood checked again within 5 years. Mention that cholesterol levels tend to increase with age in our society, especially in women after menopause.

Those individuals with cholesterol levels in the acceptable range of 160 to 200 mg/dl (4.1–5.2 mmol/L) should be advised to keep their cholesterol at or below this range. Although not required by the NCEP, I recommend that participants whose cholesterol levels fall in the 180 to 200 mg/dl (4.65 to 5.2 mmol/L) range who also have two or more risk factors be given the same advice as those in the borderline category of 200 to 240 mg/dl. Regular cholesterol checks are recommended every 5 years as a minimum. These individuals should be given basic information about healthy eating patterns and perhaps some nutrition handouts. Choose from the inexpensive government publications listed in the Resources section of this book.

If a participant has previously had his or her cholesterol tested and finds a difference, explain that normal physiology can affect test values by as much as ±20 mg/dl (0.5 mmol/L). Also, stress has a profound influence on some individuals, raising cholesterol levels by as much as 50 mg/dl (1.3 mmol/L) or more.

Persons with cholesterol results between 200 and 240 mg/dl (5.2–6.2 mmol/L) and who have no or only one additional risk factor are classified as borderline high risk. They should be given dietary advice and more detailed handouts. Recommend that they see their usual medical provider for a complete lipid profile within 3 months. If other risk factors or symptoms of coronary disease are present, this should be done sooner. Emphasize that screenings are *not* a substitute for regular medical care.

Reassure those at borderline high risk that the majority of people in their category are able to reduce cholesterol to safer levels without using drugs. If other risk factors are present, these will also need attention.

Participants with high-risk cholesterol levels of over 240 mg/dl (6.2 mmol/L) should be given detailed handouts and referred to their physicians as soon as possible, preferably within a month. Included in the high risk group are those testing borderline high who have clinical disease or two or more other risk factors. Any child or adolescent with a total cholesterol level over 170 mg/dl (4.4 mmol/L) also deserves a referral. The physician will do a fasting lipid panel and possibly other tests.

A referral mechanism for treatment after the testing date must be available for those with high blood cholesterol and for those with borderline levels and two or more risk factors. Be prepared for the high-risk group because they frequently comprise one third or more of all participants. A list of dietitians and physicians in the area interested in treating elevated cholesterol levels should be compiled in advance and available to these individuals. Any participant who does not have a physician will need a referral from this list. Counselors should be emphatic that high-risk persons obtain a follow-up but should not cause alarm. Hypercholesterolemia warrants immediate attention but does not constitute an emergency.

More and more people today desire health information even though they are not at high risk. Distribute educational materials and inform participants of any upcoming nutrition classes. If at all possible, have them register for the course at the screening when their motivation is high.

Follow-Up

Screening should augment, not replace, regular medical care. After the screening, the high-risk individuals who have been referred to physicians or dietitians should be contacted by mail or phone. If staffing permits, an ideal follow-up also includes those with borderline blood cholesterol levels. Determine the following:

- Have any participants undergone further testing? If so, where?
- Have any participants contacted their physician?
- Have any participants initiated the recommendations of their treating physicians, especially dietary, drug, or other interventions?
- Have any participants obtained nutritional counseling?

Public screening participants found to be in need of further evaluation do in fact see their physicians. Up to two thirds have reportedly done so after attending well-managed screenings. A reasonable goal of follow-up should be to determine that at least half of those referred to their medical providers see them within the suggested time period.

Interface With the Medical System

Maintain and foster a close relationship with local sources of medical care. If all participants with plasma cholesterol levels over 200 mg/dl (5.2 mmol/L) are referred to their physicians, the area's medical system could easily be overwhelmed.

To encourage smooth referrals, inform local physicians in personal letters of the upcoming cholesterol screening and your recommendations for physician follow-up. Give them samples of the cholesterol literature that will be distributed to participants and the criteria for physician referral. Invite them to attend the screening or perhaps give a presentation on cholesterol.

The medical director for the screening should inquire as to the willingness of physicians to guide patients toward desirable and ideal cholesterol levels. Recent surveys indicate that physician attitudes are changing rapidly to keep in step with the advances in cholesterol management.

If at all possible, the screenings's medical director should present a program on cholesterol and the value of screening to the local medical society, at the hospital's grand rounds, or at a similar physician education meeting. The American Heart Association has an excellent training program for physician education, complete with slides to facilitate and standardize the important message to local doctors.

An unfortunate and sometimes major stumbling block to cholesterol management in some communities is physicians' attitudes regarding acceptable levels. Physicians have been reluctant to diagnose hyper-cholesterolemia for values less than the 95th percentile, or nearly 300 mg/dl (7.8 mmol/L). Even reference laboratories frequently do not label values as abnormal unless they are above the 95th percentile. Yet studies have determined that there is a fivefold increase in risk within these "normal" limits (6, 19, 20).

Public screenings are an important first step in controlling cholesterol because they can reach large segments of the community. Trained staff, frequent calibration of equipment, and quality assurance measures will ensure accurate results.

SCREENING SUPPLIES CHECKLIST[3]

Registration Area
- [ ] tape, thumbtacks, paper clips
- [ ] file boxes
- [ ] triplicate labels
- [ ] capillary tubes
- [ ] cash box with start-up cash
- [ ] pens, pencils
- [ ] registration forms, handouts, notepads, waiver forms
- [ ] tables, table skirts, plastic covers, chairs
- [ ] blood pressure cuffs

Phlebotomy Station
- [ ] tables, chairs, reading materials
- [ ] lancets (sterile razor-tipped device for obtaining a drop of blood)
- [ ] autoclix (spring-loaded lancet plunger)
- [ ] bleach solution (a 1:10 dilution of household bleach with water is sufficient to kill bacteria, AIDS virus, etc.)
- [ ] cotton balls (to stop bleeding and wipe off the first drop of blood)
- [ ] bandages (use even if bleeding has apparently stopped)
- [ ] vinyl disposal gloves of medical quality (need not be sterile; these are used for all personnel who come in contact with blood, such as the phlebotomists and analyzing machine operators)
- [ ] alcohol wipes, chem wipes
- [ ] hazardous waste containers, trash cans
- [ ] capillary tubes or vials, labels
- [ ] ammonia inhalants

---

[3]The assistance of Zoë Rabinowitz in the preparation of this list is greatly appreciated.

Analyzing Station and Results Table

☐ tables, skirts, plastic covers, chairs
☐ pens, pencils, thumbtacks
☐ analyzer equipment (enough machines to minimize waiting)
☐ cholesterol slides or cassettes (1 for each participant)
☐ chem wipes (to clean equipment)
☐ pipettes
☐ bleach solution (to clean table)
☐ trash cans with plastic liners

Counseling and Referral Station

☐ tables, chairs
☐ pens, pencils
☐ file boxes (for registration forms)
☐ educational literature (see *Handouts* in Resources section at end of this book)

References

1. National Heart, Lung, and Blood Institute (NHLBI). (1985). NHLBI Consensus Development Conference on lowering blood cholesterol to prevent heart disease. *Journal of the American Medical Association,* **253**, 2080-2090.
2. Sempos, C., Fulwood, R., Haines, C., Carroll, M., Anda, R., Williamson, D.F., Remmington, P., & Cleeman, J. (1989). The prevalence of high blood cholesterol among adults in the United States. *Journal of the American Medical Association,* **262**, 45-52.
3. Wilson, P.W.F., Christiansen, J.C., Anderson, K.M., & Kannel, W.B. (1989). Impact of national guidelines for cholesterol risk factor screening. *Journal of the American Medical Association,* **262**, 41-44.
4. Expert Panel of the National Cholesterol Education Program (NCEP). (1988). Report of the Expert Panel of the NCEP on detection, evaluation, and treatment of high blood cholesterol in adults. *Archives of Internal Medicine,* **148**, 36-39. (Also available from the National Cholesterol Education Program, NIH Publication No. 88-2925)
5. Levy, A.S. (1988, November). *Recent trends in public beliefs about fat and cholesterol. NCEP/Food and Drug Administration Survey.* Presented at the First National Cholesterol Conference, Washington, DC.
6. Castelli, W.P., Garrison, R.J., Wilson, P.W.F., Abbott, R.D., Kalousdian, S., & Kannel, W.B. (1986). Incidence of coronary heart disease and lipoprotein cholesterol levels: The Framingham Study. *Journal of the American Medical Association,* **256**, 2835-2842.
7. Wynder, E.L., Field, F., & Haley, N.J. (1986). Population screening

for cholesterol determination. *Journal of the American Medical Association*, **265**, 2839-2842.

8. Boerma, G.J.M., van Gorp, I., & Liem, T.L. (1988). Revised calibration of the Reflotron cholesterol assay evaluated. *Clinical Chemistry*, **34**, 1124-1127.

9. Greenland, P., Bowley, N.L. French, C.A. Meiklejohn, B., Gagliano, S., & Sparks, C.E. (1990). Precision and accuracy of a portable blood analyzer system during cholesterol screening. *American Journal of Public Health*, **80**, 181-184.

10. Kaufman, H.W., McNamara, J.R., Anderson, K.M., Wilson, P.W.F., & Schaefer, E.J. (1990). How reliably can compact chemistry analyzers measure lipids? *Journal of the American Medical Association*, **263**, 1245-1249.

11. Pearson, J.R., Dusenbury, L.J., & Byyny, R.L. (1988). Worksite screening for hypercholesterolemia. *American Journal of Medicine*, **85**, 369-374.

12. McManus, B.M., Toth, A.B., Engel, J.A., Myers, G.L., Naito, H.K., Wilson, J.E., & Cooper, G.R. (1989). Progress in lipid reporting practices and reliability of blood cholesterol measurement in clinical laboratories in Nebraska. *Journal of the American Medical Association*, **262**, 83-88.

13. College of American Pathologists. (1985). *Comprehensive chemistry survey* (set C-D). Skokie, IL: College of American Pathologists.

14. Laboratory Standardization Panel, National Cholesterol Education Program. (1988). Current status of blood cholesterol measurement in clinical laboratories in the United States. NIH Publication No. 88-2928, Bethesda, MD.

15. Naughton, M.J., Luepker, R.V., & Strickland, D. (1990). The accuracy of portable analyzers in public screenings programs. *Journal of the American Medical Association*, **263**, 1213-1217.

16. Farquhar, J.W., Fortmann, S.P., Maccoby, N., Haskell, W.L., Williams, P.T., Flora, J.A., Taylor, C.B., Brown, B.W., Soloman, D.S., & Hulley, S.B. (1985). The Stanford Five-City Project: Design and methods. *American Journal of Epidemiology*, **122**, 323-334.

17. Hagen, R.D., Upton, S.J.V., Avakian, E.V., & Grundy, S. (1986). Increases in serum lipid and lipoprotein levels with movement from the supine to standing position in adult men and women. *Preventive Medicine*, **15**, 18.

18. Myers,G.L., & Cooper, G.R. (1989). Laboratory performance in cholesterol testing. *Cardiovascular Reviews and Reports*, **10**, 14-26.

19. Multiple Risk Factor Intervention Trial Research Group. (1982). Multiple Risk Factor Intervention Trial: Risk factor changes and mortality results. *Journal of the American Medical Association*, **148**, 1465-1477.

20. Martin, J.J., Hulley, S.B., Browner, W.S., Kuller, L.H., & Wentworth, D. (1986). Serum cholesterol, blood pressure, and mortality: Implications from a cohort of 361,662 men. *Lancet*, **2**, 933-936.

Suggested Readings

Blair, S.N., Piserchia, P.V., Wilbur, C.S., et al. (1986). Worksite health promotion: A public health intervention model for worksite health promotion. *Journal of the American Medical Association, 255*, 921-926.

Bly, J.L., Jones, R.C., & Richardson, J.E. (1986). Impact of worksite health promotion on health care costs and utilization: Evaluation of Johnson & Johnson's Live for Life program. *Journal of the American Medical Association, 256*, 3235-3240.

Brink, S.C. (1987). *Health risks and behavior: The impact on medical costs.* Brookfield, WI: Milliman and Robertson.

Bruno, R., Arnold, C., Jacobsen, L., et al. (1983). Randomized controlled trial of a non-pharmacologic cholesterol reduction program at the worksite. *Preventive Medicine, 12*, 523-532.

Carpenter, R.A. (1988). Heart at work: The evolution and evaluation of a low-cost worksite health promotion program. *Health Values, 12*, 34-40.

Fielding, J.E. (1984). Health promotion and disease prevention at the worksite. *Annual Review of Public Health, 5*, 237-265.

Glanz, K., & Seewald-Klein, T. (1986). Nutrition at the worksite: An overview. *Journal of Nutrition Education, 18*, S1-S11.

Merrill, B.E. (1983). Evaluating a health promotion program by examining health care claims. *Priorities in health statistics: Proceedings of the 19th National Meeting of the Public Health Conference on Records and Statistics* (pp. 75-79) (DHHS Publication No. PHS 81-1214).

O'Donnell, M.P. (1986). *Design of workplace health promotion programs.* Royal Oak, MI: *American Journal of Health Promotion.*

Parkinson, R.S. (1982). *Managing health promotion in the workplace.* Palo Alto, CA: Mayfield.

Taylor, R.B., Ureda, J.R., & Denham, J.W. (1982). *Health promotion principles and clinical applications.* Norwalk, CT: Appleton-Century-Crofts.

Chapter

12

Cholesterol Education Programs

More than a third of all American adults are at high risk for heart attacks based on their serum cholesterol levels. And over 60 million Americans need intensive dietary and even drug intervention to lower their cholesterol levels (1). Worse, most of them do not even know what their cholesterol values are. And according to at least one survey, 60% of American men and women with known heart disease or high-risk cholesterol levels have not received any cholesterol counseling (2). Clearly we are in desperate need of comprehensive cholesterol-control programs— in our hospitals, communities, schools, and work sites.

Developing a health-oriented culture is more cost-effective in the long run than individual case-finding and personal health instruction. It facilitates frequent, ongoing reinforcement of positive health habits from one's peers and from the organization. Most important, perhaps, is that once in place, a wellness culture will be health-enhancing for future members as they enter the system.

Cholesterol management encompasses a tri-level hierarchy of approaches beginning with attempts to simply increase the general awareness of diet and cholesterol. The first level includes conveying health messages via posters and newsletters and sponsoring screenings (discussed in chapter 11) to identify people at high risk of having hypercholesterolemia. The second level aspires to effect behavior changes through health education. Classes about nutrition, exercise, stress management, and so forth are most effective when they are integrated. An exercise program, for example, assists in weight loss and smoking cessation, and stress management aids in changing inappropriate eating behaviors. The highest tier of prevention builds on the previous two in developing a cultural environment that fosters a wellness lifestyle (3). Together, all three levels of intervention can drastically reduce a person's chance of developing one of our society's major killer diseases (see Figure 12.1).

Establishing a cholesterol control system on any of these levels involves four basic steps: program design, marketing and promotion, implementation, and evaluation. Each of these steps is discussed in the following sections. A special section addressing the format and techniques for teaching a cholesterol-lowering class is included at the end of this chapter.

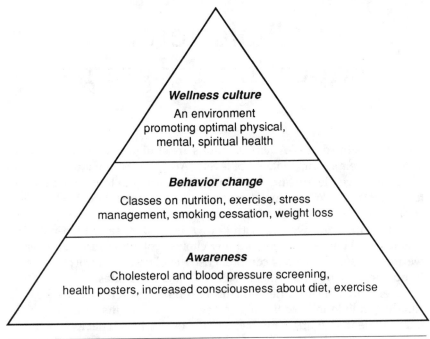

Figure 12.1   The hierarchy of approaches to cholesterol control.

Step I Program Design

Planning is the most important phase of any health promotion program. A detailed design that includes clear objectives, careful record-keeping, and a preset evaluation strategy is essential for management personnel to accept the proposal. Slighting this stage is most often responsible for a subsequent breakdown in efficiency or effectiveness. Key areas in program design include assessing needs, support, and resources; setting goals and policies; and using this information to select programs and evaluation criteria.

The first priority is assessing the needs of the group seeking a prevention program. What do members need, and what does the sponsoring organization intend to achieve? Is mere detection of elevated cholesterol levels desired, or will the organization orchestrate health education, provide nutritional guidance, and manage the medical aspects of cholesterol control? Is the group seeking to achieve immediate gains in morale and productivity or a healthy culture for long-lasting health benefits and reduced absenteeism and medical costs?

Successful programs enlist support and interest from many different levels of an organization. Though experience has shown that endorsement from top management is crucial, participation in the design process should be shared by people at all levels. Assessing the needs of the different groups enables you to employ effective marketing and behavior modification tactics and increases the likelihood for everyone's cooperation in implementing the program. Staff and managers may also share in making decisions about policies and physical facilities and help with the ongoing process of program evaluation and modification. In corporate wellness programs, responsibility rests with personnel departments (35.1%), top management (20.5%), the safety group (18.2%), the medical department (14.3%), health benefits (7.4%), employees (1.3%), and unions (0.2%) (4).

Resources for technical expertise, communication, education, and program costs must be determined and kept clearly in mind. Adequate funds and sufficient staff must be available to write, teach, and disseminate information throughout the organization. Consultants in health promotion can help immensely in advising the steering committee or top management in various aspects of the program.

Technical resources are needed to manage the cholesterol tests, blood pressure measurements, and exercise devices. Personnel within the community or in hospitals, county health departments, the American Heart Association, or volunteer nursing organizations can supplement an institution's resources. Representatives from medical and exercise equipment suppliers will help train personnel in the proper use of their equipment.

Communication resources, including the offices of employee health, personnel, benefits, and public relations, are needed to promote the cholesterol management program in general and to announce upcoming events. People with special skills are needed to design and produce attractive, simple, and effective flyers, posters, and audiovisual pieces to announce upcoming projects and courses.

Educational resources include physicians, nurses, dietitians, psychologists, and fitness instructors who are knowledgeable about diet, cholesterol, and health. If none of these people are already within the organization, you may be able to seek them out from the community. Contact local health clubs, hospitals, or the health department for help.

The amount of money each participant pays for the program will vary with the type of sponsoring organization and the characteristics of the prospective participants. A certain level of copayment is desirable in health education classes, perhaps with a reimbursement (cash or other) to participants who meet the goals. Grants are available from a number of government and private sources.

Some of the costs of implementing a health promotion program may be immediately offset by lowered insurance premiums. An increasing number of insurers, such as Blue Cross/Blue Shield, are adopting this policy for groups instituting wellness programs. They will even help develop the program. Later, as employee medical claims decrease, insurance premiums will be adjusted even lower. Sometimes the best option is to share a program with one or more other organizations to spread out the costs.

Goals and Policies

Both long-term and short-term goals for the cholesterol program must be clearly defined and written down. Don't assume everyone has identical expectations for the risk-reduction program. Each department in the organization will have a different agenda, such as facilitating recruitment, improving employee health and morale, or decreasing staff turnover. The ultimate goal, of course, is to curb the alarmingly high rate of atherosclerosis. The medical costs and loss of productivity associated with atherosclerosis remain unsurpassed by any other disease.

Policies need to be set early and clearly. For example, who is eligible for the program—the community, a company's employees, employees' families? Who will pay for the program and how? Will copayment be required for cholesterol tests or for classes? Will the classes be held during company time, personal time, or a mixture of both?

Finally, what specific program can be offered within the budgetary constraints? Examples include cholesterol screenings and medical follow-up for those at high risk; classes on nutrition; an exercise facility; or auxiliary programs targeting weight loss, stress management, and smoking cessation. Cholesterol screening was discussed thoroughly in chapter 11, and nutrition classes and program evaluation are discussed in Steps III and IV, which follow. Addressing these and the next Step will ensure a pertinent and effective program.

Step II Marketing and Promotion

Central to any marketing plan is an accurate understanding of the prospective audience. This may be obtained through the marketing departments of local hospitals, which frequently survey their surrounding populations. Ask for a demographic data base and a mailing list. A hospital usually requests a fee for this information unless the program is closely affiliated with the hospital. Alternative sources for demographic data bases include private marketing companies, many of which can provide selective lists of a particular zip code or age bracket.

Another option, especially if the target audience is specific, is to complete a new marketing survey. Questions should include demographics (age, sex, home address), cholesterol awareness and concern, interest in a cholesterol course in general, and specific aspects such as the topics discussed in Step III.

Billboards, memos, circulars, leaflets, and general mentions in meetings can serve to advertise the program. Details are best introduced at a special session. This may take place in a large group, or in smaller ones broken up by department. Allow up to an hour to announce the rationale and goals for the heart-health initiative, and give a detailed explanation of what will be available. A health fair can be used to kick off the program—this can feature cholesterol screening; height, weight, and blood pressure measurements; and dissemination of health education materials. This is also an excellent way to encourage involvement of other family members.

Once the program is initiated, advertisement and promotion are essential to encourage participation and maintain interest over time. If the institution has a marketing or public relations department, enlist its assistance. The staff can incorporate announcements about upcoming events into existing communication lines and publicity styles. They can assist in working with the local media to get positive press releases.

Step III Program Implementation

Changing eating behaviors requires a program of instruction and behavior modification tailored to the educational levels, age, gender, and learning styles of the participants. The format may include any combination of lectures, cooking demonstrations, audiovisual instruction, assigned readings, or group discussion.

I recommend five sessions that meet once a week for 60 to 90 minutes. Few people can realistically commit to longer periods, and 5 weeks is just long enough for people to break dietary habits. Between sessions, assignments and goals provide continuity and reinforcement of the topics.

The ideal group size is 10 to 16 participants, each committed to attending all five sessions. Group dynamics, which are powerful in the course's total impact, are inhibited when fewer than 6 or more than 25 enroll. Sustained behavior change is fostered when couples attend the workshop together.

The course requires a room to be set up as a real or staged kitchen, complete with shelves, plastic food models, food scales, and food packages. A stove, dishes, and cooking utensils add realism and help with instruction. Audiovisual equipment, if used appropriately, enhances learning and enlivens the presentation. (Suppliers of relevant audiovisual tapes, food models, and scales are listed in the Resources section at the end of this book.)

Instructors should collect packages and cans of a wide variety of standard and healthy food products. Particularly useful are items with misleading labels such as saturated vegetable oils that are labeled "no cholesterol," "lite," or "reduced cholesterol." Also bring in those hard-to-find alternatives such as canola oil, soy "cheese" and "mayonnaise," and high-fiber, low-fat snack items. The packages can be used throughout the course to provide a comparison of ingredients, increase participants' familiarity with nutritious foods, and reinforce intelligent shopping habits.

Decide which modified recipes to cook and serve during the final session and have recipes ready for distribution. Each recipe should provide nutritional information by way of a table or pie chart of fat, protein, and carbohydrate, or a list of how many fat calories or equivalent pats of butter it contains.

Develop a format for participants' notebooks. These will contain all the material covered in the course as well as food intake records, relevant articles, research findings, label comparisons, and recipes. The design should encourage ongoing use after the course, especially for recording subsequent levels of cholesterol, blood pressure, and body weight. I prefer to distribute material on a weekly basis as a topic is discussed rather than give out complete notebooks at the beginning of the course.

Third-party payment for the course generally requires a referral from the participant's primary care physician. The referring physician must request hyperlipidemia treatment, not simply dietary counseling, on the referral form.[1] Most insurance companies require that the instructor be a registered dietitian, physician, nurse, or health educator.

Few organizations outside of health departments, hospitals, or very large corporations have staff who are already qualified to teach cholesterol-lowering classes. First-time instructors can study the material in this and preceding chapters, attend special workshops, or utilize local registered dietitians. The teacher may use the chapters of this book to prepare weekly topics and reading assignments.

---

[1]Reimbursement is optimized when the specific medical ICD code is utilized, such as 272.0 for pure hypercholesterolemia, 272.1 for hypertriglyceridemia, and 272.2 for mixed hyperlipidemia. The most general code is 272.4, which refers to unspecified hyperlipidemia.

Step IV Program Evaluation

Program evaluation serves the vital function of measuring the benefits that have occurred as a result of the program. This may be done in terms of enhanced health knowledge and/or reduced health care costs. Feedback about each facet of the cholesterol management system deserves critical review in order to recognize the specific program modifications that may be necessary. The overall goal is to evaluate the effectiveness of the program in terms of lifestyle improvements.

To address this evaluation issue, a government conference on priorities in health statistics met in 1981. One of the results of this important meeting was the determination that healthy lifestyles did result in fewer medical claims, and that this was statistically significant (5). With the high expense of tracking individuals' health care costs, organizations should be encouraged to follow changes in risk factors because favorable trends will likely result in cost savings over time.

Evaluating the outcome of the program can be as straightforward as looking for improved scores on nutrition education tests or surveys for positive changes in lifestyle behavior patterns (6). Consider the feedback to the following questions before and after the course begins.

- What diet or other lifestyle changes have occurred as a direct result of the course?
- Was the screening enough to change habits known to be unhealthy?
- To what extent did classes, posters, and other educational materials assist in making improvements in health habits?
- Were changes in the corporate environment, such as nutritious cafeteria food and designation of nonsmoking areas, helpful?

Questionnaires may also be used to evaluate the quality of participants' lives. Supervisors and associates could comment on any performance or mood changes that they noted in participants after the program. Asking the individuals themselves or their spouses may be the best method of evaluating subjective improvements because they can identify what educational tools bolstered achievement, morale, or joie de vivre. Companies may choose to monitor employee job satisfaction, productivity, turnover, and absenteeism.

Another measurement of strategy effectiveness is the trend (ideally a lowering) in blood cholesterol or blood pressure. This data can indicate what percentage of participants versus nonparticipants are lowering their levels and by how much. Individual values, like all medical information, must be confidential.

Although improvements in serum cholesterol levels, morale, and absenteeism begin within weeks, rates of heart attack and stroke will not decline appreciably for 5 to 10 years. Consistent data from several international studies show that we can expect at least a 2% reduction in coronary heart disease for every 1% reduction in serum cholesterol (7). Thus, cholesterol control should be viewed as a long-term project, requiring a 5- to 10-year period to appreciate the major cost savings and health benefits.

Cost-effectiveness is rated as the primary goal of health promotion programs by leaders in corporate health affairs (3). However, the time required to collect and analyze the large amount of data used to identify reductions in health care expenses, heart attacks, strokes, and the like can prove prohibitive. Yet institutions that have the resources to complete such analyses have reported positive health enhancement for such programs as cholesterol levels (8, 9), blood pressures (10), smoking rates (11), absenteeism (12, 13), medical claims (14), activity level (15), obesity (16), job performance (17), and overall cost effectiveness (18, 19).

Organizations without such data-processing resources can track major risk factors, such as cholesterol, blood pressure, and smoking. They can infer from this information that their own in-house program will be cost-effective if employees' cholesterol levels, blood pressures, and so forth are lowered. The health risk appraisal is another inexpensive alternative for evaluation.

Health Risk Appraisal

A valuable tool for assessing the medical impact of health promotion programs is the health risk appraisal (HRA). This is a computer-scored questionnaire about lifestyle characteristics such as serum cholesterol level, blood pressure, weight, smoking, drinking, seat belt use, and others. The data base for most of these software programs was compiled from the national statistics by the Centers for Disease Control. A wide variety of HRA formats are available from public and private organizations.

For the corporate client, a group summary is a valuable option to include with the HRA. The summary tabulates the percentage of employees in each age and sex category who have elevated cholesterol, blood pressure, or other characteristics. Then it calculates the potential years of life saved by improving lifestyles. These calculations may be compared at yearly intervals to estimate the reduction in risk factors within various departments, across organizational strata, or in the company as a whole.

Teaching a Cholesterol-Lowering Class

Poor dietary habits are difficult to break, and to do so requires modern constructive behavioral techniques. The nutrition course described in this section incorporates practical applications of a variety of such techniques. Examples include self-monitoring (using diet logs), contingency contracting (writing a personal contract for behavior change), stimulus control (keeping unhealthy food out of the house), cognitive restructuring (practicing positive imagery and affirmations), and positive reinforcement (rewards for successes).

In addition, effective nutritional group counseling requires a well-organized lesson plan. Keeping to a simple course outline prevents participants from feeling overwhelmed by all the available (and frequently confusing) nutritional information. The salient points of the dietary approach focus on restricting cholesterol and fat, particularly saturated fat, while consuming more fiber, particularly soluble fiber. Additional benefits come from eating fish rich in omega-3 fatty acids, but stress that this does not preclude lean red meats or skinned poultry from one's diet. The background information found in chapters 7, 8, 9, and 10 can be reviewed by the instructor and discussed.

The instructor should explain the material in a simple and concrete fashion—For example: "I recommend no more than two eggs a week" rather than, "Limit your cholesterol intake to a maximum of 300 milligrams a day." Pictures, drawings, or food models are valuable in demonstrating proper serving sizes and combinations for attractive, heart-healthy meals.

Like all wellness measures, cholesterol control should emphasize the positive aspects of health enhancement. Eating for health can and should be delicious as well as nutritious. Participants must be made aware that "diet" is not a four-letter word for deprivation and denial, but rather is a plan to eat naturally. This means choosing a wide variety of foods that are low in fat, salt, sugar, and additives yet high in protein, fiber, vitamins, and minerals.

Incremental changes in diet are more likely to be sustained and appreciated than sudden, drastic changes. A useful motto to begin with is this: "First things first: Avoid the worst." Both participant and instructor must be tolerant of a sluggish start and occasional setbacks. A 3- to 6-month trial is necessary before it is decided that the plan has failed or that the participant has not followed instructions.

The instructor's energetic, positive attitude and effective communication skills are indispensable in leading class members to lower their cholesterol levels. The group's cultural background must be understood, especially their favorite dishes, cooking methods, and eating traditions. Demonstrating how nutrition is important to them as individuals and to their families will instill a sense of relevancy and thus the motivation to change.

During the course instructors should give participants frequent positive feedback to reinforce healthy behaviors. Because atherosclerosis develops over decades, it is vital that participants make a lifelong commitment to healthy eating. Such a resolution involves ongoing effort and dedication so that the overall goal is not abandoned after inevitable splurges or slip-ups. Involving spouses or significant others can help build a supportive environment.

Repetition also promotes retention. Some key points are so critical that they deserve reiteration throughout the course:

- There is a distinction between dietary cholesterol and blood cholesterol levels.
- For blood cholesterol, the lower, the better.
- Lowering blood cholesterol levels lowers one's chances of a heart attack; every 1% decrease in blood cholesterol corresponds to a 2% decrease in CHD risk.
- This eating pattern also helps control diabetes, hypertension, stroke, obesity, and certain cancers.
- Dietary changes and, if necessary, the use of cholesterol-lowering drugs can control cholesterol even in people with greatly elevated levels. In fact, those with the worst cholesterol problems stand to gain the most from this course.
- Eating heart-healthy foods must continue for life, not just until cholesterol falls into a safe range.

Lesson Plan

The following 5-week plan[2] has been used successfully in teaching diverse community groups about cholesterol control. For each 60-to 90-minute session I have developed a list of objectives, an explanation of critical points, an outline, teaching aids, a group activity, and an assignment.

Session 1: What Is Cholesterol and How Is It Controlled?

The challenge at this first session is to present the background information needed for further discussion. Part I of this book provides the details regarding this information. Nothing can be assumed; if necessary touch on all the basic facets of nutrition. Asking members of the group to paraphrase the important concepts in their own words frequently exposes misunderstandings. Specific questions encourage curiosity and involvement.

Objectives, Session 1. Participants will

1. understand the basics of cholesterol physiology and the role cholesterol plays in coronary heart disease and stroke;

---

[2]The assistance of Mary Montgomery, R.D., and Mary Taylor in the preparation of this section is greatly appreciated.

2. know how a healthy diet both limits the amount of cholesterol that is absorbed and increases the number of LDL receptors, helping the liver to perform its cleanup job;
3. realize that, traditionally, "normal" values for cholesterol have been set far too high for optimal health;
4. become aware of other lifestyle factors relevant to the prevention and treatment of atherosclerosis;
5. be able to state the major dietary components that affect blood cholesterol levels;
6. learn how to maintain a food intake log; and
7. make at least one goal that will initiate dietary change and/or exercise habits.

Outline, Session 1.

1. Introduction of facilitator, participants, and course outline (10 minutes)
2. Major points of atherosclerosis (5 minutes)

    (a) High prevalence in advanced societies
    (b) Contributing risk factors
    (c) Gradual progression from childhood and possible reversal

3. The effect of dietary cholesterol on serum cholesterol (5 minutes)
4. The effects of saturated and unsaturated fat on serum cholesterol (5 minutes)
5. The effects of soluble and insoluble fiber on digestion and cholesterol metabolism (5 minutes)
6. The many positive effects of fish, especially those with a high omega-3 content (5 minutes)
7. Keeping an accurate food record (15 minutes)
8. Group activity: Goal setting (20 minutes)
9. Questions and answers

Teaching Aids, Session 1. Blackboard and chalk, or poster paper and markers; extra pens; tables; and chairs.

Activity, Session 1. At the end of this meeting instructors need to discuss goal setting. Involve the participants in defining their own problem areas and setting personal goals for the next 6 months. This promotes empowerment (internal locus of control) and confidence in their abilities to manage cholesterol. Stress that gradual change is not only acceptable but preferred; sudden alterations in eating patterns are unlikely to be sustained.

Dietary goals should be personal, specific, and measurable. Initially one to three goals should be set, with at least one of them targeting a weak spot. Some participants may prefer to set a relatively easy goal at first, to ensure success and build confidence and momentum. Participants can fill out a personal contract, such as the one in Figure 12.2, and post it in a conspicuous place.

Examples of initial goals include the following:

- To limit all meat portions to 3-1/2 ounces
- To enjoy a fish meal at least twice each week
- To prepare a meatless entree, such as a bean casserole or soup, twice each week
- To eat vegetables, fruit, and grains at least twice a day

Assignment, Session 1.   Select a reading from the list of resources. Choose from the wide assortment of publications according to the participants' needs (see the Resources section at the end of this book). Prepare a goal statement and behavior-change contract, complete with a reward and consequence for achieving or not achieving the goal.

Sample Behavior Change Contract

I, _____ contract to

eat_____

(food groups, amounts, frequencies, etc.)

_____

_____

_____,

stop smoking by _____, exercise _____ times per week, and

(date)

practice relaxation exercises _____ times per day.

If I achieve my goal for a full month, I will reward myself with

_____.

If the goal has not been met I will place $_____ into a reward fund for later successes and try again.

Signed _____

(patient)

_____

(professional)

_____

(family member)

Figure 12.2   Sample of a personal contract for behavior change.

Session 2: Implementing Dietary Change

This week's objective is to translate the knowledge of cholesterol physiology from the first session into an understanding of the Step One and Step Two eating plans. Members need the tools and structure to select their foods from within these boundaries:

Step One: 30% of total calories from fat with a maximum of 10% each from saturated and polyunsaturated, and 10% to 15% from monounsaturated fat; 300 mg of cholesterol a day; 40 gm of fiber (both soluble and insoluble); and 2 gm of sodium.

Step Two: 25% of total calories from fat, including a maximum of 7% saturated, 10% from polyunsaturates, and 10% to 15% from monounsaturates; 200 mg of cholesterol a day; and 50 to 60 gm of total fiber.

A critical part of this session is teaching participants how to read food labels with a discriminating eye. Careful scrutiny is essential because misleading advertising by the food industry is rampant. The most conspicuous marketing ploys are placed on the front of a package, which is dedicated to advertising. An individual must turn to the side or back of the package to find any true nutritional information.

Legislation calling for more uniform and accurate labeling guidelines is desperately needed. Unfortunately, such changes are slow to occur, and the consumer is normally left with misleading phrases such as the following:

- *No cholesterol*. This means simply that the product contains no animal products, not that it is healthy. It may well contain saturated vegetable oils, additives, preservatives, salt, sugar, or other unhealthy ingredients.
- *Cholesterol reduced*. Foods carrying this label are reformulated or processed to lower cholesterol by 75% or more below the level of the original product. The product may still be too high in cholesterol. This should not be confused with "Low cholesterol," which means that the product contains 20 mg or less.
- *Contains one or more of the following*. This is called flexi-labeling, and it allows the producer to use whatever fat or oil has the lowest current market price. Because tropical oils (coconut, palm, and palm kernel) are inexpensive, these highly saturated oils are used to a great extent in some foods.
- *Made with 100% vegetable oil*. This phrase is a tipoff that the product may contain tropical oils or hydrogenated oils.
- *83% fat-free*. This usually refers to the product's fat percentage by weight, not by calories. This downplays the apparent health risk of these foods because fat provides twice the calories of protein or carbohydrates. Cold cuts that are 83% fat-free by weight still derive 70% of their calories from fat (due to water content).

Consumers should be encouraged to follow the changes that occur within the food industry and to support legislation that requires more stringent labeling criteria for all food products.

Knowing one's upper limit for grams of saturated fat facilitates sizing up a food item at a glance. Table 12.1 can be used as a reference for maximum recommended daily saturated fat intake. Emphasize that this is only a guide to the *average* daily consumption and may be exceeded on some days if compensated for on others. Recall the limit for fat in the Step One eating plan is 30% of total calories and for Step Two, 25%.

Table 12.1 Saturated Fat Quotas

Daily calorie allowance	Daily limit of saturated fat Step One	Step Two
1,000	<11 gm	< 8 gm
1,500	<17 gm	<12 gm
2,000	<22 gm	<16 gm
2,500	<28 gm	<19 gm
3,000	<33 gm	<23 gm
4,000	<44 gm	<31 gm

Note. For a given caloric intake, the recommended maximum intake of saturated fat can be determined in grams. (A gram can be compared to the weight of a standard paper clip.)

If participants are willing to go a step further, they can calculate the percentage of calories a product derives from fat using the grams of total and saturated fat from the label. Because every gram of fat contains 9 calories, multiply the grams of fat by 9 to get the number of fat calories. Divide this by the total calories that are from fat:

% fat calories = (grams of fat × 9)/total calories × 100%

Example: A brand of low-fat cottage cheese lists that each 4-ounce (110 gm) serving contains 100 total calories and 2 gm of fat. These 2 gm will give 18 fat calories, which make up only 18% of the total calories (18/100). In contrast, a Brie cheese label lists 95 total calories in a 1-ounce (28.3 gm) serving and 8 gm of fat. Dividing the 72 fat calories into 95 shows that 76% of the Brie's calories are derived from fat, most of which is saturated.

One point to emphasize is the ratio of polyunsaturated to saturated fats, or the P/S ratio, in foods such as margarines and spreads. Heart-healthy brands have a P/S ratio greater than 2.5. Unfortunately, the products that have the worst P/S ratios do not usually list it. Explain to class members that monounsaturated fats are not included in the P/S ratio and are usually not mentioned on food labels. The quantity of monounsaturates can be calculated by subtracting polyunsaturated and saturated fats from the total fat content. Olive oil and canola oil can be used as examples of oils rich in monounsaturates.

Another approach to explaining fat content is to list foods according to their equivalent "pat of butter," because the lunch-room butter pat is familiar to nearly everyone. One pat equals 5 gm or 45 calories. A list of common foods and their butter pat equivalents can be compiled from food tables. Attributing 25 or so pats to certain fast-food sandwiches is certainly graphic.

A third way of determining fat content is to use a paper calculator or wheel that has the values printed for various food items. These can be obtained from a variety of sources (see the Resources section at the end of this book).

Objectives, Session 2. Participants will be able to

1. explain the relationship of dietary cholesterol and saturated fat to blood cholesterol,
2. state the goals of the Step One and Step Two eating plans,
3. determine whether their present diets are heart-healthy,
4. be able to critically read a food label and obtain nutrient information,
5. calculate a product's percentage of fat calories from food labels (optional),
6. differentiate between regulated labeling and "buzz word" advertising, and
7. know their average daily limit in terms of grams of saturated fat.

Outline, Session 2.

1. Introduction to the Step One and Step Two eating plans (20 minutes)

    (a) Dietary cholesterol
    (b) Percent of total calories from fat
    (c) Percent of total calories from saturated fat
    (d) Total and soluble fiber
    (e) Sodium limits

2. Reading food labels (20 minutes)

    (a) Ingredients listed by weight
    (b) Evaluation of fat content
    (c) Calculation of percent of calories from fat
    (d) Fiber, minerals, and vitamins
    (e) Detecting misleading phrases

3. Ranking different brands of food item as to overall nutrition (15 minutes)
4. Group activity: Reading food labels and evaluating food records (30 minutes)
5. Questions and answers

Teaching Aids, Session 2.

- Food labels or entire packages, boxes, and cans of a variety of food products, both healthy and unhealthy. Especially important are food products with hidden saturated fat such as nondairy creamers, coconut oil, saturated vegetable shortening, cookies, and certain crackers. Also display modern alternatives to butter, eggs, fat, and cheese to increase participants' familiarity with these items.
- Fat-calculator wheel
- Projector and slides of food labels, or an overhead projector and transparencies
- For the discussion of food records, have on hand some food models available from a variety of sources (see Resources) or homemade models such as a deck of cards to demonstrate a 3.5-ounce (100 gm) piece of meat or a matchbox to demonstrate 1 ounce of cheese. Squares of yellow cardboard can represent pats of butter in demonstrating an entire meal's fat content. Measuring cups and spoons can be used to demonstrate a serving size, and a food scale can be used for weight.

Activity, Session 2.

- Have participants gather around the selected examples of food products and discuss the effect of different ingredients on serum cholesterol, blood pressure, body weight, and so forth.
- Rank several brands of a particular food item (such as margarine) according to overall nutritional value.
- Discuss participants' successes and any difficulties they have encountered in keeping the dietary goals they set in the first session. This encourages group support, a vital aspect of the course's success.
- With the group, discuss and evaluate the food records of a few members. Critique each day as a unit for intake of fat, fiber, fish, calories, protein, vitamins, and minerals. If the instructor(s) can perform a computer analysis of food records, participants can turn in their food records at the end of this session.

Assignment, Session 2.   Instruct each participant to keep individual food records for at least two weekdays and one weekend day. The record must include all important ingredients of complex dishes, serving sizes, and brand names, if indicated.

Session 3: Selecting Heart-Healthy Foods—Supermarket Survival

Building on the previous week's lesson on reading food labels, this session focuses on the actual selection of fresh and healthy food in the markets. The list of tasty, heart-healthy alternatives to traditional high-fat foods is growing longer. For many people, the stumbling block is simply locating them in the store.

Taking a shopping tour of a local supermarket is a fun and effective way to teach food selection. "Discovering" the health food aisle may provide participants the impetus to keep nutritious food in the pantry. The dairy case is a perfect site for a practical lesson on reading food labels. Point out produce and fish that look, feel, and smell fresh. Stop by the delicatessen and ask the clerk about the ingredients in such items as potato salad or paté. This will break the ice for many people who are timid about publicizing their health concerns.

In the classroom, generate a group discussion to rank foods based on their heart-healthiness. Include margarines, using their P/S ratios; spreads such as jams, peanut butter, and salad dressings; dairy products like cheeses, milks, and sour cream; meats and entrees, including frozen and prepared dinners; and baked goods such as cookies, crackers, muffins, and snacks. Use labels and packages collected by the instructor and group members.

Objectives, Session 3. Participants will be able to

1. utilize a modern supermarket's design to make heart-healthy food selections;
2. recognize heart-healthy food products on the shelf from an inspection of the label; and
3. recognize freshness in fish, produce, and other food products.

Outline, Session 3.

1. Finding low-fat items in the dairy and meat cases (20 minutes)
2. Selecting fresh and appropriately ripe produce (20 minutes)
3. Selecting fresh fish (20 minutes)
4. Group activity: Supermarket tour (60–90 minutes; includes all the above)
5. Return of food logs to participants with written feedback attached
6. Questions and answers

Teaching Aids, Session 3. Copies of the "poor choice," "better choice," and "best choice" food tables from chapters 7, 8, and 9 can be used as a springboard for classroom discussion or as a shopping guide in the supermarket.

Activity, Session 3. Take a supermarket tour. Then in the classroom, have participants rank different brands of the same food product according to their labels. If a tour proves too time-consuming, view a video on supermarket selections.

Assignment, Session 3. Have participants review their cupboards, pantries, and refrigerators for unhealthy food items and list them on the left side of a piece of paper. On the right side of the same page they should list healthy alternatives for each. A copy of this could be turned in to the instructor(s) as valuable feedback on participants' specific eating patterns and food choices.

Session 4: Recipe Modification

The ultimate step in controlling cholesterol is to prepare meals that are low in fat and high in fiber. The creatures of habit in your group will be relieved to learn that they can still enjoy their favorite recipes. Most can easily be altered to become heart-healthy dishes without sacrificing taste. After all, it's not the entire recipe that is unhealthy—usually only certain ingredients. Chapter 10 offers some ideas for ingredient substitutes along with three sample recipes.

Objectives, Session 4. Participants will be able to

1. understand the concepts and techniques needed to improve the overall nutritional quality of recipes;
2. modify some of their favorite recipes to lower total fat, saturated fat, and cholesterol;
3. increase the soluble fiber in recipes, and
4. learn healthy ways to prepare fish.

Outline, Session 4.

1. Identify problem ingredients in recipes (5 minutes)
2. Present methods to improve the recipe (10 minutes)

    (a) Decrease the amount of the ingredient
    (b) Replace the ingredient with a heart-healthy alternative
    (c) Eliminate the ingredient without replacement

3. Discuss common substitutions (5 minutes)
4. Discuss difficult substitutions (5 minutes)
5. Discuss how new foods enter our lives, either passively through family tradition, or actively by consciously trying new or modified recipes (5 minutes)
6. Group activity: Cooking demonstration of recipe modification with taste sampling; review (50 minutes)
7. Recommend cookbooks, magazines, and newsletters

Teaching Aids, Session 4. Ingredients for recipe, stove, cooking utensils, nonstick pans, vegetable spray coating, baking racks.

Activity, Session 4. Do a cooking demonstration utilizing as many of the concepts of recipe modification as possible. An instructor who is unfamiliar with the recipe may prepare a side dish, such as a salad, along with the main entree. Encourage questions during the preparation and as much assistance in preparation as is convenient.

Assignment, Session 4. Have each class member adjust three of his or her favorite recipes during the following week to make them more nutritious, even if only minor changes are indicated. Members should select at least one that utilizes a different cooking method, such as baking instead of frying. Ask them to bring photocopies of the recipes, before and after the changes, to distribute to the other participants.

Session 5: Menu Planning

The final session brings together all the information from previous lessons to show participants how to develop menu planning skills and choose healthy meals in restaurants. Eating patterns and taste preferences develop over many years and are partially determined by physiological, psychological, and social needs. Planning is essential to change such deeply ingrained habits; otherwise, food choices fall prey to these habits or to the whims of a rumbling stomach.

A balanced diet includes foods from all food groups and in correct proportion. Participants should be concerned with the entire day's intake, not just one meal or one food item. High-fat foods should be coupled with lower fat items so that the overall percentage in a day's consumption approximates the 25% to 30% goal.

A simple method for basic menu planning is to base decisions on three-meal clusters. Have class members think about their last meals and projected future meals as well as their taste preferences at the time. A light lunch, for example, is a good idea for someone anticipating a rich dinner in a restaurant that evening. This three-meal-cluster technique is easy to teach and simple to apply. Many nutritionists find that they use this method almost automatically.

For participants willing and able to go further into menu planning, an optional lesson plan could include the menu planning material from chapter 10. Program leaders familiar with it will be able to answer questions from the group during this final session.

Restaurant Resourcefulness. Because one in three meals in America today is eaten away from home, a discussion on dining out is also warranted. Dining out is one of the most difficult situations in which to maintain healthy eating habits. Peer pressure, use of alcoholic beverages, and the ''special occasion'' mentality are areas that deserve attention.

Although improvements are fortunately taking place, only a minority of restaurants have low-fat menu items. It is always wise to call ahead or preview the menu before eating at an unfamiliar establishment. The local chapter of the American Heart Association or health department may have a list of restaurants or hotels that offer special heart-healthy menu items. Restaurants can usually provide healthy alternatives, even though these may not be on the menu, such as a cottage cheese and fruit plate or a yolkless omelette.

Encourage class members to ask the table server about ingredients and methods of preparation and insist that all sauces and salad dressings be served on the side. If asked, most cooks will agree to lighten up on the cream, butter, oil, and spreads. Discuss low-fat alternatives such as baked potatoes or rice instead of French fries. Another idea is sharing a high-fat entree or high-calorie dessert with another person.

Objectives, Session 5. Participants will

1. understand the essential components of heart-healthy meal planning,
2. know their individual daily limits in grams for total and saturated fat and milligrams for dietary cholesterol,
3. write a heart-healthy and balanced menu plan for three meals (or one week),
4. obtain healthy foods in restaurants,
5. feel in control of food selection and exert their influence in improving our food supply, and
6. recognize and modify situations when dining out that adversely affect healthy food selection.

Outline, Session 5.

1. Components of meal planning (30 minutes)

   (a) Daily totals of saturated and total fat
   (b) Servings from different food groups
   (c) Balancing menus

2. Putting it all together (10 minutes)
3. Sample menu (5 minutes)
4. Restaurant menu evaluation (10 minutes)

   (a) Identifying high-fat foods (fried foods, sauces, etc.)
   (b) Understanding adverse and preferred cooking methods

5. Questions to ask about menu items (10 minutes)

   (a) Ingredients used: specific type of oil, amount and type of cheese, leanness of meat
   (b) Methods used in preparation and cooking

6. Discussion of problems likely to arise when dining out (5 minutes)

   (a) Social situations and peer pressure

   (b) "Special occasion" mind-set that results in overindulging

7. Group activity: Potluck dinner (45 minutes)

8. Final questions and answers, distributing a list of recommended local restaurants and the course evaluation

Teaching Aids, Session 5. Examples of necessary and convenient cooking equipment, such as a steamer, pastry brushes, salad spinner, cheese plane, sharp knives, and nonstick cookware. Include restaurant menus to inspire a lively discussion on the nutritional value of various items and relevant questions to ask the waitperson. Many restaurants have copies of their menus for outside distribution; others will often give a copy if they understand its usefulness to the course.

Activities, Session 5.

• Using the week's assignment, share recipes that have been modified; distribute photocopies of the recipe before and after the changes. Individual members can discuss the problems they encountered during the early trials with their modified recipes.

• A potluck dinner is an excellent finale to the course. This brings together all the aspects of healthy eating and helps solidify peer support. Have members bring in modified recipes, share their difficulties in preparation, and mention any changes in taste or texture.

• An alternative to the potluck is meeting for dinner at a local restaurant. Discuss difficulties in ordering, peer pressure, and temptations to overeat.

Assignment, Session 5. Distribute an evaluation designed to test the retention of important concepts and also to give feedback to the instructors. The latter is vital to improvements in course content, teaching techniques, and future marketing.

Removing the Most Common Behavior Change Barriers

An unfortunate but common block to behavior change is conflicting information in the lay press regarding cholesterol and diet. There have been and probably always will be authors who negate the beneficial effect that a healthy diet has on serum cholesterol or health in general. But it is no myth that nearly half of our citizens die from cholesterol clogged arteries. Extensive evidence indicates that diet is intimately involved with atherosclerosis and other chronic, killer diseases. After reviewing tremendous amounts of data from many types of studies, the National Research Council had this comment in their 1989 report (20): *"The evidence that the intake of saturated fatty acids and cholesterol are causally related to atherosclerotic cardiovascular disease is especially strong and convincing."*

One point of contention raised about the cholesterol intervention studies is the claim that they have not demonstrated an improvement in life expectancy. This is true about most studies, including the Lipid Research Clinics study (7), because they were not designed to study life expectancy. They were only designed to study the effect of diet on CHD. To evaluate death rate, or mortality, the studies would have had to be redesigned with a much longer follow-up time and much higher budget.

Three studies were extended 5 to 10 years beyond the original time frame and have, in fact, demonstrated a reduction in mortality with lowering blood cholesterol. These include the Coronary Drug Project (21), the Stockholm Ischemic Heart Disease Study (22), and the Oslo Study Diet and Antismoking Trial (23). The reduction of mortality in these studies with cholesterol lowering was 11%, 26%, and 40%, respectively.

Misconceptions also exist regarding healthy eating practices, and some are likely to be voiced during the cholesterol course. These fallacies must be dispelled because the confusion and hesitation they engender undermine the motivation needed to change habitual eating patterns. Here are the most common sources of misunderstanding and suggested answers to clarify them:

Q: *Do I have to give up my favorite foods?*
A: Only rarely are favorite recipes and foods entirely off-limits. Your favorite recipes may need some modification but not elimination. Poor-choice foods will, however, need to be eaten less frequently and in smaller quantities. Furthermore, this change should be gradual, so that improved eating patterns become established for life.

Sometimes we only need to switch to a different brand, such as from a regular egg-based mayonnaise to a canola or soy spread. The tables of heart-healthy food alternatives in chapter 7 will guide your food selection.

Q: *Why should I accept a lifetime of boring and tasteless meals?*
A: Meals will be boring only if your taste buds are in a rut. Switching to a new eating pattern will be stimulating. If you take this program to heart, you'll experience and learn a great deal over the next 3 months and beyond. Unlimited possibilities exist for catering to individual tastes.

Q: *Aren't health foods more expensive?*
A: A nutritious eating pattern is not dependent on gourmet *"natural"* foods that are sold only in specialty shops. Many healthy foods are actually less expensive than canned, prepared, and adulterated foods. A reduced

fat and cholesterol diet can save a typical person several hundred dollars a year (24). Lean stew meat and select cuts, for example, are much more affordable than marbled prime steak, which will only prime you for a heart attack. Bean dishes can be prepared for literally pennies a serving. Healthy food is an excellent long-term investment in your health.

Q: *What do I do if my family and friends don't want to eat the new foods?*
A: Diet is implicated in America's top three causes of death—CHD, cancer, and stroke—so good nutrition should not be restricted to a select few. Even schoolchildren are adversely affected by our high-fat, high-salt diet (24). Your family and friends will be influenced by your decision to eat healthy foods even though it may take them months or years to follow your example.

Q: *Should I stop following my weight-reducing diet?*
A: The Step One and Step Two eating plans are naturally weight reducing. By lowering your fat intake you will lose weight as long as other aspects of your diet remain unchanged. If you need to lose considerable weight, just use the same food tables, but select fewer servings each day and exercise more.

References

1. Sempos, C., Fulwood, R., Haines, C., Carroll, M., Anda, R., Williamson, D.F., Remington, P., & Cleeman, J. (1989). The prevalence of high blood cholesterol among adults in the United States. *Journal of the American Medical Association, 262*, 45-52.
2. Harris, L., & Associates. (1988). Bristol Laboratories' Cholesterol Awareness Survey. Poll No. 871041. Available through Citizens for Public Action on Cholesterol. Washington, D.C.
3. Walsh, D.C., & Egdahl, R.H. (1989). Corporate perspectives on work site wellness programs: A report on the seventy Pew Fellows conference. *Journal of Occupational Medicine, 31*, 551-556.
4. Fielding, J., & Breslow, L. (1983). Health promotion programs sponsored by California employers. *American Journal of Public Health, 73*, 538-541.
5. Merrill, B.E. (1983). Evaluating a health promotion program by examining health care claims. *Priorities in Health Statistics: Proceedings of the 19th National Meeting of the Public Health Conference on Records and Statistics* (pp. 75-79) (DHHS Publication No. PHS 81-1214).
6. University of Iowa College of Medicine. (1980). Model workshop on nutrition counseling in hyperlipidemia. NIH Publication No. 80-1666, p. 95.

7. Lipid Research Clinics Program. (1984). The Lipid Research Clinics Coronary Primary Prevention Trial results II. The relationship of reduction in incidence of coronary heart disease to cholesterol lowering. *Journal of the American Medical Association, 251*, 365-374.

8. Bruno, R., Arnold, C., Jacobsen, L., Winick, M., & Wynder, E. (1983). Randomized controlled trial of a non-pharmacologic cholesterol reduction program at the worksite. *Preventive Medicine, 12*, 523-532.

9. Quigley, H. (1986). L.L. Bean cholesterol reduction program. *Journal of Nutritional Education, 18*, S54-S57.

10. Suggs, T.F., Cable, T.A., & Rothenberger, L.A. (1990). Results of a work-site educational and screening program for hypertension and cancer. *Journal of Occupational Medicine, 32*, 220-225.

11. Jackson, S.E., Chenoweth, D., Glover, E.D., Holbert, D., & White, D. (1989). Study indicates smoking cessation improves workplace absenteeism rate. *Occupational Health and Safety*, December, 1989. pp. 13-18.

12. Jones, R.C., Bly, J.L., & Richardson, J.E. (1990). A study of a worksite health promotion program and absenteeism. *Journal of Occupational Medicine, 32*, 95-99.

13. Lynch, W.D., Golaszewski, T.J., Clearie, A.F., Snow, D., & Vickery, D. (1990). Impact of a facility-based corporate fitness program on the number of absences from work due to illness. *Journal of Occupational Medicine, 32*, 9-12.

14. Bly, J.L., Jones, R.C., & Richardson, J.E. (1986). Impact of worksite health promotion on health care costs and utilization: Evaluation of Johnson & Johnson's Live for Life program. *Journal of the American Medical Association, 256*, 3235-3240.

15. Shephard, R., Corey, P., & Renzland, P. (1983). The impact of changes in fitness and lifestyle upon health care utilization. *Canadian Journal of Public Health, 74*, 51-54.

16. Brownell, K., Cohen, R., & Stunkard, A. (1984). Weight loss competitions at the work site: Impact on weight, morale, and cost-effectiveness. *American Journal of Public Health, 74*, 1283-1285.

17. Bernacki, E.J., & Baun, W.B. (1984). The relationship of job performance to exercise adherence in a corporate fitness program. *Journal of Occupational Medicine, 26*, 529-531.

18. Bowne, D., Russell, M., & Morgan, J. (1984). Reduced disability and health care costs in an industrial fitness program. *Journal of Occupational Medicine, 26*, 809-816.

19. Fielding, J. (1982). Effectiveness of employee health improvement programs. *Journal of Occupational Medicine, 24*, 907-916.

20. National Research Council, Committee on Diet and Health. (1989). *Diet and health. Implications for reducing chronic disease risk*. Washington, D.C.: National Academy Press.

21. Canner, P.L., Berge, K.G., Wenger, N.K., Stamler, J., Friedman, L., Prineas, R.J., & Friedwald, W. (1986). Fifteen year mortality in Coronary Drug Project patients: Long-term benefit with niacin. *Journal of the American College of Cardiology, 8*, 1245-1255.
22. Carlson, L.A., & Rosenhamer, G. (1988). Reduction of mortality in the Stockholm Ischaemic Heart Disease Secondary Prevention Study by combined treatment with clofibrate and nicotinic acid. *Acta Medica Scandinavia, 223*, 405-418.
23. Hjermann, I., Holme, I., & Leren, P. (1986). Oslo Study Diet and Anti-smoking Trial. Results after 102 months. *American Journal of Medicine, 80*, 7-11.
24. Berwick, D.M., Cretin, S., & Keeler, E.B. (1980). *Cholesterol, children, and heart disease: An analysis of alternatives.* New York: Oxford University Press.

Chapter

13

The Call for Prevention

We have come to take the seemingly miraculous cures of modern medicine almost for granted. And we tend to forget that our improved health has come more from preventing disease than from treating it once it strikes. Our fascination with the more glamorous "pound of cure" has tended to dazzle us into ignoring the often more effective "ounce of prevention."

Jimmy Carter

A comprehensive, societal approach to cholesterol control will be the most powerful in promoting health, longevity, and the quality of life. A strong public policy with effective government intervention and accurate media reporting is essential to reach all sectors of the population. Education about nutrition, exercise, and smoking must be disseminated to all citizens, especially children and health professionals. The food industry must develop healthy products and clearly label them with honest nutrient information. Finally, these approaches must be complemented by a personal commitment to improve one's own health habits.

According to the Surgeon General's report on health promotion and disease prevention, only about 1% to 2% of health expenditures are spent on preventive programs (1). Yet undeniable evidence has established that healthy lifestyles can prevent the bulk of our nation's premature deaths and disabilities (2). The time is ripe for a major wellness campaign—in particular, a program of cholesterol control.

Because of its central role in our major killer diseases, cholesterol is a key player in prevention. Population studies, metabolic and animal experiments, autopsy reports, and now even clinical trials have provided strong and consistent proof that serum cholesterol can be controlled and that this in turn can prevent CHD (3). Dietary changes alone could prevent an estimated 80% of heart attacks, sparing 450,000 American lives each year (4).

Evidence that we have already begun to curtail atherosclerosis is potent testimony to the efficacy of health education and lifestyle changes. Heart attack rates in the United States dropped about 35% in the years between 1970 and 1987 after adjusting for an aging population. Coincident with an advancing national wellness movement, the decline has been most marked in recent years (5, 6). Stroke rates have declined to less than half the rates recorded during the early 1960s (see Figure 13.1).

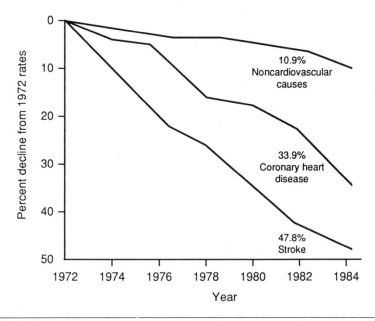

Figure 13.1 Death rates from CHD and stroke have been decreasing since the mid-1960s, most rapidly since the late 1970s. The percentage decline has been age-adjusted, a calculation that compensates for the increased number of older persons in our population today.

Note. From "1990 Heart and Stroke Facts," p. 4. Copyright 1989 by American Heart Association. Reprinted by permission of the American Heart Association, Inc.

Lifestyle Changes

Most of the credit for our dramatic downturn in atherosclerosis over the past 30 years must be given to improvements in lifestyle rather than medical treatment. Public consciousness and knowledge about cholesterol is rapidly increasing. The number of Americans who had had their cholesterol levels checked in 1983 was only 35%, compared with 46% in 1986 and 59% in 1988. The percentage of the population that knew their cholesterol numbers increased from 3% in 1983 to 7% in 1986 and to 17% in 1988. Only 29% believed that dietary fat was important in causing heart disease in 1983, compared with 43% in 1986 and 55% in 1988 (7).

Shoppers are demanding healthy foods, and these foods are becoming more universally available. The amount of saturated fat and cholesterol in the U.S. diet has been falling since 1959 (8). Butter, egg, and total fat consumption has decreased 20% to 30% whereas consumption of poultry and unsaturated fats has increased. Average daily cholesterol intake has fallen from 600 mg in 1959 to a more reasonable (though still excessive) 400 mg today.

Parallel with these dietary changes, a comparison of two large national surveys found that cholesterol levels abated 10 to 20 mg/dl between the 1950s and the 1970s (9). This single element can account for at least a third of the fall in CHD (10).

Other lifestyle-related risk factors have also played a major role in driving down the rates of atherosclerotic diseases. Once the world leader in the use of tobacco products, America now has one of the lowest rates of all developed countries. During the 1950s, more than half of all U.S. adults smoked cigarettes, compared to less than a third today (11). The declines in cholesterol levels and smoking rates account for over half of the total decrement in CHD (10).

William Strong and co-workers in New Orleans have followed the effect of these lifestyle changes on atherosclerosis (12). They have examined coronary arteries at autopsy for over 20 years and found that the average amount of plaque indeed decreased. White males between the ages of 25 and 44 showed half as much surface area involvement in the 1969 to 1978 period as compared with the years from 1959 to 1964. Unfortunately, in black men the reverse was true—even more atherosclerosis was present than previously, suggesting that black men's diets have deteriorated.

Although the cholesterol epidemic has affected nearly all the Western industrialized countries, the United States is presently the pacesetter in trying to reverse it. Most Western European countries are only beginning to introduce heart-healthy foods and adequate nutritional labels. Most Eastern European countries are even experiencing an increase in CHD, as higher standards of living result in greater consumption of cigarettes and rich foods. Figure 13.2 compares changing rates in CHD in men and women in 22 countries (13).

Note that these are age-adjusted CHD death rates, meaning that statistical adjustments have been made to account for different numbers of persons in various age categories. Rates in each country are adjusted to fit the age spread of a standard population, allowing valid comparisons to be made between the countries. Although the age-adjusted CHD rates in the United States have fallen, the actual (or crude) rate has remained stable at about 550,000 deaths a year because of the aging of our population.

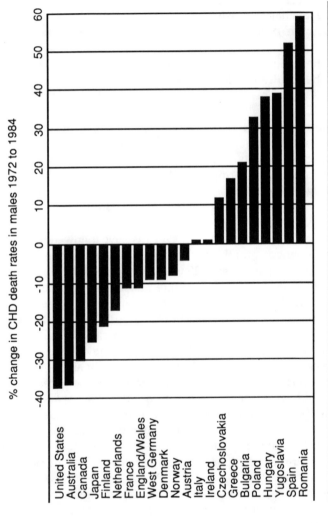

Figure 13.2 CHD rates have been falling in many countries, especially in the U.S., which had the second-highest rate in the world in the 1960s. Other countries, especially in Eastern Europe, are still experiencing a rise in cholesterol-related deaths. *Note.* Reproduced, by permission, from *World Health Statistics Annual 1987*, Geneva, World Health Organization, 1987, page 8.

Advances in Medical Technology

Overshadowed by lifestyle changes, medical advances have been less instrumental in stemming the tide of atherosclerosis. Most of the relevant technological innovations were developed after the heart attack rate had already begun to decline. Also, the greatest achievements have been in reducing the number of initial heart attacks and sudden cardiac deaths, which are least under the influence of advancing technology (14, 15).

Furthermore, although in-hospital CHD deaths seem to be reduced in some studies (16), other studies failed to show any benefit from hospital coronary care units (CCUs) (17). Some investigators even doubt that routine hospitalization helps most heart attack patients (18, 19). Careful record keeping after hospitalization has determined that overall life expectancy of heart attack victims has not changed in 20 years (20-23). At most, CCUs could be responsible for 10% of the total reduction in CHD deaths, mostly due to drugs used to correct dangerous heart rhythms (10).

One characteristic of CHD that obviously limits critical care medicine is that it strikes so suddenly and unpredictably. At least one third of people who suffer their first heart attack never make it to the emergency room alive. More than half of those beset with their second, third, or fourth attacks are dead on arrival. Sixty percent of CHD deaths, or about 350,000, occur each year before the patient ever reaches the hospital (5). Only the 40% who die within the hospital might have been saved by present or future medical advances.

Perhaps the greatest medical achievement in cardiology has been increased public awareness and control of blood pressure. When the National High Blood Pressure Education Program was inaugurated in 1972, only one in eight Americans with hypertension was adequately treated. Fully half were not even diagnosed. Today, at least three quarters of American adults have had a blood pressure check within the past 2 years, and at least half of the hypertensives are controlled (24). Approximately 8% of our CHD decline and an even greater percentage of the drop in strokes have been attributed to medical and dietary measures to control hypertension (10).

Children and Atherosclerosis

Perhaps our most worrisome national trend is the deteriorating health of our children. By 1 year of age, many U.S. children are already eating nearly as much cholesterol as the maximum recommended limit for adults—250 mg a day. As in adults, a statistically significant relationship exists between children's saturated fat and cholesterol intakes and their blood cholesterol levels (25). By 1 year of age, the average cholesterol level

288 Understanding and Managing Cholesterol

has reached that of normal adults, 150 mg/dl (3.9 mmol/L). About 5% of U.S. children age 5 to 18 already have cholesterol levels over 200 mg/dl (5.2 mmol/L) and 20% have levels over 185 mg/dl (4.8 mmol/L) (26).

To study the early stages of atherosclerosis in children, a government-sponsored study in Bogalusa, Mississippi, has been following cholesterol levels and blood pressure of children beginning at birth. The results have been both informative and frightening. Children with high risk factors tend to have high risk factors as adults; this is a process known as *tracking* (27, 28). Further, the cholesterol and blood pressure levels in these children correlate with the amount of plaque already present in their young arteries (29, 30).

The surprising fact that atherosclerosis has its origins in infancy has been confirmed by autopsies on children who died in accidents (31). Pathologists find fatty streaks, the precursors to plaque, in the arteries of most toddlers. The more serious fibrous plaques are already initiated in essentially all of the aortas and three quarters of the coronary arteries of teenagers (32,33). Studies of Korean and Vietnam War casualties demonstrated that most men in their early 20s have serious plaque already established in their coronary arteries (34, 35).

The younger age groups have unfortunately been bystanders to America's fitness craze. The President's Council on Physical Fitness and Sports and the National Children and Youth Fitness studies found shockingly poor fitness levels in children between the ages of 6 and 18 (36-38). Physical education receives less and less emphasis in the schools (39). Meanwhile, television viewing has skyrocketed, now averaging 20 to 30 hours a week in children over age 3 (40). This unhealthy pastime reaches its peak in fourth grade, when children average an incredible 6 hours of television a day. A direct correlation has been found between the amount of television viewing and childhood obesity (41).

Television viewing also has a detrimental indirect effect on diet. An average child is exposed to 22,000 commercials, many of which are for unhealthy, high-calorie foods. Seventy percent of the commercials interrupting Saturday-morning cartoons are for food, and 80% of these are for "junk" foods (42).

In conjunction with diminishing activity, childhood obesity and its health risks are escalating (36, 43). Childhood obesity has increased by over 50% over the past 15 years. The National Institutes of Health estimate that a fourth of our school-age children and a third of our adolescents are overweight (44). Fully half are completely sedentary.

Excessive weight gain is more of a health hazard and more difficult to treat when it develops in children because the obesity is associated with hypercellularity, an increase in the number of fat cells (45). Stunkard has estimated that fully 80% of overweight children will become overweight adults (46).

As with adults, childhood obesity correlates with higher LDL and tri-glyceride concentrations and lower HDL levels (27). In a group of over-weight adolescents, Becque found that 97% had four or more risk factors for CHD in addition to their obesity (47). Overall, 30% to 60% of U.S. children have at least one risk factor for heart disease by age 10. Worse, this figure is increasing, not decreasing (48).

Preventive efforts must begin in childhood, when health habits and plaque growth originate. Time and money for better physical fitness programs are urgently needed, as are teachers and courses in nutrition, cooking, and stress management. Learning these valuable tools will provide students with alternatives to drug abuse, indolence, and a diet of fast foods. Parents, too, must know and practice sound nutritional principles to help their children establish healthy lifestyles.

A variety of instructional materials are available to teach nutrition and other aspects of heart health. An example is the Heart Treasure Chest by the American Heart Association. This kit, developed for children ages 3 to 6, contains a curriculum guide, games, stethoscope, and certificates. Audiovisual aids include filmstrips, recipe cards, and booklets. It is avail-able through the national office or local chapters.

Cholesterol screening should be initiated in childhood, by the schools if not by local physicians. Opinions vary on the age at which testing should begin, but my recommendation is at 5, or sooner if the family is prone to CHD. (Five is also the recommended age for initial blood pressure measurement and is the usual time for the final series of childhood immunizations.) As with adults, the frequency of retesting depends on the initial level and associated risk factors. If serum cholesterol is normal at age 5 (110 to 140 mg/dl or 2.8 to 3.6 mmol/L), a recheck every 5 or 10 years will suffice until age 20.[1]

Where Do We Go From Here?

Health professionals are in an excellent position to help their clients enhance their health, performance, and quality of life. In a 1978 Harris poll, 70% of American adults reported that their physicians were poten-tially the most reliable and useful sources of health information (49). Registered dietitians (RDs) can also play a major role in stemming the tide of atherosclerotic diseases. Other health professionals too, including nurses, exercise physiologists, health educators, and wellness personnel,

---

[1]The NCEP has assigned an expert committee to review the literature on children and lipids and make recommendations. The report, which is due in 1991, will address issues such as the age for initial screening, safe cholesterol levels, and treatment.

can fill a vital gap in our health care delivery system and should be reimbursed by insurance companies for their valuable services.

Health care providers must be informed of the recent breakthroughs in cholesterol research. Many do not yet realize that lowering cholesterol makes a difference in health risks. Definite proof of this was not obtained until results of the Lipid Research Clinic study were released in 1984 (50). Medical staff should emphasize the importance and effectiveness of reducing cardiovascular risk factors and motivate their clients to assume responsibility for their own health.

To enhance patient interest, motivation, and awareness, every office and exam room should provide educational brochures and handouts. Each year the National Heart, Lung, and Blood Institute updates its "NHLBI Kit," which contains a current list of publications and educational materials for professionals and the public. The American Heart Association has developed a comprehensive program entitled "Heart Rx." It includes handouts and modules for instruction in the areas of nutrition, smoking cessation, high blood pressure, and the warning signs of disease. (See the Resources section at the end of this book.)

As a matter of routine, health professionals may begin by asking all patients if they know their cholesterol numbers. People today really appreciate this simple demonstration of concern, and they respect those who are attuned to this timely and critical topic. If the individual's cholesterol level has not been recently determined, the medical provider should arrange for a test.

Time constraints cannot be ignored, and the standard 15-minute office visit provides too little time to adequately cover nutrition. Physicians may need assistance from their staff and better utilization of patient education materials. As a rule, I believe they should refer more patients to RDs if they do not have the time or experience to do nutritional counseling. RDs assume active roles in this respect by helping clients select proper foods through experiences such as supermarket tours. RDs can also advise and assist clients with preparation of heart-healthy meals.

In dealing with time limitations, health professionals can schedule appointments more frequently. Allow time for the most pressing questions during each visit. Most of the following salient points can be made in only a few minutes:

- Half our citizens are still dying from cholesterol-clogged arteries, and most of the remainder barely escape this fate.
- Lowering blood cholesterol levels lowers one's chances of a heart attack; every 1% decrease in cholesterol corresponds to a 2% decrease in risk.
- For blood cholesterol, the lower, the better.
- With dietary changes and, if necessary, the use of cholesterol-lowering drugs, even people with greatly elevated cholesterol can control it.

- Heart-healthy foods are not part of a special diet but rather a normal diet that should be continued for life.
- A healthy eating plan will not only control cholesterol but will also help lower weight and blood pressure and reduce the risk of diabetes and certain cancers.
- Eat less fat, especially saturated fat, by cutting down on meats, eggs, and full-cream dairy products.
- Eat more fiber, especially soluble fiber.
- Eat more fish, especially cold-water fish.

Based on these points, then, health professionals can conduct formal counseling sessions to help clients achieve healthier lifestyles. Such sessions involve setting behavioral goals and designing a plan to reach the target cholesterol level. The individual, not the medical staff, should determine the strategy to achieve the goal. Goals should be easily attainable and approached in a gradual, stepwise fashion. Although a positive attitude is essential, dramatic changes should not be expected or even encouraged in most cases. The professional/client partnership should strive for a unique, incremental, and permanent trend toward healthier habits.

To assist clients with the inherent difficulties of behavioral change, create a *personal health contingency contract* for the client. In this contract define the desired activity goal and the method of self-monitoring. Determine, with the client, what will be the rewards for meeting the goal and the consequences for failing. At the onset, identify attitudes and beliefs that contribute to risk-taking behavior. These must be critically examined and corrected to avoid an inner struggle and eventual subconscious sabotage of the behavioral goals. The contract should be signed by the health professional, the client, and anyone else who will provide moral support, such as a spouse. (See page 268.)

Wellness professionals lend sustenance to the prevention program by maintaining an open rapport and a caring relationship with the client. Frequent positive reinforcement and the creation of a supportive family and peer environment helps ensure ongoing success. Finally, the credibility of the health promotion program is bolstered by wellness professionals themselves leading exemplary lifestyles.

Health Institutions

Hospitals, medical schools, and research units are all too frequently captivated by advanced disease and dramatic technological treatment (51). A widespread preventive orientation is just beginning to take root and should be fostered and expanded. More research is needed in cholesterol metabolism, in early detection of disease, and in nutritional and pharmacological approaches to treatment. Social scientists must continue to explore what motivates people to change and how they acquire the skills to maintain new health habits for a lifetime. Improved techniques are needed in social marketing and behavior modification to engage and influence the populace.

Hospital laboratories must begin defining normal cholesterol levels in terms of health rather than disease. The traditional values used to define "normal" cholesterol have been set far too high, missing the majority of people at risk for atherosclerotic diseases. As a result, physicians frequently intervene only for those at the highest risk for CHD. Even greatly elevated cholesterol levels are frequently ignored, sometimes by cardiologists (52).

Few of the millions of people who have undergone coronary artery bypass grafting or balloon angioplasty have received adequate information or assistance in changing lifestyle habits. It is deplorable that coronary care patients in many hospitals are still served bacon, eggs, and cream as they lie recovering from a heart attack that was induced by the very same diet. Not too long ago they were allowed to smoke as well.

Unfortunately, many physicians feel that discussing diet will not have sufficient impact, that people just won't change their diets. In their defense, it is true that only 30% of people comply with even modest dietary advice (53). Nonetheless, all patients deserve to know the chances that they are taking with their lives.

In one review of hospitalized patients with cholesterol levels between 351 and 1,060 mg/dl (9.05–27.4 mmol/L), hypercholesterolemia was diagnosed in only a third. Many of these already had documented vascular disease. Only a quarter of the patients were put on a cholesterol-lowering diet, and only a fifth had repeat cholesterol tests within a year (54).

In spite of diet's close link to many common diseases, the nutritional knowledge base of most physicians tends to be scant at best. Very few medical schools include more than a cursory nutrition seminar in their curricula. In a 1983 government survey, only 28% of surveyed physicians thought that a high-fat diet was very important in causing coronary heart disease. In 1986, the survey was repeated and still only 40% of physicians responded correctly. In both surveys, the public's awareness of the importance of nutrition to coronary disease was greater than the doctors', though physicians are closing the gap (55).

To help remove these stumbling blocks, a professional education committee was formed as part of the NCEP. The committee's mission is to increase physician awareness of the importance and effectiveness of cholesterol control. The American Heart Association has also spearheaded a progressive physician's cholesterol education program to update doctors on recent findings and therapeutic measures. Dramatic changes are needed in physician awareness and effectiveness in primary prevention—that is, before symptoms develop.

Business and Industry

Employers are contributing an increasing portion of the health care dollar, and cardiovascular diseases make up a lion's share of these costs. Escalating medical expenditures and insurance premiums impose severe financial constraints on businesses, and many are discontinuing health insurance benefits to their employees. An alternative is to structure insurance coverage and other benefits to encourage employees to maintain healthy lifestyles. In this way benefits can be maintained and health care costs stabilized without affecting the company's bottom line. Research has shown that employees with healthy lifestyles not only have lower cholesterol levels, but they have lower health care costs as well (56, 57). Companies that offer health promotion programs or have a healthy culture should demand preferential group premium rates.

A more aggressive and effective step is to initiate health promotion activities in the workplace (58, 59). Cholesterol screening at the workplace is particularly effective in reaching high-risk men, who seldom seek medical care without symptoms. Nutrition education and cholesterol management in particular have been shown to be both effective and cost-efficient (60-62). A current national health promotion objective is to have at least 50% of work sites with 50 or more employees offer cardiovascular prevention programs (an increase from only 17% in 1985) (70).

Perhaps the most crucial element of corporate health promotion is the development of a wellness-oriented corporate culture or environment. A health-conscious environment is important because consistent effort on the part of the individual is usually not sufficient to sustain better health habits. In the words of Judd and Robert Allen of the Human Resources Institute (Morristown, NJ) (53)

> The best global predictor of health behavior and long-term success in lifestyle change efforts is culture. In our American cultures, it is too frequently the norm not to exercise, to eat a fat laden non-nutritious diet, to binge on alcohol and other drugs, to use tobacco, to have dissatisfying interpersonal relationships, and to mismanage stress. Studies show that while these norms for health risk behavior can be violated for a short period of time, and, by a few for a lifetime, the overall tendency is to revert to the norm even after diligent efforts to change. (p. 41)

A positive corporate culture helps instill a desire for change via peer pressure, a sense of group responsibility, or economic incentives. Typical features of a heart-healthy culture include nutritious food in the cafeteria and vending machines, an effective smoking policy, a fitness room, health-oriented posters and films, and special events such as cholesterol screenings and "fun runs." Challenges within a department or competitions between departments are very effective in improving group compliance rates with desired health habits.

Creating a healthy environment not only has its own impact on lifestyles but also greatly enhances the long-term effectiveness of behavior change programs, such as nutrition or smoking cessation classes. As an example, Pacific Northwest Bell had little success in encouraging employees to enroll in a smoking cessation class. Then in 1985, a company-wide smoking ban was instated. During the first 6 months of the smoking ban, a quarter of all smokers enrolled in the class, over three times the level achieved during the previous attempt (63).

Most large corporations are self-insured today for health care costs. Economic incentives for healthy lifestyles can be built into the benefits package (64). Incentives such as "wellness days off," cash bonuses, or lower copayments or deductibles can be given to those who choose to lead a healthy lifestyle (or choose to participate in a risk-reduction program).

Another alternative is for the company to offer free or reduced-rate participation in outside classes on nutrition, weight control, smoking cessation, and the like. For companies that need outside expertise in health promotion, the American Heart Association has developed "Heart at Work," a low-cost set of awareness and prevention programs for the work site. It is designed to help a wide range of businesses prevent heart attack and stroke in their employees (see the Resources section for more information).

Some of the most ambitious and successful corporate health promotion programs include Johnson & Johnson's *Live for Live*, Control Data's *Total Life Concept*, IBM's *A Plan for Life*, Kellogg's *Feeling Gr-r-reat Program*, AT&T's *Total Life Concept*, Kodak's *Life Enhancement Plan*, Kimberly Clark's *Health Management Program*, Tenneco's *Health and Fitness Program*, and wellness programs at PepsiCo, General Mills, Ford, General Motors, L.L. Bean, Procter and Gamble, and many insurance companies (65).

Although there are still ethical and legal questions, the rising cost of health care will soon push the benefits-lifestyle connection into the financial forefront. Unless risk factors decline or medical care improves, the annual cost of CHD is projected to increase 40% by 2010 (66).

Public Policy Makers

Cholesterol control is relevant to everyone, not only those at the highest risk for CHD. Half of those stricken with CHD have cholesterol levels under 225 mg/dl (5.8 mmol/L); a third are below the national average of 215 mg/dl (5.6 mmol/L). For this reason, cardiovascular crusaders such as Jeremiah Stamler, Paul Dudley White, and Ancel Keys have advocated a population or public health approach to atherosclerotic diseases. For several decades they have championed mass educational efforts and effective legislation (67). The successes of the National Smoking Education Program and the National High Blood Pressure Education Program attest to the effectiveness of this cultural strategy. The National Heart, Lung, and Blood Institute's National Cholesterol Education Program poses new challenges to health professionals as well (68).

Between 1917 and 1989, 14 government documents appealed to the American people to decrease their intake of fat and increase their intake of fiber (69). Lending his support, the former Surgeon General Dr. C. Everett Koop identified fat intake as the dietary public enemy number one in his 1988 report on nutrition and health (69). The Public Health Service's nutrition objectives for the year 2000 focus on education about dietary fat and cholesterol (70). The goal is to have at least 60% of those with high cholesterol taking action to reduce their levels (presently this figure is 11%). They should understand the relationship between dietary saturated fat and cholesterol and CHD. All states are encouraged to include nutrition education as part of the required curriculum in elementary and secondary schools. The average serum cholesterol level in adults should be at or below 200 mg/dl (5.2 mmol/L).

Other organizations, such as the American Heart Association, the American Health Foundation, the Centers for Disease Control, the American Medical Association, and the American Dietetic Association, are joining forces to combat the unnecessary death and disability due to atherosclerosis. The major emphasis from these groups has been to increase professional and public awareness of cholesterol and the role that diet, exercise, and smoking cessation play in preventing cardiovascular disease. They sponsor conferences for continuing medical education, coordinate public screenings, and distribute a variety of literature on heart health.

Figure 13.3 illustrates the beginnings of our society's control of cholesterol and, it is hoped, its direction for the future. During the last three decades, our average cholesterol levels have fallen from 235 to 215 mg/dl (6.2 to 5.6 mmol/L), but we can and should move toward even healthier levels. If our average cholesterol levels fall into the 160 mg/dl (4.1 mmol/L) range, as is still the case in Japan, heart attack and stroke will once again become rare diseases.

Government and Legislation

The Surgeon General's report *Healthy People* summarizes the role of government in this way (1):

> Federal and State governments have other important responsibilities in disease prevention and health promotion: to provide

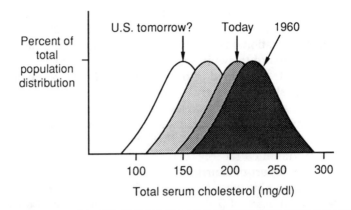

Figure 13.3   Modest changes in diet and blood cholesterol have already had an effect on blood cholesterol levels in the United States, shifting the distribution curve to the left. Further effort is needed to get a greater percentage of our citizenry into the ideal cholesterol range of 160 mg/dl (4.1 mmol/L) and below.

leadership in setting priorities and goals for prevention activities; to help expand the knowledge base through research and data collection; to assure that preventive services are provided to high risk groups on a priority basis; to determine and enforce health and safety standards protecting people; and, if necessary, *to provide economic incentives to encourage health and safety* [italics added]. (p. 144)

A practical example of the latter goal would be for unhealthy food products to be taxed appropriately for their contribution to our staggering national health bill. Another is to reverse the present policy of subsidizing the tobacco industry. Cigarettes should be restricted from minors and be heavily taxed. The tobacco farmer should be aided in transferring to another cash crop or occupation.

Lawmakers can assist in meeting our health objectives by enforcing standards of laboratory quality and encouraging health promotion efforts in the private sector. Several states are wrestling with issues surrounding cholesterol screening, including the training and licensing of personnel and certification requirements of the laboratory procedure. Their statutes must be supportive of responsible health promotion and not unnecessarily restrictive or cumbersome.

Legislation may be necessary to mandate insurance coverage for preventive measures such as cholesterol testing and nutritional counseling. At present these services are sadly undercompensated and thwart efforts to improve the health of insured individuals. Privately, citizens and companies can insist on health promotion services and discounts for healthy lifestyles.

Food industry regulations calling for healthier ingredients and standardized package labeling have been struggling in Congress for years with minimal success. Heavy lobbying efforts by some of the food manufacturers have limited the strength of any requirements. However, the public health implications of a nutritious food supply are enormous.

Local governments can implement an effective plan of cholesterol awareness and control, perhaps in conjunction with regional health system agencies and county health departments. Programs may include cholesterol and blood pressure screening, lecture series, fitness facilities, and sporting events; or they may sponsor nutritional counseling, smoking cessation, and other self-help groups. Community campaigns using multiple mass-media sources, such as those used by the Stanford Five Cities Project and the Pawtucket Heart Health Project, can influence food selection and impact the health of an entire region (see the Resources section).

Other community organizations can be recruited to assist, such as the local medical society, the American Heart Association, and the Red Cross, as well as chambers of commerce, churches, HMOs, or service and fraternal groups. In some communities, private initiatives by health-food stores and restaurants have had tremendous impact. The help of health promotion consultants can be enlisted as needed. The Resources section at the end of this book has more ideas.

The Food Industry

From a public health standpoint, heart-healthy eating is for everyone, not just for those with advanced coronary disease. The human body has not been designed for the highly processed and adulterated products that many of us consume in excess. Small wonder that the top three causes of death in America—CHD, cancer, and stroke—all have strong causal links to nutritional factors.

It will become easier to maintain healthy diets as the quality of our food supply improves. Research has already resulted in the development of two types of fat substitutes, Olestra and Simplesse, and lower-fat beef and dairy products. The food industry should develop tasty, low-cost, convenient foods rich in fiber, complex carbohydrates, and vitamins but low in cholesterol, total fat, and saturated fats. Better means of preservation for unsaturated fats also must be found. Consumers must demand higher nutritional quality in all food staples and exercise their purchasing power when these products arrive on the shelves.

Food manufacturers should routinely label their products in a clear and honest fashion. Regulations should allow for nutritious products to state reasonable health claims that are backed by medical authorities. But until labeling standards are upgraded, only mass education can expose and discredit producers that use misleading slogans such as "contains no cholesterol," or vague terms such as "lite" on unhealthy products. The present movement toward reducing tropical oils from packaged baked goods and fast-food restaurants is a welcome beginning. The FDA has conducted hearings across the United States to develop minimum standards for labeling information and format (71).

Restaurant managers and chefs must become better informed about nutrition. At present, few chefs are trained to cook for health, and most culinary education programs exclude nutrition science.

Fortunately a new health consciousness is just beginning to surface in a few cooking schools. In addition, a small but growing number of restaurants are offering heart-healthy menus endorsed by health groups such as the American Heart Association. This is crucial because of the inherent difficulty in discerning what ingredients and cooking methods are used in public kitchens.

The Media

In *Healthy People 2000*, the first step to meeting the national nutrition objectives calls for a "marked improvement in accessibility of nutrition information and education for the general public" (70).

Community health education has been shown to be an effective and necessary step toward alleviating chronic diseases (72, 73). People who receive information about cholesterol are twice as likely to make changes in lifestyles as those who don't.

Mass media such as newspapers, magazines, radio, and television will continue to have great potential for disseminating health information. Though the efforts and successes of these sources can be applauded, some areas are neglected. The paucity of articles on the dangers of smoking is a glaring example. The print media's single biggest advertisement revenue source is tobacco companies.

I contend that the media has a social responsibility to present accurate and relevant material. Editorial personnel should screen sources for their credentials and make sure information is credible. Many newspaper and magazine stands abound with sensationalistic headlines and articles that present distorted views of health topics. The sudden and unwelcome rise in fish-oil capsule consumption was a by-product of such journalism. Many books, too, contain partially correct and misleading information, unqualified claims of fast and easy cures, and recommendations based on outdated or unfounded theories. Not only can they be harmful in themselves (by omitting important details such as contraindications to a "cure"), but they can also make it nearly impossible for the general public to sort through the deluge of conflicting reports. Sadly, many individuals abandon their health goals in confusion and a sense of futility.

Social Responsibility

A personal commitment to health will continue to be the ultimate issue in cholesterol control. Superhuman efforts by the government, business, private agencies, and medical institutions are doomed to failure if their advice remains unheeded. It is up to each one of us as individuals—we either take responsibility for our lives or run a sizable risk of dying a premature and preventable death.

By its nature, the insidious growth of plaque breeds complacency. Because atherosclerosis is silent until its terminal stages, we must intervene in earlier stages—much earlier. A quarter of initial heart attack deaths occur without any prior symptoms—the first symptom of cholesterol buildup is the last. Routine electrocardiograms reveal that up to 30% of heart attacks occur without any chest pain. This is especially common in diabetics and the elderly. Clearly, a wait-and-see approach cannot curtail a disease process that lies concealed until its terminal stage.

For several decades now, government and private organizations have been espousing the benefits of a prudent diet, exercise, and smoking cessation. The pervasiveness of unhealthy lifestyle habits is in large part due to a lack of self-responsibility for well-being. In the words of John Knowles, former president of the Rockefeller Foundation, Americans "want a treat, not a treatment" (74). A 1978 Harris poll revealed that 71% of the public agreed with this statement (49): "I myself, and most people, just go on doing the things that make us less healthy, even when we know we shouldn't." Similarly, over 90% of respondents agreed with this statement: "If we Americans lived healthier lives, ate more nutritious food, smoked less, maintained proper weight and exercised regularly, it would do more to improve our health than anything doctors and medicine could do for us." Finally, in a 1986 government survey, 70% of 4,000 adults questioned believed that high cholesterol is caused by diet, yet only 23% had made any dietary changes (7).

A healthy lifestyle and environment is essential for the prevention of atherosclerosis. In fact, we have no real choice but prevention. Although atherosclerosis is nearly always preventable, once it is established it has no cure. Medically, all we have are temporizing treatments and palliative procedures. These after-the-fact measures are expensive, dangerous, and variable in their effectiveness.

On the positive side, it is reassuring that by taking charge of our lifestyles we can have a tremendously positive impact on our health. Responsible self-care can and does alleviate most of the risk factors for atherosclerosis, and it has largely been through these personal decisions to eat healthier foods, exercise, and avoid tobacco that we are curtailing cholesterol death. As individuals and as a society, we are winning.

References

1. U.S. Department of Health, Education, and Welfare, Public Health Service. (1979). *Healthy people: The Surgeon General's report on health promotion and disease prevention* (U.S. DHEW, PHS Publication No. 79-55071A). Rockville, MD.
2. Committee on Diet and Health, Food and Nutrition Board, Commission on Life Sciences, National Research Council. *Diet and Health. Implications for Reducing Chronic Disease Risk.* Washington, DC: National Academy Press, 1989.
3. Expert Panel of the National Cholesterol Education Program (NCEP). (1988). Report of the NCEP Expert Panel on detection, evaluation, and treatment of high blood cholesterol in adults. *Archives of Internal Medicine,* **148**, 36-39.
4. Hopkins, P.N., & Williams, R.R. (1986). Identification and relative weight of cardiovascular risk factors. *Cardiology Clinics,* **4**, 3-32.
5. American Heart Association. (1988). *1989 heart facts.* Dallas: American Heart Association.
6. National Heart, Lung, and Blood Institute. (1987, February). *The fourteenth report of the NHLBI Advisory Council* (U.S. Department of Health and Human Services Publication No. NIH 87-2729). Rockville, MD.
7. Levy, A. (1988, November). FDA/NCEP Cholesterol Awareness Survey: Recent trends in public beliefs about fats and cholesterol. First National Cholesterol Conference, Washington, DC.
8. Brown, W.V., Ginsberg, H., & Karmally, W. (1984). Diet and the decrease in coronary heart disease. *American Journal of Cardiology,* **54**, 27C-29C.
9. Beaglehole, R., LaRosa, J., Heiss, G., Davis, C.E., Williams, D.D., Tyroler, H.A., & Rifkind, B.M. (1979). Serum cholesterol, diet, and the decline in coronary heart disease mortality. *Preventive Medicine,* **8**, 538-547.
10. Goldman, L., & Cook., E.F. (1984). The decline in ischemic heart disease mortality rates. *Annals of Internal Medicine,* **101**, 825-836.
11. Consensus Development Conference. (1989). *Reducing the health consequences of smoking: 25 years of progress—a report of the Surgeon General, 1989* (U.S. Department of Health and Human Services, Public Health Service Publication No. CDC 89-8411). Rockville, MD: U.S. Department of Health and Human Services
12. Strong, J.P., Dalmann, M.C., Newman, W.P., Tracy, R.E., Malcom, G.T., Johnson, W.D., McMahan, L.H., Rock, W.A., & Guzman, M.A.

(1984). Coronary heart disease in young black and white males in New Orleans: Community pathology study. *American Heart Journal*, **108**, 747-759.

13. World Health Organization. (1987). *World health statistics annual (1987)* (p. 8). Geneva: World Health Organization.

14. Pell, S., & Fayerweather, W.E. (1985). Trends in the incidence of myocardial infarction and in associated mortality and morbidity in a large employed population, 1957-1983. *New England Journal of Medicine*, **312**, 1005-1011.

15. Stamler, J. (1985). The marked decline in coronary heart disease mortality rates in the United States, 1968-1981: Summary of findings and possible explanation. *Cardiology*, **72**, 11-22.

16. Levy, R.I. (1981). The decline in cardiovascular disease mortality. *Annual Review of Public Health*, **2**, 49-70.

17. Goldberg, R. (1977). Time trends in prognosis of patients with myocardial infarction—a population based study. *Johns Hopkins Medical Journal*, **144**, 73-80.

18. Hill, J.D., Hampton, J.R., & Mitchell, J.R.A. (1978). A randomized trial of home-versus-hospital management for patients with suspected myocardial infarction. *Lancet*, **1**, 837-841.

19. Mather, H.G., Morgan, D.C., Pearson, N.G., Reed, K.L., Shaw, D.B., Steed, G.R., Thorne, M.G., Lawrence, C.J., & Riley, I.S. (1976). Myocardial infarction: A comparison between home and hospital care for patients. *British Medical Journal*, **1**, 925-929.

20. Gillum, R.F., Folsom, A.R., & Blackburn, H. (1986). Decline in coronary heart disease mortality: Old questions and new facts. *American Journal of Medicine*, **76**, 1055-1065.

21. Goldman, L., Cook, F., Hashimoto, B., Stone, P., Muller, J., & Loscolzo, A. (1982). Evidence that hospital care for acute myocardial infarction has not contributed to the decline in coronary mortality between 1973-1974 and 1978-1979. *Circulation*, **65**, 936-942.

22. Weinblatt, E., Goldberg, J.D., Ruberman, W., Frank, C.W., Monk, M.A., & Chaudhary, B.S. (1982). Mortality after first myocardial infarction: Search for a secular trend. *Journal of the American Medical Association*, **247**, 1576-1581.

23. Friedman, G.D. (1979). Decline in hospitalizations for coronary heart disease and stroke: The Kaiser-Permanente experience in Northern California, 1971-1977. In *Proceedings of the Conference on the Decline in coronary Heart Disease Mortality* (U.S. Department of Health, Education, and Welfare Publication No. NIH 79-1610). Rockville, MD.

24. Stamler, R., Stamler, J., Riedlinger, W.F., Algera, G., & Roberts, R.H. (1978). Weight and blood pressure: Findings in hypertension screening of 1 million Americans. *Journal of the American Medical Association*, **240**, 1607-1610.

25. Berenson, G.S., Blonde, C.V., Farris, R.P., Foster, T.A., Frank, G.C., Srinivasan, S.R., Voors, A.W., & Webber, L.S. (1979). Cardiovascular disease risk factor variables during the first year of life. *American Journal of Diseases of Children, 133*, 1049-1057.

26. Freedman, D.S., Srinivasan, S.R., Cresanta, J.L., Webber, L.S., & Berenson, G.S. (1987). Cardiovascular risk factors from birth to 7 years of age: The Bogalusa Heart Study: Serum lipids and lipoproteins. *Pediatrics, 80*, 789-796.

27. Freedman, D.S., Burke, G.L., Harsha, D.W., Srinivasan, S.R., Cresanta, J.L., Webber, L.S., & Berenson, G.S. (1985). Relationship of changes in obesity to serum lipid and lipoprotein changes in childhood and adolescence. *Journal of the American Medical Association, 154*, 515-520.

28. Webber, L.S., Cresanta, J.L., Voors, A.W., & Berenson, G.S. (1983). Tracking of cardiovascular disease risk factor variables in school-aged children. *Journal of Chronic Diseases, 36*, 647-660.

29. Newman, W.P., Freedman, D.S., Voors, A.W., Gard, P.D., Srinivasan, S.R., Cresanto, J.L., Williamson, G.D., Webber, L.S., & Berenson, G.S. (1986). Relation of serum lipoprotein levels and systolic blood pressure to early atherosclerosis: The Bogalusa Heart Study. *New England Journal of Medicine, 314*, 138-144.

30. Aristimuño, G.G., Foster, R.A., Voors, A.W., Srinivasan, S.R., & Berenson, G.S. (1984). Influence of persistent obesity in children on cardiovascular risk factors: The Bogalusa Heart Study. *Circulation, 69*, 895-904.

31. Cresanta, J.L., Hyg, M.S., Burke, G.L., Downey, A.M., Freedman, D.S., & Berenson, G.S. (1986). Prevention of atherosclerosis in children. *Pediatric Clinics of North America, 33*, 835-858.

32. Vetican, D., & Vetican, D. (1980). Atherosclerotic involvement of the coronary arteries of adolescents and young adults. *Atherosclerosis, 36*, 449-460.

33. Strong, W.B. (Ed.) (1978). *Atherosclerosis: Its pediatric aspects.* New York: Grune & Stratton.

34. McNamara, J.J., Molot, M.A., Stremple, J.F., & Cutting, R.T. (1971). Coronary artery disease in combat casualties in Vietnam. *Journal of the American Medical Association, 216*, 1185-1187.

35. Enos, W.F., Holmer, M.J., & Beyer, J. (1953). Coronary disease among US soldiers killed in action in Korea. *Journal of the American Medical Association, 152*, 1090-1093.

36. Ross, J.G., Pate, R.R., & Delpy, L.A. (1987). National Children and Youth fitness Study II. Office of Disease Prevention and Health Promotion, Public Health Service. *Journal of Physical Education, Recreation, and Dance*, 50-96.

37. Reiff, G.G., Dixon, W.R., & Jacoby, D. (1986). *The President's Council*

on *Physical Fitness and Sports 1985 National School Population Fitness Survey*. Washington, DC: U.S. Department of Health and Human Services, Office of the Assistant Secretary for Health.
38. Ross, J.G., & Gilbert, G.G. (1985). National Children and Youth Fitness Study: A summary of findings. *Journal of Physical Education, Recreation, and Dance*, **56**, 45-50.
39. American Academy of Pediatrics. (1987). Physical fitness and schools. *Pediatrics*, **80**, 449-450.
40. Nielson, A.C. (1968-1970 and 1976-1980). Nielson Reports on Television. Northbrook, IL: A.C. Nielson Co.
41. Dietz, W.H., Jr., & Gortmaker, S.L. (1985). Do we fatten our children at the TV set? Obesity and television viewing in children and adolescents. *Pediatrics*, **75**, 807-812.
42. Cotugna, N. (1988). TV ads on Saturday morning children's programming—What's new? *Journal of Nutrition Education*, **20**, 125-127.
43. Gortmaker, S.L., Dietz, W.H., Sobol, A.M., & Wehler, C.A. (1987). Increasing pediatric obesity in the United States. *American Journal of Diseases in Children*, **141**, 535.
44. U.S. Department of Health and Human Services, Public Health Service. (1985). Health implications of obesity. National Institutes of Health Consensus Development Conference Statement. Vol. 5, No 9. Bethesda, MD.
45. Dustan, H.P. (1985). Obesity and hypertension. *Annals of Internal Medicine*, **103**, 1047-1049.
46. Stunkard, A.J., & Burt, V. (1967). Obesity and the body image. II. Age at onset of disturbances in the body image. *American Journal of Psychiatry*, **123**, 1443-1447.
47. Becque, M.D., Katch, V.L., Rocchini, A.P., Marks, C.R., & Moorehead, C. (1988). Coronary risk incidence of obese adolescents: Reduction by exercise plus diet intervention. *Pediatrics*, **81**, 605-612.
48. Berenson, G.S., Frank, G.C., Hunter, S.M., Srinivasan, S.R., Voors, A.W., & Webber, L.S. (1982). Cardiovascular risk factors in children: Should they concern the pediatrician? *American Journal of Diseases in Children*, **136**, 855-862.
49. Harris, L., & Associates. (1978). Health maintenance. S2818 available from Pacific Mutual Life Insurance Co., P.O.Box 9000, Newport Beach, CA 92660.
50. Lipid Research Clinics Program. (1984). The Lipid Research Clinics Coronary Primary Prevention Trial results. I. Reduction in incidence of coronary heart disease. *Journal of the American Medical Association*, **251**, 351-364.
51. Ginzberg, E. (1990). High-tech medicine and rising health care costs. *Journal of the American Medical Association*, **263**, 1820-1822.
52. Gutowski, T., Adelson, R., & Cohen, M.V. (1988). Poor acceptance

of blood lipids as treatable risk factor among cardiologists [Abstract]. *Circulation*, **78**, II-384.

53. Allen, J., & Allen, R.F. (1986). From short term compliance to long term freedom: Culture-based health promotion by health professionals. *American Journal of Health Promotion*, **1**, 39-47.

54. Nash, D.T. (1986). Hypercholesterolemia during hospitalization: The case for closer surveillance. *Postgraduate Medicine*, **79**, 303.

55. Schucker, B., Bailey, K., Heimbach, J.T., Mattson, M.E., Wittes, J.T., Haines, C.M., Gordon, D.J., Cutler, J.A., Keating, V.S., & Goor, R.S. (1987). Change in public perspective in cholesterol and heart disease. Results from two national surveys. *Journal of the American Medical Association*, **258**, 3527-3531.

56. Brink, S.C. (1987). *Health risks and behavior: The impact on medical costs*. Brookfield, WI: Milliman and Robertson.

57. Merrill, B.E. (1983). Evaluating a health promotion program by examining health care claims. Priorities in Health Statistics: Proceedings of the 19th National Meeting of the Public Health Conference on Records and Statistics. (DHHS, PHS Publication No. 81-1214).

58. Blair, S.N., Piserchia, P.V., Wilbur, C.S., & Crowder, J.H. (1986). A public health intervention model for work-site health promotion. *Journal of the American Medical Association*, **255**, 921-926.

59. Fielding, J.E. (1984). Health promotion and disease prevention at the worksite. *Annual Review of Public Health*, **5**, 237-265.

60. Glanz, K., & Seewand-Klein, T. (1986). Nutrition at the worksite. *Journal of Nutrition Education*, **18**, S1-S12.

61. Joseph, H.M., & Glanz, K. (1986). Cost-effectiveness and cost-benefit analysis of worksite nutrition programs. *Journal of Nutrition Education*, **18**, S12-S16.

62. Bruno, R., Arnold, C., Jacobsen, L., Winik, M., & Wynder, E. (1983). Randomized controlled trial of a non-pharmacologic cholesterol reduction program at the worksite. *Preventive Medicine*, **12**, 523-532.

63. Martin, M.J., Fehrenbach, A., & Rosner, R. (1986). Ban on smoking in industry. *New England Journal of Medicine*, **315**, 647-648.

64. Warner, K.E., & Murt, H.A. (1984). Economic incentives for health. *Annual Review of Public Health*, **5**, 107-133.

65. Pritchard, R.E., & Potter, G.C. (1990). *Fitness Inc. A guide to corporate health & wellness programs*. Homewood, IL: Dow Jones-Irwin.

66. Weinstein, M.C., Coxson, P.G., Willians, L.W., Pass, T.M., Stason, W.B., & Goldman, L. (1986). Coronary heart disease morbidity, mortality, and cost for the next quarter-century. *Clinical Research*, **34**, 386A.

67. Stamler, J. (1978). Lifestyles, major risk factors, proof, and public policy. *Circulation*, **58**, 3-19.

68. Lenfant, C. (1986). A new challenge for America: The National Cholesterol Education Program. *Circulation*, **73**, 855-856.

69. U.S. Department of Health and Human Services, Public Health Service. (1988). The Surgeon General's Report on Nutrition and Health. [DHHS (PHS) Publication No. 88-50210]. Washington, DC: U.S. Government Printing Office.

70. U.S. Department of Health and Human Services, Public Health Service. (1990). Healthy people 2000: National health promotion and disease prevention objectives. [DHHS, PHS Publication No. 017-001-00474-0 (full report) or 017-001-00473-1 (summary report)]. Washington, DC: U.S. Government Printing Office.

71. U.S. Department of Health and Human Services, Food and Drug Administration. (March 7, 1990). Food Labeling Reform. Washington, DC: Author.

72. Public Health Service. (1983, September/October). Promoting health/preventing disease: Public Health Service implementation plans for attaining the objectives for the nation. *Public Health Report* (Suppl.), pp. 132-155.

73. Farquhar, J.W., Maccoby, N., Wood, P.D., Alexander, J.K., Breitrose, H., Brown, B.W., Jr., Haskell, W.L., McAlister, A.L., Meyer, A.J., Nash, J.D., & Stern, M.P. (1977). Community education for cardiovascular health. *Lancet*, **1**, 1192-1195.

74. Knowles, H.J. (1977). The responsibility of the individual. *Daedalus, Journal of the American Academy of Arts and Sciences*, **106**, 57-80.

Appendix A
Guidelines for
Maximal Exercise Testing

Age and health category	Age at which maximal exercise testing is recommended
Apparently healthy	Males over age 45, females over age 55
No symptoms but borderline or high-risk in terms of cholesterol, blood pressure, smoking, family history, etc.	Over age 35
Symptoms of heart or lung disease	Any age
Known heart or lung disease, diabetes, hypertension, or other serious disease	Any age

In spite of the near-universal benefit of exercise, some medical and physical problems preclude exercise testing and training. These contraindications to exercise are listed on the following page.

Target Heart Rates for Exercise[a]

Average maximum heart rate	Age	Initial target heart rates (60% to 75% of maximum)		Advanced target heart rates (85% of predicted maximum)
		Heart rate per minute	Heart rate per 10 sec	
195	25	117-146	20-24	166
190	30	114-143	19-24	162
185	35	111-139	19-23	157
180	40	108-135	18-23	153
175	45	105-131	18-22	149
170	50	102-128	17-21	145
165	55	99-124	17-21	140
160	60	96-120	16-20	136
155	65	93-116	16-19	132
150	70	90-113	15-19	128

[a]Target heart rates are based on the individual's (predicted) maximal heart rate according to age. This is roughly equal to 220 minus the age in years. The initial training heart rate for someone 50 years old, for example, would lie between 119 to 145 beats per minute, or 20 to 24 beats every 10 seconds.

Exclusions for Entry into Exercise Programs

1. Unstable angina pectoris (uncontrolled by medication)
2. Resting systolic blood pressure over 200 mmHg or resting diastolic blood pressure over 100 mmHg
3. Significant drop (20 mmHg or more) in resting blood pressure from the patient's average level that cannot be explained by medications
4. Moderate to severe aortic stenosis
5. Acute infection or fever
6. Uncontrolled atrial or ventricular arrhythmias (irregular heartbeats)
7. Uncontrolled tachycardia (heart rate over 100 beats per minute at rest)
8. Symptomatic congestive heart failure
9. Third-degree heart block
10. Active pericarditis or myocarditis (inflammation around the heart)
11. Recent blood clot in a vein or artery
12. ST displacement (abnormal ECG) greater than 3 mm at rest
13. Uncontrolled diabetes
14. Bone or joint problems that prohibit exercise

Note. Data from American College of Sports Medicine. *Guidelines for exercise testing and prescription.* Edition 3. Philadelphia, Lea & Febiger, 1986, p. 55.

Appendix B
Treatment Guidelines

A blood cholesterol determination is warranted for every adult over age 20 and for children by the age of 5, earlier in high-risk families. The average of 2 or 3 measurements, taken 1 to 8 weeks apart, should be used. (Use 3 measurements if the initial two values differ by more than 30 mg/dl, or .8 mmol/L.) A nonfasting total cholesterol measurement is adequate for initial evaluation.

If total cholesterol (TC) is less than 180 mg/dl (4.65 mmol/L), recheck cholesterol at least every 5 years, and sooner if the individual's diet changes significantly, if hypertension develops, or if a female enters menopause.

If TC is 180 to 200 mg/dl (4.65-5.2 mmol/L), recheck total nonfasting cholesterol within 6 months. If it is still higher than 180 mg/dl, discuss with the person a basic healthy diet (such as the Step One eating plan) and a reduction or elimination of other modifiable risk factors.

For TC higher than 200 mg/dl, the NCEP recommends doing a fasting lipid profile to determine LDL levels. I also recommend lipid profiles to patients with TC of 180 to 200 mg/dl (4.65-5.2 mmol/L) who have two or more other risk factors.

Note: LDL rather than total cholesterol is used for classifying people into borderline and high-risk categories and for determining treatment. The goal of treatment is to maintain LDL levels below 130 mg/dl (3.36 mmol/L).* But for convenience and to reduce costs, TC can be used for periodic rechecks; a TC level of 200 mg/dl (5.2 mmol/L) would be the surrogate for an LDL of 130 mg/dl (3.36 mmol/L) and 240 mg/dl (6.2 mmol/L) for an LDL of 160 mg/dl (4.1 mmol/L). If TC ever rises higher than 130 mg/dl, determine LDL level using a fasting lipid profile and follow the appropriate algorithm (to be described).

If LDL cholesterol is between 130 and 160 mg/dl (3.36-4.1 mmol/L) and the person is free of atherosclerosis or any two of the other risk factors, he or she falls into the borderline high-risk category. Follow Algorithm 1.

---

*The NCEP accepts an LDL goal of 130 to 160 mg/dl (3.36-4.1 mmol/L) if the individual is free of clinical atherosclerosis and has no other or only one other risk factor. But I believe these LDL levels are unhealthy and are generally unwarranted, even in the absence of other risk factors, and thus I have included more stringent recommendations here. Ultimately, treatment decisions lie with the individual and his or her physician, according to special circumstances and how aggressively they wish to prevent atherosclerosis.

If LDL is higher than 160 mg/dl (4.1 mmol/L), the individual is in the high-risk category (as are 26% of American adults). Also in the high-risk group are an additional 10% of adults with LDL cholesterol between 130 and 160 mg/dl and with existent atherosclerosis (history of a heart attack, angina, or stroke) or any two other risk factors. For any person determined to be high-risk, do a complete blood count, urinalysis, and blood sugar, creatinine, and thyroid function tests to rule out secondary causes of hypercholesterolemia. See Algorithm 2 for other recommendations.

Algorithm 1:
Treating Borderline High-Risk Individuals

Begin treatment for anyone in this group by initiating a Step One eating plan and controlling other risk factors. Recheck cholesterol in 4 to 6 weeks. If the LDL cholesterol goal of less than 130 mg/dl (3.36 mmol/L) is achieved, recheck cholesterol in 6 months and annually thereafter.

If that goal is not achieved after 6 months, consult with a registered dietitian (RD) if you have not already done so. The dietitian can analyze the person's diet to determine whether the Step One eating plan is being followed and whether to proceed to the Step Two eating plan. Reevaluate the exercise program and other approaches to controlling risk factors. Recheck TC in 4 to 6 weeks and obtain a fasting lipid profile at 3 months.

If the goal of maintaining LDL at less than 130 mg/dl (3.36 mmol/L) is now achieved, follow the individual's progress, taking TC values four times the first year and twice a year thereafter. TC should remain below 200 unless HDL is very high. At least once a year do a fasting lipid profile to ensure that LDL remains below 130 mg/dl.

If LDL persists above 130 mg/dl in spite of an adequate RD-supervised Step Two eating plan, consider a genetic cause for hypercholesterolemia. Other family members should be encouraged to have lipid profiles. Follow Algorithm 2 for any person whose LDL remains above 130 with a Step Two diet. Drug therapy (see Algorithm 3) may be warranted after 6 months if the Step Two eating plan is unsuccessful, especially when other risk factors are present.

Algorithm 2: Treating High-Risk Individuals

Begin the Step One eating plan and other risk factor modification, if such have not already been instituted (Figure B.1). Consultation with a physician is strongly recommended to test for secondary causes of hypercholesterolemia. Evaluate immediate family members for lipid disorders.

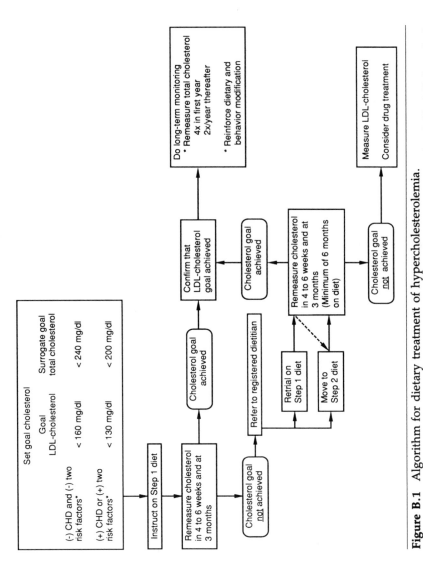

Figure B.1 Algorithm for dietary treatment of hypercholesterolemia.
Note. From *NCEP Report of the Expert Panel on Detection, Evaluation, and Treatment of High Blood Cholesterolemia in Adults,* DHHS Publication No. 88-2925, (p. 45) by National Cholesterol Education Program, 1987, Bethesda, MD: Author.

311

Recheck total (nonfasting) cholesterol in 4 to 6 weeks, and do a complete lipid profile in 3 months.

The goal is to keep LDL below 130 mg/dl (3.36 mmol/L). If that is achieved, recheck cholesterol 4 times the first year and at least twice a year thereafter. If TC later rises above 200 mg/dl (180 mg/dl, or 4.65 mmol/L, if other risk factors are present), do a complete fasting lipid profile and follow the appropriate algorithm.

If the cholesterol goal is not met in 3 months, consult with a registered dietitian, who can reanalyze the individual's eating plan and either try Step One again or proceed to Step Two. The person should decrease dietary cholesterol and saturated fat as much as possible and eat more fish and soluble fiber. Recheck TC in 4 to 6 weeks and LDL in 3 months. If LDL remains over 190 mg/dl (4.9 mmol/L) after 6 months, medication may be needed (see Algorithm 3).

If LDL below 130 mg/dl is achieved with these additional measures, recheck TC four times the first year and twice a year thereafter. Include a fasting lipid profile at least once a year.

Algorithm 3: Treating Through Drug Therapy

For anyone whose LDL cholesterol remains above 160 mg/dl (4.1 mmol/L) after Algorithm 2 treatment, first maximize the non-drug approaches to cholesterol control and eliminate other modifiable risk factors. Review the medical history with an emphasis on liver or kidney disease, hypertension, or other cardiovascular disease. If LDL remains over 190 mg/dl (4.9 mmol/L) for 6 months, select an initial drug. Consider all the lipid fractions (LDL, HDL, and triglycerides), the person's age, other diseases, medications, and the ability to tolerate side effects. Recheck TC in 4 to 6 weeks and take a complete lipid profile in 3 months.

If the LDL goal of 130 mg/dl (3.36 mmol/L) is achieved, recheck TC every 3 months and take a fasting lipid profile once a year. If the goal is not achieved with the optimal dosage, either choose a different drug or add another for combination therapy. A lipid specialist may need to be consulted.

Triglyceride Management

Triglyceride levels in the blood should ideally remain below 150 mg/dl (1.7 mmol/L), and certainly below 250 mg/dl (2.8 mmol/L). Levels higher than 250 mg/dl should be treated by a change in diet, especially in women, diabetics, and those with a positive family history for coronary heart disease. If the levels remain above 500 mg/dl (5.6 mmol/L) despite 4 to 6 months of an RD-supervised dietary trial, consider drugs such as niacin or gemfibrozil. Extremely high triglyceride levels (more than 1,000 mg/dl or 11.3 mmol/L) can cause serious inflammation of the pancreas (pancreatitis) and deserve immediate attention. Levels this high may be due to elevated chylomicron or VLDL and will probably require referral to an endocrinologist or lipid specialist.

Resources

Organizations

American Dietetic Association
216 W. Jackson Blvd. #800
Chicago, IL 60606-6995
Tel: 800-877-1600

American Heart Association
7320 Greenville Ave.
Dallas,TX 75231
Tel: 214-750-5300

American Hospital Association
Center for Health Promotion
840 N. Lake Shore Dr.
Chicago, IL 60611
Tel: 312-280-6000

Association for Fitness in Business
310 N. Alabama St., Ste. A100
Indianapolis, IN 46204
Tel: 317-636-6621

Bureau of Health Education
Centers for Disease Control
Bldg. 14
Atlanta, GA 30333
Tel: 404-329-3111

Consumer Information Center
Superintendent of Documents
P.O. Box 100
Pueblo, CO 81002
Tel: 719-948-3334

National Cholesterol Education Program
National High Blood Pressure Education Program
NHLBI Smoking Education Program
Information Center
4733 Bethesda Ave., Ste. 530
Bethesda, MD 20814
Tel: 301-951-3260

National Dairy Council
6300 N. River Rd.
Rosemont, IL 60018
Tel: 708-696-1020

National Heart, Lung, and Blood Institute
Office of Prevention, Education, and Control
Bldg. 31, Rm. 4A21
Bethesda, MD 20892
Tel: 301-951-3260

National Live Stock and Meat Board
444 N. Michigan Ave.
Chicago, IL 60611
Tel: 312-467-5520

National Wellness Institute
South Hall
1319 Fremont St.
University of Wisconsin at Stevens Point
Stevens Point, WI 54481
Tel: 715-346-2172

Nutrition Foundation
888 17th St. NW, Ste. 300
Washington, DC 20006
Tel: 202-872-0778

Office of Health Information and Health Promotion
Office of the Surgeon General
Department of Health, Education, and Welfare
Rm. 721BHHH
200 Independence Ave. SW
Washington, DC 20003
Tel: 202-472-5370

President's Council on Physical Fitness and Sports
Department of Health, Education, and Welfare
Rm. 3030, Donohoe Bldg.
400 Sixth St. SW
Washington, DC 20201
Tel: 202-755-7947

U.S. Department of Agriculture
Human Nutrition Information Service
6505 Belcrest Rd.
Hyattsville, MD 20782
Tel: 301-436-5724

U.S. Government Printing Office
Superintendent of Documents
Washington, DC 20402-9325
Tel: 202-783-3238

Washington Business Group on Health
922 Pennsylvania Ave. SE
Washington, DC 20003
Tel: 202-547-6644

Wellness Councils of America (corporate programs)
Historic Library Plaza
1823 Harney St., Ste. 201
Omaha, NE 68102
Tel: 402-444-1711

General Nutrition References

Anderson, J.W. (1990). *Plant fiber in foods*. Lexington, KY: HCF Nutrition
  Research Foundation.
Committee on Diet and Health, Food and Nutrition Board, Commission
  on Life Sciences, National Research Council. (1989). *Diet and health:
  Implications for reducing chronic disease risk*. Washington, DC: National
  Academy Press.
Grundy, S.M., Bilheimer, D., Blackburn, H., Brown, W.V., Kwiterovich,
  P.O., Mattson, R., Schonfild, G., & Weidman, W.H. (1982). Rationale
  of the diet-heart statement of the American Heart Association. Report
  of Nutrition Committee. *Circulation, 65*, 839A-854A.
National Research Council. (1989). *Recommended dietary allowances* (10th
  ed.). Washington, DC: National Academy Press.
Nutrition Committee, American Heart Association. (1988). Dietary guide-
  lines for healthy Americans: A statement for physicians and health
  professionals. *Arteriosclerosis, 8*, 218A-221A.
Pennington, J., & Church, H. (1985). *Food values of portions commonly used*
  (14th ed.). Philadelphia, PA: Lippincott.
Rinzler, C.A. (1987). *The complete book of food—A nutritional, medical, and
  culinary guide*. New York: World Almanac.
Surgeon General. (1988). *The Surgeon General's report on nutrition and health*
  (DHHS, Publication No. 88-50210). Washington, DC: Public Health
  Service.

Nutrition References
From the United States Government

Available from the Human Nutrition Information Service, U.S. Department of Agriculture, or U.S. Government Printing Office:

- *Nutritive value of foods: Home and garden bulletin 72.*
- *Provisional table on the fatty acid and cholesterol content of selected foods.*
- *Provisional table on content of omega-3 fatty acids and other fat components of selected foods.*

Cookbooks

Connor, S.L., & Connor, W.E. (1986). *The new American diet.* New York: Simon and Schuster.

Cooley, D.A. & Moore, C.A. (1987). *Eat smart for a healthy heart.* Woodbury, N.Y.: Barron's Educational Series, Inc.

Goor, R., & Goor, N. (1987). *Eater's choice: A food lover's guide to lower cholesterol.* Boston: Houghton Mifflin Co.

Grundy, S. (Ed.) (1989). *American Heart Association's low-fat, low-cholesterol cookbook.* New York: Times Books.

Piscatella, J.C. (1982). *Don't eat your heart out cookbook.* New York: Workman.

Nutrition Newsletters

Cholesterol Update (intended for professional audience)
Citizens for Public Action on Cholesterol
888 17th St. NW
Washington, DC 20006
Tel: 202-466-4553

Diet and Nutrition Letter (professional and lay audience)
Tufts University
P.O. Box 57857
Boulder, CO 80322-7857
Tel: 800-525-0643

Environmental Nutrition (consumer oriented)
2112 Broadway
New York, NY 10023

Heart News Digest (lay audience)
National Center for Cardiac Information
8001 Forbes Pl., Ste. 105
Springfield, VA 22151
Tel: 703-321-0534

Nutrition Action (professional and lay audience)
Center for Science in the Public Interest
1501 16th St. NW
Washington, DC 20036-1499
Tel: 202-332-9110

Nutrition and the M.D. (professional)
PM, Inc.
14349 Victory Blvd. #204
Van Nuys, CA 91401

Nutrition Forum (addresses food quackery)
JB Lippincott, Co
Downsville Pike, Rt. 3, Box 20-B
Hagerstown, MD 21740

Handouts for Patients, Clients, or Screening Participants

Available From the American Heart Association

Cholesterol and your heart. (11 pp)

Dining out. (15 pp)

Recipes for low-fat, low-cholesterol meals. (47 pp)

Dietary treatment of hypercholesterolemia: A manual for patients. (110 pp)

Salt, sodium, and blood pressure. (20 pp)

The American Heart Association diet. (poster)

Grocery guide. (70 pp)

Available From National Cholesterol Education Program

So you have high blood cholesterol . . . . (1987). (NIH Publication No. 87-2922; 26 pp).

Eating to lower your high blood cholesterol. (1987). (NIH Publication No. 87-2920; 51 pp).

Facts about blood cholesterol. (1987). (NIH Publication No. 87-2696; 3 pp).

Healthy heart handbook for women. (1987). (NIH Publication No. 87-2720; 32 pp).

Test your healthy heart I.Q.—A self quiz. (NIH Publication No. 2724; 1 p).

Dietary guidelines for Americans: Avoid too much fat, saturated fat, and cholesterol. (1986). (NIH Publication No. NN171; 12 pp).

Eating for life. (1988). (NIH Publication No. 3000; 23 pp).

Available From the Consumer Information Center

Making bag lunches, snacks, and desserts using the dietary guidelines. (1989). 124-W (32 pp).

Preparing foods and planning menus using the dietary guidelines. (1989). 125-W (32 pp).

Shopping for food and making meals in minutes using the dietary guidelines. (1989). 126-W (36 pp).

Eating better when eating out using the dietary guidelines. (1989). 123-W (20 pp).

Other Sources

Other materials are available through an increasing number of food producers, including Arrowhead Mills, Coleman Natural Beef, Fantastic Foods, General Mills, Hain, Health Valley, Kellogg, Mori-Nu Tofu, Mountain Son, Quaker, R.W. Knutsen, Santa Cruz, Spectrum Natural, Westbrae Natural.

Professional Materials

Available From the American Heart Association

Diet in the healthy child. (4 pp).

Physicians' cholesterol education handbook: Recommendations for the detection, classification, and treatment of high blood cholesterol. (28 pp).

Dietary treatment of hypercholesterolemia: A handbook for counselors. (83 pp).

1990 heart and stroke facts. (44 pp).

Heart Rx. (Developed for physicians' offices, this program includes modules for instruction and handouts in the areas of nutrition, smoking, high blood pressure, and warning signs of disease.)

Available From National Cholesterol Education Program or the National Heart, Lung, and Blood Institute

NHLBI kit. (Annual). (This packet contains ideas and materials for preventing heart disease, lung disease, and stroke. Intended for a wide audience including hospitals, work sites, physicians' offices, and community health departments.)

The dietary management of hyperlipoproteinemia: A handbook for physicians and dieticians. (1980). (USDHHS, NIH Publication No. 80-110).

Report of the expert panel in detection, evaluation, and treatment of high blood cholesterol in adults. (1988). (USDHHS, NIH Publication No. 88-2925).

Highlights of the report of the expert panel in detection, evaluation, and treatment of high blood cholesterol in adults. (1987). (NIH Publication No. 87-2926).

Raab, C., & Tillotson, J.L. (1984). *Heart to heart: A manual on nutritional counseling for the reduction of cardiovascular disease risk factors.* (USDHHS, NIH Publication No. 85-1528).

With every beat of your heart: An ideabook for community heart health programs. (1987). (USDHHS, NIH Publication No. 87-2641).

Model workshop on nutrition counseling in hyperlipidemia. (1980). (USDHHS, NIH Publication No. 80-1666).

Play your cards right . . . stay young at heart: A heart healthy nutrition education program. (1988). (USDHHS, NIH Publication No. NN-314).

Available From the Consumer Information Service

Good sources of nutrients. (1989). (Publication No. 171-W, 17 pp).

Nutritional Education Video Resources

The heartcare program—Four videotapes totaling 46 minutes on the dietary management of cholesterol. Available from:
Hall-Foushee Productions, Inc.
1313 5th St. SE, Ste. 214B
Minneapolis, MN 55414
Tel: 612-379-3829

Eat to your heart's content—A 30-minute video on recipe modification.
Available from:
National Health Video, Inc.
12021 Wilshire Blvd., Ste. 550
Los Angeles, CA 90025
Tel: 213-472-2275

Healthy nutrition—A 20-minute video and educational pamphlet developed
as part of the WellAware series by Whole Person Associates. Available
from:
Whole Person Press
P.O. Box 3151
Duluth, MN 55803
Tel: 800-247-6789

Lower your cholesterol now—A video by Leni Reed, and *Cholesterol count-
down*—slides and visual aids by Jane Andrews. Available from:
The National Wellness Institute, Inc.
South Hall, 1319 Fremont St.
Stevens Point, WI 54481
Tel: 715-346-2172

Videos, food models, food scales, written materials, fat calculator wheels,
and other teaching aids available from:
Nasco
901 Janesville Ave.
Fort Atkinson, WI 53538
Tel: 414-563-2446

or

1524 Princeton Ave.
Modesto, CA 95352
Tel: 209-529-6957

Resource Materials for Corporate Programs

It's your business: A guide to heart and lung health at the workplace. (1986).
(USDHHS, NIH Publication No. 86-2210; 59 pp).

"Heart at Work" (program covering nutrition and weight control, blood
pressure, smoking, exercise, and signs of and emergency procedures for
a heart attack). American Heart Association.

Make worksite wellness programs work for your company. (1990). (USDHHS,
NIH Publication No. 2648).

Community Programs

Community guide to cholesterol resources. (NIH Publication No. 2927; 31 pp).
Community guide to high blood pressure control. (NIH Publication No. 2333; 137 pp).
With every beat of your heart: An ideabook for community heart health programs. (1987). (NIH Publication No. 2641; 59 pp).

Free radio spots and other public service announcements are available from NHLBI's Office of Prevention, Education, and Control.

National Innovators in Community Heart Health

Bloomington Heart & Health Program
(Minnesota Heart Health Program)
1900 W. Old Shakopee Rd.
Bloomington, MN 55431
Tel: 612-887-9603

Pawtucket Heart Health Program
Memorial Hospital of Rhode Island
111 Brewster St.
Pawtucket, RI 02860
Tel: 401-728-7591

Project LEAN (Low-Fat Eating for America Now)
Henry J. Kaiser Family Foundation
2400 Sand Hill Rd.
Menlo Park, CA 94025
Tel: 415-854-9400

Stanford Five-City Project
Distribution Center
Stanford Center for Research in Disease Prevention
1000 Welch Rd.
Palo Alto, CA 93404-1885
Tel: 415-723-0003

Laboratory Support Publications

Laboratory Standardization Panel, National Cholesterol Education Program, National Heart, Lung, and Blood Institute. (1988). A report on current status of blood cholesterol measurement in clinical laboratories in the United States. *Clinical Chemistry,* **34**, 193.

Laboratory Standardization Panel, National Cholesterol Education Program, National Heart, Lung, and Blood Institute. (1990). *Recommendations for improving cholesterol measurement.* (NIH Publication No. 90-2964). Bethesda, MD: NCEP Information Center/Publications. [The Executive Summary is NIH Publication No. 90-2964a.]

Institutions Supporting Screenings

American Health Foundation
320 E. 43rd St.
New York, NY 10017
Tel: 212-953-1900
(This organization offers assistance to communities desiring cholesterol screenings. They will train personnel and provide the analyzers, press releases, and participant handouts.)

Eastman Kodak
255 East Ave.
Rochester, NY 14604
Tel: 800-828-6316

Boehringer-Mannheim
9115 Hague Rd.
Indianapolis, IN 46250
Tel: 800-428-5074

Abbott Laboratories
1 Abbott Park Dr.
Dept. 921, Bldg. AP6C
Abbott Park, IL 60064
Tel: 800-323-9100

Technical Support

The Commission on Office Laboratory Assessment
8701 Georgia Ave, Ste. 610
Silver Spring, MD 20910
Tel: 301-588-5882

G.L. Myers, G.R. Cooper
Division of Environmental Health Laboratory Sciences
Center for Environmental Health and Injury Control
Centers for Disease Control
1600 Clifton Rd.
Atlanta, GA 30333

National Institute of Standards and Technology
  (formerly, the National Bureau of Standards)
Dr. Michael Welch
Chemistry Bldg., Rm. A113
NIST
Gathersburg, MD 20899
Tel: 301-975-3100

Excel
College of American Pathologists
P.O. Box 1234
Traverse City, MI 49685
Tel: 800-333-4004

Laboratory Standardization Panel on Blood Cholesterol
Measurement of the National Institutes of Health
National Cholesterol Education Program
National Heart, Lung, and Blood Institute
P.O. Box C-200
Bethesda, MD 20892

Reference Laboratories

David J. Hassemer, M.S.
Chief, Clinical Chemistry
State Laboratory of Hygiene
University of Wisconsin
Center for Health Sciences
465 Henry Mall
Madison, WI 53706
Tel: 608-263-3692

Leonard Sideman, Director
Division of Chemistry and Toxicology
Bureau of Laboratories
Pennsylvania State Department of Health
Rickering Way and Welsh Pool Rd.
Lionville, PA 19353
Tel: 215-363-8500

Ivan D. Frantz, Jr., M.D.
Director, Minnesota Lipid Research Clinic
Department of Medicine
Box 192, Mayo Memorial Bldg.
420 Delaware St. SE
Minneapolis, MN 55455
Tel: 612-626-1900

G. Russell Warnick
Director, Lipoprotein Laboratory
Northwest Lipid Research Clinic
Rm. 732, Harborview Hall
326 Ninth Ave.
Seattle, WA 98104
Tel: 206-223-3236 or -3148

Wolfgang Patsch, M.D.
Baylor College of Medicine
Mail Station F-701, Rm. F-740
6565 Fannin
Houston, TX 77030
Tel: 713-790-4351

Herbert K. Naito, Ph.D.
Head, Section of Lipids, Nutrition, and Metabolic Diseases
Department of Biochemistry, L-11
The Cleveland Clinic Foundation
9500 Euclid Ave.
Cleveland, OH 44106
Tel: 216-444-5744

Robert Rej, Ph.D.
Head, Clinical Chemistry Laboratory
Division of Laboratories and Research
New York State Department of Health
Empire State Plaza
Albany, NY 12201
Tel: 518-473-7130

Thomas Cole, Ph.D.
Lipid Research Center
Washington University School of Medicine
4566 Scott Ave., Box 8046
St. Louis, MO 63110
Tel: 314-362-3522

Dr. E.J. Schaefer
USDA Human Nutrition Research Center on Aging at Tufts University
711 Washington St., Rm. 501
Boston, MA 02111
Tel: 617-556-3104

Index